**Eleventh Edition**

# Chamberlain's Symptoms and Signs in Clinical Medicine

## An Introduction to Medical Diagnosis

**Colin Ogilvie** MD FRCP
Consultant Physician to the Royal Liverpool Hospital,
the Liverpool Regional Cardiothoracic Centre
and the King Edward VII Hospital, Midhurst

**Christopher C. Evans** MD FRCP
Consultant Physician to the Royal Liverpool Hospital and
the Liverpool Regional Cardiothoracic Centre

WRIGHT
1987        Wright, Bristol

Published under the Wright Imprint by
IOP Publishing Limited
Techno House, Redcliffe Way, Bristol BS1 6NX

First Issued, April 1936
Reprinted, November 1936
Second Edition, September 1938
Reprinted, February 1940
Reprinted, November 1941
Third Edition, June 1943
Reprinted, May 1944
Reprinted, May 1945
Fourth Edition, June 1947
Reprinted, October 1948
Reprinted, October 1950

Fifth Edition, October 1952
Sixth Edition, March 1957
Seventh Edition, May 1961
Reprinted, June 1964
Eighth Edition, November 1967
Ninth Edition, September 1974
Reprinted, June 1977
Reprinted, April 1978
Reprinted, July 1979
Tenth Edition, June 1980
Reprinted, April 1983
Eleventh Edition, 1987

*British Library Cataloguing in Publication Data*
Chamberlain, Ernest Noble
    Chamberlain's Symptoms and signs in
    clinical medicine : an introduction to
    medical diagnosis.—11th ed.
    1. Diagnosis
    I. Title   II. Ogilvie, Colin   III. Evans,
    C.C.
    616.07'5     RC71

    ISBN 0 7236 0864 4

Typeset, printed and bound in Great Britain by
Hazell Watson & Viney Limited
Member of the BPCC Group
Aylesbury, Bucks

# Chamberlain's Symptoms and Signs in Clinical Medicine

## Preface
## to the Eleventh Edition

It is half a century since this book was first published and, until now, there have been only two principal authors; for this edition, a third joins the team.

We believe that the technological advances in medicine since the last edition have in no way diminished the need to hear the patient's own story and to record with accuracy all symptoms and signs. We also recognize that the demands of modern medicine have inevitably encroached upon the time the physician can actually spend with his patient. We have therefore tried to make parts of our book less discursive, especially the introductory chapter, where we now aim to bring the student more quickly to the patient's bedside.

The chapter dealing with fever has been removed, because most of the subject is covered in the chapter on tropical diseases and elsewhere in the book. The chapter on the endocrine system has been completely re-written and expanded, with a series of new illustrations, and for this we are most grateful to Dr Paul Belchetz.

Although a detailed description of laboratory and radiographic techniques is outside the scope of this book, we have continued our policy of illustrating cardiac signs with phono- and echocardiographs because these can provide a direct visual display and explanation of the abnormal sounds heard. We are again indebted to Dr Norman Coulshed for providing a series of new tracings and for helping in the revision of this chapter.

The remaining chapters have all been revised with the advice of our colleagues. We are especially grateful to Professor Frank Harris (The Examination of Children), Professor Herbert Gilles (Symptoms and Signs in Tropical Diseases), Dr Ian Gilmore (The Digestive System), Dr Michael Mackie (The Haemopoietic System) and Dr Ronald Finn (Renal, Urinary and Genital Systems).

There are some 100 new illustrations, many in colour, and for these we are indebted to colleagues who helped with the revision of the book and to many others, especially Dr Tony Ellis, Dr Susan Evans and Mr Stephen Gill and his staff in the Department of Medical Illustration, Royal Liverpool Hospital. Mrs Barbara Mann has patiently undertaken the tedious task of typing, without error, the many revisions of this new edition.

C. M. O.
C. C. E.

## Contributors

**H. M. Gilles** BSc MD FRCP FFCM MD Hon. Causa
Karolinska Institute, Stockholm
Dean and Professor of Tropical Medicine
Liverpool School of Tropical Medicine

**Frank Harris** MD MMED (Paed) FRCP(Ed)
Professor of Child Health
University of Liverpool

# Contents

## Chapter 7

## Chapter 8

## Chapter 9

**Chapter 12**

**Chapter 13**

# The history and general principles of examination

## ■ INTRODUCTION: THE STUDENT'S APPROACH TO THE PATIENT

It is natural for the student to be apprehensive when first approaching a patient. He fears that sick people will not welcome a nervous and clumsy beginner and that he can be of no help to them. This is the time for him to remember that many patients find comfort in the knowledge that their own suffering may serve, through the observations of students, to ease the burden of those who follow, perhaps even their own children. But the student has more than this to offer the patient. He can be a 'friend at court', a messenger between the fearful patient and the awesome doctor. Time and again, students have discovered facts vital to diagnosis or management that had previously been withheld because of the patient's fear, the doctor's haste or the forbidding retinue that accompanies the physician on his round. The student should approach his patient with humility and gratitude, but also with quiet confidence and pride in the responsibility which will be his for the remainder of his life.

Clinical medicine is above all a matter of communication between people, and the quality of the student's relationship with patients and colleagues could decide his success or failure as a physician. It is no exaggeration to say that even facial expression, tone of voice and manner of movement can all affect the ability to elicit the patient's story and to lead him back to health. For it is in such outward signs that we display those attitudes of mind—impatience, boredom, embarrassment, disbelief and reproach—which act as a barrier to communication with others. In the presence of his patient the student must master his emotions, clear his mind of distracting thoughts and avoid all appearances of haste. His manner should be alert and attentive, yet gentle and sympathetic. Without these qualities, he will neither obtain the facts needed for diagnosis nor effectively convey the advice essential to management.

Before confronting the patient, the student must not only have composed his own attitude but he should also have anticipated, so far as possible, the likely attitude of the particular patient he has come to see. He must be ready for the resigned and sometimes resentful manner of the patient with chronic incurable disease, the frightened questioning from those with recent alarming symptoms, the desperate pleading of the patient in acute pain, the inattention and unresponsiveness of the seriously ill. He must also adapt himself to the patient's ethnic, social, educational and intellectual background and use forms of speech which he can understand.

Whether in a hospital ward or the patient's home, it is wise to speak first to those who are looking after the patient. The nurse or relative in charge will indicate whether the patient is available for examination. So far as possible, patients should not be disturbed during meal times, when they have visitors or while they are undergoing diagnostic or therapeutic procedures. The attendant will also be able to say whether, because of the patient's present mental or physical state, any special precautions are needed. The student can thus be forewarned of language difficulty, emotional traits or any defects of memory, concentration, hearing or speech which might call for some modification of his approach.

Before attempting to obtain a formal clinical history, the student should introduce himself and ask if he may put some questions about the illness which took the patient to his doctor. He should then make sure that the patient is as free as possible of any immediate physical or mental discomfort. Except in urgent cases, it is preferable to postpone the interview rather than try to elicit the history of a patient who is drowsy from drugs, or feeling sick, or wanting to visit the toilet. In general, it is best to interview the patient alone and to call later upon a relative for information which is not obtainable from the patient. When it comes to the physical examination, an attendant should be present to help the patient undress or change position or, where appropriate, to act as chaperone.

■　　　　　　GUIDE TO HISTORY RECORDING

### The presenting problem

Some patients come out at once with their story; others remain silent. The former must not be interrupted except to steer them away from irrelevancy. The latter should be gently encouraged rather than questioned. In other words, the patient's history should whenever possible be received, not taken.

Most patients expect the doctor to make the first move. After a few words to put the patient at his ease, he must find out why the patient has come. The conventional opening question 'What do you complain of?' is not always suitable. Some patients have no real symptoms but feel obliged to mention a minor discomfort in answer to this question when in fact they have come with a problem rather than a pain. The more sympathetic question 'What can I do to help you?' sometimes brings a more revealing answer. However, more than one approach may have to be made before the appropriate response is obtained; a list of suggested alternatives is given below.

Whether the patient is presenting with a symptom or a problem, this should be recorded in *the patient's own words*, along with a note of its duration. If the patient's own words consist of a diagnosis (e.g. bronchitis, angina) rather than a symptom (e.g. cough, chest pain), he must be asked to indicate how this condition affects him. The symptoms and not the 'diagnosis' are then recorded, thus: Cough: 3 months. Chest pain: 1 week.

*Questionnaire*

> *What do you feel wrong with yourself?*
> *In what way do you feel ill?*
> *What can I do to help you?*
> *Tell me why you've come to see me.*
> *What took you to the doctor? (for patients who have already seen another doctor)*

## The antecedent history

The aim of this part of the history is to sketch in the patient's personal and family background. Although it is chronologically appropriate to record this antecedent history before the history of the present condition, it may be best to take the main history first, especially from patients who have come with their story well prepared; if the flow is interrupted, they could easily forget what they had intended to say. On the other hand, reticent or frightened patients may be put at ease by answering a few simple questions about home and family before attempting to describe the illness for which they are seeking help.

The facts elicited in this part of the history may have bearing on management as well as diagnosis. For example, the physical fitness of a relative or the presence of stairs in the patient's house may determine whether he can be nursed at home while a previous illness can sometimes contraindicate the use of a drug for the present illness.

The antecedent history includes *past health*, *family history* and *social or personal history*.

**Past health** Patients often omit trauma (accidents and operations) or mishaps in pregnancy (miscarriages, 'toxaemia') when asked about previous illnesses. Specific inquiry should therefore be made about these. Patients may also forget transient minor illness which, though unimportant to them at the time, may have a significant relationship to their present problem. Typical examples of this are a minor dental procedure prior to the onset of subacute bacterial endocarditis or an episode of diplopia in a patient presenting years later with paraplegia due to multiple sclerosis. Where a direct link between past and present illness is clear, it is better to record the earlier illness as part of the history of the present condition than to relegate it to past health.

*Questionnaire*

> *Have you had any serious illness in the past? How did it affect you?*
> *Any operations or bad injuries?*
> *Any stillbirths, miscarriages or problems in pregnancy?*
> *Have you ever been to a hospital?*
> *Have you missed time from work because of illness?*
> *Have you ever visited your doctor before?*
> *Have you ever had . . .* (here list illnesses possibly relevant to present complaint)

**Family history** The main purpose here is to find out whether there are in the family any diseases relevant to the patient's own illness. The possible causes for a disease affecting more than one member of a family are:

1. Environmental: transmission of infection, poverty, common dietary or smoking habits, poor hygiene, etc.

2. Coincidental, as in the case of common diseases, such as cancer.

3. Heredity: many diseases 'run' in families but most of those transmitted by known modes of inheritance are relatively rare.

Fear of acquiring or transmitting a family disease is a common cause for seeking medical advice and these patients may have anxiety symptoms simulating the illness which they dread.

The past and present health and, where applicable, the age and cause of death of all first-degree relatives, are recorded and the patient should also be asked whether any relative has had symptoms similar to his own. Inquiry about consanguinity may be relevant in certain rare inherited diseases.

*Questionnaire*

> *Are you married?*
> *Is your wife/husband well?*
> *Do you have children?* (record age and sex). *Have they ever been seriously ill?* (record details)
> *Have you lost any children?* (record age and cause of death)
> *Do you have brothers and sisters?* (record age and sex). *Have they ever been seriously ill?* (record details)
> *Have you lost any brothers or sisters?* (record age and cause of death)
> *Are both your parents living?* (if not, give age and cause of death)
> *Have they ever been seriously ill?* (record details)
> *Do you know of anyone in the family with symptoms like yours?*
> *Do you know of any disease affecting more than one member of your family?*

**Social history** The questions asked under this heading are designed to uncover anything in the patient's personal life relevant to either the cause or management of his illness. We need, therefore, to know about his work, hobbies, habits, environment at home, visits abroad, domestic and marital life and any potential source of mental stress.

*Questionnaire*

> *Are you working?*
> *What exactly do you do?* (record hours, physical activity, potential hazards, travelling)
> *How long have you done this job?*
> *What jobs have you done before, starting when you left school?* (record as above)
> *What do you do in your spare time?* (Hobbies, sport, etc.)
> *Are your meal-times regular? When is your main meal?*

*Do you or did you smoke?* (record duration, number of cigarettes/ cigars/pipes per day)
*Do you or did you take alcohol?* (record type and amount)
*Do you or did you take drugs of any kind?* (record type and amount)
*Have you been abroad?* (record where and when)
*Tell me about your home* (rooms, stairs, toilet facilities, state of repair)
*Who is living in the same house? Have any been ill recently?*
*Do you keep animals at home?*
*Is all well at home and at your work?*
*Have you had any recent worries or stresses?*

**History of present condition**  The patient is now encouraged to tell his story in his own words. Questions should be confined to those needed to establish the date and mode of onset of each symptom, its chronological development to the present day (*see Fig.* 1.1) and its precise nature along with any associated phenomena. Leading questions must not be asked, although alternatives can be offered. For example: 'Did your pain come suddenly or gradually?' is permitted; 'Did your pain come suddenly?' is not.

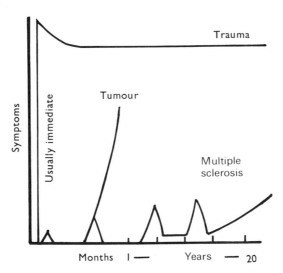

**Fig. 1.1** Time factor in development of spinal cord symptoms.

When the patient has finished his story and answered 'No' to the question: 'Have you any other symptoms at all?', he may then be asked leading questions to ensure that no symptom has been forgotten. A list of symptoms that may be elucidated is given in *Table* 1.1.

| Table1.1 | **Symptom review** | | | |
|---|---|---|---|---|
| | *Gastrointestinal* | *Cardio-respiratory* | *Neurological* | *Others* |
| | Appetite | Cough | Blackouts | Urinary symptoms |
| | Indigestion | Sputum | Vertigo | Menstrual |
| | Nausea | Haemoptysis | Headaches | symptoms |
| | Vomiting | Dyspnoea | Visual changes | Skin rashes |
| | Dysphagia | Palpitations | Hearing changes | Joint pains |
| | Constipation | Leg swelling | Pareses | Swellings |
| | Diarrhoea | Chest pain | Paraesthesiae | Weight change |
| | Abdominal pain | | Tremors | |
| | Bleeding | | | |

*Questionnaire*

*Onset* (record for each symptom in chronological order)
> *When did your (symptom) first start?*
> *Were you perfectly well before then?*
> *Have you ever had anything like this before?*
> *Did your (symptom) come suddenly one day or gradually?*
> *What were you doing when it came on?* (if onset sudden)

*Development* (record for each symptom in chronological order)
> *What has happened to your (symptom) since then?*
> *Coming and going?* (record frequency, duration and relationship if any to physiological or environmental factors)
> *Getting worse or better?* (record whether the change has been gradual; if not, when it occurred and whether related to physiological or environmental factors)

*Description* (pain given here as an example)
> *Show me where you feel your pain.*
> *Does it move anywhere?*
> *What kind of pain is it? Aching, stabbing, throbbing, gripping?*
> *How bad is it? Does it make you stop what you're doing?*
> *How often do you get it?* (record whether continuous or number of times per day, week, month or year)
> *How long does it last?*
> *Does it come at any special times?*
> *Does anything bring it on or make it worse?*
> *Does anything relieve it? What do you do when it comes on?*
> *Do you feel anything else wrong at the same time?*

■   **THE PHYSICAL EXAMINATION**

The physical examination begins during the taking of the history because certain abnormalities—of mood, speech, posture and movement, for example—are then more evident than when the patient is asked to lie still and silent on a couch. The history usually points to the system or part of the body to be examined first and in greatest detail. Systematic examination follows and should comprise the following:

1. *General inspection* of the whole body for external evidence of disease: wasting, dehydration, obesity, jaundice, pallor, cyanosis, rashes, swellings, abnormal stature or development, abnormal facial characteristics and pathological changes in the skin, hair, nails, limbs or joints.

2. *The respiratory system*: nose, paranasal sinuses, throat, airways, lungs and sputum.

3. *The cardiovascular system*: heart, peripheral veins and arteries and blood pressure.

4. *The digestive system*: mouth, oesophagus, stomach and intestines, liver, gallbladder, hernial orifices, rectum, faeces and vomitus.

5. *The haemopoietic system*: lymph nodes, spleen, liver and blood.

6. *The genito-urinary system*: kidneys, bladder, genitalia, breasts and urine.

7. *The nervous system*: cerebration, speech, cranial nerves and motor and sensory systems.

8. *The special sense organs*: eyes, ears, nose.

9. *The psychological state*.

Although the physical findings are recorded in systems, the examination should be adapted for the patient's convenience. For example, the neck, spine and loins can be examined as well as the lungs when the patient sits up.

## ■ SOME IMPORTANT AND COMMON SYMPTOMS

### Pain

**Pathways and causation** Pain is transmitted through the free nerve endings via the posterior nerve roots and the spinothalamic tracts to the thalamus and ascending bulbar reticular system, and there is evidence to suggest that recognition of pain and the associated emotional disturbances lies in the thalamus, though the localization of pain may be a function of the cerebral cortex.

The stimuli productive of pain are several, and an understanding of them contributes to the interpretation of pain as a symptom of disease. It is unnecessary here to deal with physiological responses to painful stimuli, e.g. a pin-prick or burn, but sensory nerve endings in the skin and mucous membranes are so rich that pain is easily evoked and easily localized, whereas in some viscera, e.g. the gastrointestinal tract and heart, the nerve endings are more scattered and this may account partly for the less precise distribution of the pain and its deep character. Further, some tissues, e.g. the lung and visceral pleura and the alimentary tract, are normally insensitive to stimuli that affect the skin (cutting, burning), though an inflamed organ, as in appendicitis or gastric ulceration, may be painful to the touch or squeezing. On the other hand, colicky pain in the digestive tube may be caused by distension or obstruction which may act through the sensory nerve endings or by pulling on mesenteric vessels, for it is well established that pain may be caused by traction or distension of arteries. Such visceral sensations are probably carried by the sympathetic nervous system.

Whether physical causes act by producing chemical changes is difficult to prove in short-acting stimuli such as a cut, but there is no doubt that they do so when the pain persists after the physical agent has been removed, e.g. after a blow or irradiation. More certainly, some types of pain are essentially due to chemical agents, noxious or rendered so by the condition of the tissue upon which they act.

Thus substances such as histamine, acetylcholine and 5-hydroxytryptamine are responsible for pain in allergic processes, and HCl, when introduced experimentally into the stomach, can be shown to aggravate the pain of an active peptic ulcer.

The pain of ischaemic origin, as in angina or intermittent claudication, is presumed to be due to metabolites resulting from oxygen insufficiency, though the nature of the metabolites is not yet known.

In interpreting the origin of pain it must be realized that while the skin is very sensitive and pain is easily localized to the affected segments of the spinal cord, this is not so in visceral and deep somatic pains (muscles and periosteum) in which the painful stimuli may be received by many segments of the cord and even affect neighbouring segments. This is seen in conditions such as perforation of an ulcer, angina or even intestinal colic in which the pain may be widespread.

Pain may also be 'referred' to other areas of the body which are innervated from the same segments as the viscus involved. Pleural pain may radiate to the abdominal wall, biliary colic pain may spread to the scapular area, and central diaphragmatic lesions may cause shoulder-tip pain (4th cervical segment).

It may be noticed that the position of the pain does not always decide the organ from which it is arising, but factors that modify the pain may do so. Thus a central chest pain is not always anginal and if it is constantly provoked by swallowing suggests an oesophageal lesion. Similarly, a hypogastric pain may suggest a vesical origin if it is associated with dysuria, a uterine origin if it is related to menstruation, or an intestinal pain if it is modified by bowel action.

**Clinical aspects** One of the commonest of complaints, pain can vary in significance from diagnostic certainty to misleading confusion.

The patient who describes a band-like sensation across the chest which occurs on walking and which is quickly relieved by rest leaves little doubt that he is suffering from angina pectoris. On the contrary, the individual who changes the description from pain in the chest to a throbbing or bumping sensation and cannot even place his hand with accuracy over the area of discomfort does little to help in the diagnosis. None the less, there are few of us who have not experienced pain and have realized that it is not always easy to find suitable adjectives to describe it or even to locate it precisely.

Tolerance must be shown (as in all questioning) and questions framed in differing ways to make sure whether the answers are the same.

The duration of the pain and whether it is continuous or wavelike may also be significant.

Then the severity should be ascertained. It may vary from degrees expressed by such words as 'terrible', 'agonizing' or 'excruciating' to 'slight' or 'annoying'. Wrong usage of words by patients is common. Thus 'acute' is often used to mean severe rather than of short duration, and 'chronic' may imply very bad instead of prolonged.

Allowance must also be made for the variation in the threshold of pain. The same painful stimulus whether in health or disease may be regarded merely as an annoyance by one, but as intolerable by another. This may also be bound up with anxiety connected with the cause and seriousness of the pain, and often if the patient can be reassured that the underlying pathology is trivial he will cease to complain so much. In these days of widespread (though sometimes inaccurate) familiarity with coronary artery disease, any pain in the chest is regarded with more alarm than, say, a pain in the lumbar region, though the former may be no more serious and even less severe. It is very important not to regard unexplained pain as non-existent. Continued review with an open mind may sometimes eventually reveal an unexpected cause.

If this proves not to be the case, it must equally be recognized that pain can be psychogenic in origin or due to such trivial causes that the state of mind is responsible for its apparent severity.

This is particularly so in nervous apprehensive subjects and in those suffering from emotional strain, especially anxieties in the home or at work.

Psychogenic pain is rarely of constant pattern, and if the patient is seen often there will usually be considerable contradiction in the story, and the patient will often have consulted many doctors but is reluctant to believe those who blame the condition on 'nerves'.

Unlike the malingerer, a rare individual concerned solely with making profit out of his alleged pain, the psychoneurotic deserves and requires sympathetic but firm handling if he is to improve. He may have genuine pain but tends to magnify it if apprehensive or wishing to gain sympathy.

**Examination** This may be negative, as so often in peptic ulcer or angina, but it must be directed in the first place to the area of the pain. Here exploration of structures such as the skin and muscles and superficial blood vessels and nerves may supply the answer. Examples are seen in pain associated with herpes zoster, tenderness of muscles in 'rheumatism' and poor arterial pulsation in intermittent claudication.

Often the pain originates in deeper structures—notably the viscera—and care is necessary to identify the source of such pain by those methods of clinical examination and special investigations appropriate to the structure suspected, as described in subsequent chapters.

Shock is a feature of many forms of severe pain, especially the deep pain of grave visceral lesions. Cf. Shock, pp. 16–17.

*Muscle spasm* or 'guarding' in muscles supplied from the same segments of the cord is particularly common in abdominal lesions and of great diagnostic importance. It may also, as a protective measure, restrain breathing, as in pleurisy, or limit the movement of an injured joint.

*Hyperaesthesia* is also closely bound up with certain types of pain. It implies that an area of the body responds to a non-noxious stimulus with pain, or that undue pain is caused by a noxious stimulus.

The phenomenon may be observed commonly in the sensitivity of a burn to light touch, but it may also be associated with deeper lesions, e.g. superficial tenderness over the abdominal wall in inflammatory processes such as appendicitis with peritonitis.

The objectives of the questions about pain may be summarized as follows:

1. To ascertain the site and distribution of the pain and whether these are constant. This enables the observer to decide whether the pain falls into an anatomical pattern consistent with an organic origin or whether the pattern is so bizarre as to suggest a psychogenic source in a patient who is unfamiliar with anatomy and physiology.

Allowance must be made for unusual distribution of pain which is not uncommon and quite genuine and for true physical pain with a psychogenic overlay.

2. To determine the character and severity of the pain. This is often most difficult and depends on the intelligence, emotional stability and descriptive ability of the patient.

With a reliable historian many pains can give important leads to diagnosis, as witness the pain of peripheral arterial disease, renal colic and duodenal ulcer.

3. To find out what makes the pain better or worse. Familiar examples are the ease given by food and antacids in peptic ulceration, the precipitation of angina by physical effort and its relief by rest, the aggravation of pleural pain by deep breathing and its cessation if breathing is momentarily stopped.

4. To determine specific time relationships of pain, e.g. nocturnal pain in peptic ulcer, monthly pain in dysmenorrhoea, and morning headaches of cerebral tumour.

5. To assess the individual's personality and response to other discomforts of life so as to decide whether the pain might be wholly or partly psychogenic. Inquiry should be made about specific emotional disturbances and whether they are likely to be temporary or prolonged.

6. To elicit symptoms constantly associated with the pain, e.g. haematuria in renal colic or jaundice in biliary colic.

### Headache

This is one of the commonest of symptoms. Often it is harmless though distressing, but it may have serious significance.

The understanding of its mechanism is sometimes obscure, but when it has a physical basis the following factors are thought to be involved (*Fig.* 1.2).

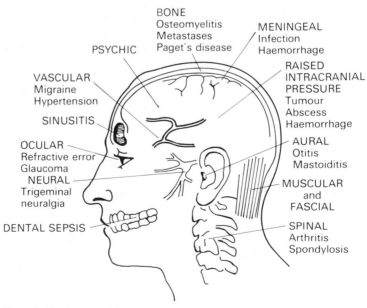

**Fig. 1.2** Headache and other pains.

1. Disorders of the cranial arteries, veins and venous sinuses. There may be alteration in tone, as in the case of migraine when there is dilatation of the external carotid artery on one side recognized by visible pulsation in the superficial temporal artery, which is relieved by arterial-constricting drugs such as ergotamine or pressure on the common carotid artery. Similar vasodilatation may be responsible for headaches resulting from hypertension, from carbon dioxide retention and from certain drugs such as nitrates. Experimentally, histamine can cause vasodilatation. Perhaps other chemical substances may also be responsible in fever and overindulgence in alcohol.

Traction on the cerebral vessels, rather than the increased intracranial pressure, may be the cause of headache in brain tumours. Essential hypertension is less commonly a cause of headache than is sometimes claimed.

2. Direct involvement of pain-sensitive structures such as those covering the cranium, e.g. the periosteum and meninges and certain nerves through which the pain is mediated, notably the 5th, 9th and 10th cranial nerves and the three upper cervical nerves. Headache caused in this way may result from local scalp lesions, tumours, malignant deposits in the skull and inflammatory processes such as meningitis and cerebral abscess.

3. Prolonged contraction of the muscles of the neck, scalp and face may cause sensations like a tight band together with stiffness of the neck. It has been suggested that this is partly due to ischaemia of the muscles and is generally psychogenic in origin, though it is possible that extracerebral lesions, as in the cervical spine, nose, nasal sinuses, eyes, ears and teeth, may cause pain in this way. It is not uncommon during car driving.

4. It is often assumed that extracranial causes may be responsible for headaches, but it is not always easy to be sure that this is the case. Local conditions of the ears and teeth may be responsible for pain but more rarely for true headache. On the other hand, pathological states of the nose and nasal sinuses which are often allergic in type may more reasonably be associated with headache.

Headaches which appear to arise in places remote from the head and neck are more difficult to explain, though from a clinical point of view they cannot be dismissed. It is common, for example, for a headache to occur in association with metabolic disorders such as uraemia and after poisoning with many drugs, including alcohol, whether taken therapeutically, pleasurably or by accident.

5. Undoubtedly, the commonest causes of headache are psychogenic. What has been said of pain in general applies to headache, especially when this is of psychological origin. It is necessary, as in all cases, to assume that the headache is physical in origin until sufficient time and repeated examination have excluded an organic basis.

The description in extravagant terms of the severity of the pain and the fact that it is never absent (though the patient may sleep) may, however, suggest a psychogenic origin. The patient's personality and emotional background will help. The detached way in which the hysterical patient describes an 'agonizing' pain is quite different from the fearful or depressed patient with an anxiety neurosis. Both differ from the patient with an expanding intracranial lesion, whose pain is bad enough to make him reluctant to talk about it but who freely rejoices in the intervals when it is absent.

**Examination** As the most important causes of headache are conditions such as cerebral tumour, cerebral abscess and meningitis, for which treatment may be available, it is wise to concentrate on the proof or exclusion of such conditions. A full neurological examination should therefore be made, but negative results at first do not necessarily exclude serious disease. Headache may precede other symptoms and signs. *See also* Chapter 10.

Physical examination in migraine occasionally shows undue pulsation of the temporal artery, but more often the diagnosis is made on the history of unilateral headache associated with visual disturbances (flashes of light, fortification figures, scotomata), and later in many cases vomiting.

Extracerebral causes may be found by examination of (1) the eyes, for glaucoma, gross refractory errors and other ocular lesions; (2) the ears, for evidence of otitis or mastoiditis; (3) the nose, for any discharge or local lesion such as a polyp; (4) the nasal sinuses, when tenderness may be found over the frontal and maxillary regions accompanied by nasal discharge, especially in chronic cases.

The whole body must of necessity be examined thoroughly for any physical disease, particularly febrile or toxic, which might link up with the headaches.

The questions to be asked of a patient complaining of headache should therefore include:

1. *The site*: Migraine, as mentioned, is usually unilateral; ocular and sinus headaches frontal; subarachnoid haemorrhage often occipital and in the neck, while neoplasms may for a time cause pain over their location.

2. *The character*: Migraine is nearly always throbbing. Cerebral tumour may also be so described, but just as often as a constant dull severe ache. Headaches associated with muscle spasm (psychogenic or due to some extracranial cause) have something of the character of a stiff neck. Neuralgic headaches, e.g. trigeminal neuralgia, are 'shooting' in type, while in headaches arising from psychogenic causes the description varies widely.

3. *The duration*: Is the headache persistent or does it come on in paroxysms? The headache of cerebral tumour often occurs in bouts and may be worse early in the morning. Similarly, migraine often starts on waking and continues for a number of hours. There may be periods of days, weeks or months free from any further attack. By contrast, psychogenic headaches are seldom absent until their cause is removed.

4. *Associated symptoms*: These are of great importance in the grosser neurological diseases such as cerebral tumour and meningitis. Alteration in behaviour, clouding of consciousness, mental confusion, vomiting, neurological signs and papilloedema are some of the more important features. The presence of albuminuria and retinopathies, hypertension, visceral disease and so forth may give the clue to the origin of the headache.

The background of psychogenic headaches is discussed in Chapter 10.

## Coma

This is defined as a state of unconsciousness from which the patient cannot be roused. It may gradually supervene in the last stages of many chronic diseases, but the present comments concern those forms which develop rapidly or unexpectedly and thus offer a problem for diagnosis in the casualty department or in the home (*see Table* 1.2 and *Fig.* 1.3).

A *history* should always be sought from relatives concerning the previous health

| Table 1.2 | **Coma: common causes and diagnostic signs** |
|---|---|
| *The cause* | *Diagnostic signs* |
| **1. Cerebral** | |
| Trauma | Skull or scalp injury |
| | Blood or CSF from nose or ears |
| Vascular | Hemiplegia; hypertension; neck rigidity (if subarachnoid haemorrhage) |
| Neoplasm | Focal CNS signs |
| | Papilloedema |
| Infections | Pus from nose or ears |
| | Neck rigidity |
| | Fever |
| Epilepsy | History or signs of convulsions |
| | Tongue scarred or bleeding |
| **2. Metabolic** | |
| Uraemia | Uriniferous breath |
| | Dehydration |
| | Twitching |
| | Retinopathy |
| | Proteinuria |
| Diabetes | Acetone on breath |
| | Dehydration |
| | Retinopathy (micro-aneurysms) |
| | Sugar and ketones in urine |
| Hypoglycaemia | Sweats |
| | Twitching |
| | Babinski's sign may be present |
| $CO_2$ narcosis | Sweats |
| | Central cyanosis |
| | Signs of lung disease |
| | Papilloedema |
| Hepatic | Jaundice |
| | Splenomegaly |
| | Haematemesis |
| | Flapping tremor |
| Myxoedema | Puffy face |
| | Dry skin |
| | Bradycardia |
| | Low temperature |
| **3. Toxic** | |
| Alcohol | Smell of breath |
| | Flushed face |
| | (Look carefully for head injury) |
| Narcotic drugs (opiates and barbiturates) | Pinpoint pupils (opiates) |
| | Shallow breathing |
| | Cyanosis |

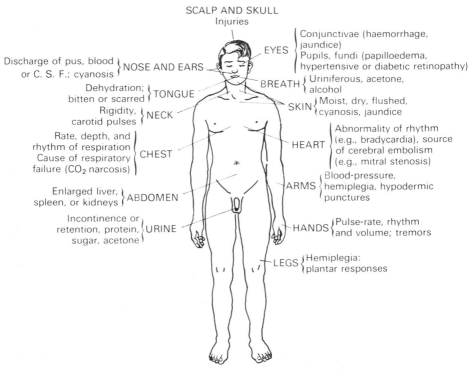

SCALP AND SKULL
Injuries

EYES — Conjunctivae (haemorrhage, jaundice)
Pupils, fundi (papilloedema, hypertensive or diabetic retinopathy)

Discharge of pus, blood or C. S. F.; cyanosis } NOSE AND EARS

BREATH { Uriniferous, acetone, alcohol

Dehydration; bitten or scarred } TONGUE

SKIN { Moist, dry, flushed, cyanosis, jaundice

Rigidity, carotid pulses } NECK

HEART { Abnormality of rhythm (e.g., bradycardia), source of cerebral embolism (e.g., mitral stenosis)

Rate, depth, and rhythm of respiration
Cause of respiratory failure (CO₂ narcosis) } CHEST

ARMS { Blood-pressure, hemiplegia, hypodermic punctures

Enlarged liver, spleen, or kidneys } ABDOMEN

Incontinence or retention, protein, sugar, acetone } URINE

HANDS { Pulse-rate, rhythm and volume; tremors

LEGS { Hemiplegia: plantar responses

**Fig. 1.3** Examination of the patient in a coma.

of the patient with special reference to hypertension, previous strokes or coronary disease, renal disease, epilepsy, diabetes and the taking of drugs such as insulin or barbiturates. If a witness of the onset is available, he should be questioned about the possibility of trauma or alcoholism, the occurrence of headaches or convulsions, and also whether the onset was sudden or gradual. In the absence of relatives, a search of the patient's personal effects may reveal clues in the form of a diabetic or epileptic card, or narcotic drugs.

*Physical examination* of the unconscious patient (*Fig.* 1.3) is obviously limited by the patient's inability to co-operate. This applies particularly to the discovery of paralysis which may be an important sign of a localized cerebral cause for the coma. However, a hemiplegia (*see also* p. 377) can usually be revealed by raising both arms or both legs and then letting them fall. The paralysed limb falls limply and heavily to the bed, the opposite side retaining sufficient normal tone to allow it to sink more gently. In lighter degrees of coma, paralysis can be detected by applying a painful stimulus to the part and observing whether there is any movement of withdrawal, e.g. flexion of the knee or screwing up of the face. It is essential that the examination should be systematic so that no important signs are overlooked. One system is to start at the top of the head looking for signs of trauma and finish at the soles of the feet by eliciting the plantar responses. This system is illustrated in *Fig.* 1.3. Certain signs, such as abolition of the tendon reflexes and incontinence or retention of urine, are common to many forms of coma, but those signs which are of value in differential diagnosis are listed in *Table* 1.2.

### Fits and faints

It is usually easy to distinguish a fit from a faint (*Table* 1.3). The former is essentially characterized by abrupt loss of consciousness and convulsive movements, though there are exceptions. The fits of *epilepsy* are described in Chapter 10, where they are contrasted with hysteria (p. 443). Here it is necessary to indicate that epilepsy can be due not only to local changes in the brain but to such indirect causes as interference with the cerebral blood supply in heart block, the effect of poisons such as alcohol and lead, and metabolic abnormalities as in uraemia and hypoglycaemia due to overdosage with insulin (or more rarely insulin-producing tumours). In infants and young children quite minor disturbances of health, as in febrile illnesses, may result in convulsions. Naturally all these causes act through the brain itself—usually the motor cells—and, although temporary cerebral ischaemia usually results in a faint, fits occur if it is prolonged.

A faint or syncopal attack is also mediated through the brain, though this organ may be normal and the effects on it are entirely vascular.

The common types of syncope are:

1. Vasovagal attacks in which a sudden fall of blood pressure, often with slowing of the heart rate, results in cerebral ischaemia.

| Table 1.3 | **Differences between fits and faints** | |
|---|---|---|
| | *Fits* | *Faints* |
| Precipitating cause | Usually none | Sudden or prolonged standing, pain, haemorrhage, fear, unpleasant sights and smells |
| Warning | Brief aura—sensory, psychic, or motor | Sense of expected loss of consciousness Nausea |
| Mode of onset | Instantaneous unconsciousness | Develops over minutes |
| Cry | Guttural on falling | None |
| Colour | Cyanosis/pallor | Intense pallor |
| Sweating | Rare | Common |
| Rigidity | Present (grand mal) | Absent |
| Convulsions | Present often (grand mal) | Rare |
| Incontinence | Common | Rare |
| Injury | Common | Occasional |
| Tongue biting | Common | None |
| After-effects | Sleep, altered behaviour, headache | Limpness and exhaustion |
| Pulse | Normal or rapid | Poor volume; slow |
| BP | Normal | Low |
| Local neurological signs | In focal epilepsy, Babinski when unconscious | |
| EEG | Abnormal | Normal |

For hysterical fits (now rare), *see* p. 443.

It is presumed that the vasomotor centres are disturbed so that blood is temporarily diverted to the splanchnic area and skeletal muscles, though obviously not to the skin, thus lowering the pressure of the circulating blood to other parts of the body, notably the brain. Another factor is the release of acetylcholine which causes pronounced vasodilatation; its destruction by choline esterase helps in the period of recovery. Such reflex disturbances can be caused by severe pain, unpleasant sights and smells, and prolonged standing or kneeling, especially in heat and sudden rising from a sitting or crouching posture. The vasomotor effects are most often psychogenic or gravitational in origin, but there may be other factors at work.

2. True cardiac syncope is less common and may be found more fully considered in Chapter 7, p. 204.

3. A number of chemical agents may cause extreme vasodilatation with a fall of blood pressure (though usually with tachycardia) and, as many of these are therapeutically employed, watch should be kept on the response of the patient to such drugs as nitrites, drugs used for hypertension, cholinergic substances, quinidine, procaine amide and beta-adrenergic blocking agents.

4. Occasional causes of fainting include hyperventilation as in hysteria, and certain organic cerebral lesions.

The features which suggest syncope rather than epilepsy are—

1. A material warning. The patient feels queer and that he must lie down. He may feel the 'colour draining away', breaks out in a cold sweat, and if he does not recline will lose consciousness, though the very act of falling may restore the cerebral circulation. He then quickly recovers, though feeling weak afterwards and inclined to faint again if he stands up too quickly.

2. The patient may observe, though more often the onlookers, that he becomes increasingly pallid and if he loses consciousness falls limply without convulsive movements or incontinence except in rare instances.

3. The pulse is feeble or absent and the blood pressure low or unrecordable. Generally the heart rate is slow. Tachycardia may be present if drugs or abnormal cardiac rhythms are responsible for syncope.

These points apply particularly to the simple vasovagal attack of psychogenic origin which is of short duration and generally harmless. When the faint is prolonged, more serious causes should be ruled out, particularly visceral catastrophes—cardiac, respiratory and abdominal—and also concealed haemorrhage. (Cf. Shock, *below*.)

*Table* 1.3 illustrates some of the points of difference between fits and faints.

### Shock

The more obvious conditions of which shock is recognized as an important feature are, of course, gross trauma, as in fractures and crushed tissues, burns and severe haemorrhage.

The syndrome as it comes to the physician's attention may have less obvious origins, as in pneumothorax, the concealed haemorrhage of duodenal ulcer or ectopic gestation, myocardial infarction, pulmonary embolism, acute abdominal catastrophes and bacteriaemia.

The accepted symptoms and signs include extreme weakness, great pallor, profuse sweating and a dramatic fall of blood pressure, often to levels of 50 mmHg or less. When the shock is less severe, allowance must be made for persons who normally have a rather low blood pressure (80–90 mmHg). The hypotension is clinically suggested by a feeble pulse generally with tachycardia. The patient is often confused and restless, but the specific features of the causal conditions may be apparent: e.g. pain in myocardial infarction; intense dyspnoea in tension pneumothorax; haematemesis or melaena in peptic ulcer.

It is important to recognize that these symptoms may be overshadowed by those of shock.

Much remains to be explained about the exact mechanisms of shock due to different causes, but the generally accepted view is that it results from circulatory collapse, particularly of the peripheral vascular system. The mechanisms include a reduction in venous return to the heart as in direct loss of blood, loss of plasma in burns and rapid removal of fluid by diarrhoea as in cholera.

In other cases there may be loss of arteriolar tonus and defective cardiac output as in myocardial infarction and in terminal stages of congestive cardiac failure in which cell metabolism is also greatly disturbed. Even so, the failure of cardiac output particularly due to infarction is often accompanied by a reflex arteriolar dilatation which aggravates the symptoms of shock. Rarer vascular causes of shock include sudden obstruction of arteries or valve orifices particularly due to pulmonary embolism or, more rarely, blockage in a major limb vessel.

Some of the features of shock are imitated by syncope, though this is generally transient.

### Loss of weight

It is not uncommon for a patient to complain of loss of weight or for his relatives and friends to notice this. It is wise to find out if throughout life the patient's weight has always fluctuated or, what is more significant, if it has remained steady over many years and has been dropping lately.

The maintenance of weight depends upon an adequate intake of suitable food, but the amount varies much from person to person. Given the right amount of food it may yet be badly digested or absorbed because of diseases affecting the digestive tract. It still remains for the digested and absorbed food to be metabolized properly and used in such a way as to rebuild the constantly breaking down tissues.

Some of the commoner causes of loss of weight can be assigned to defects in diet, impairment of digestion and absorption and variations in the state of metabolism. Psychogenic causes, such as states of anxiety, fear, depression and hysteria, may also be responsible, and are seen in an extreme form in anorexia nervosa (p. 80).

The questions that should be asked, therefore, in a patient losing weight are:

1. *How much weight has been lost and over what period of time?* It sometimes occurs that the patient merely thinks he is going 'thin' because of change of facial contours, and it is necessary to have better proof than this. The actual recording of the weight, stripped or in the same clothes and on the same scale, is clearly the most scientific method of answering the question, but without this the patient may be able to demonstrate that his clothes have become very loose.

2. *What are the habits of diet* in relation to the patient's physique, occupation and degree of physical activity?

3. *Is there loss of appetite* which will naturally lead to deficiency in food intake? This is described under Anorexia, p. 80.

4. *Is there evidence of digestive tract disease?* Conditions causing pain or difficulty in chewing and swallowing, e.g. dental disease and oesophageal obstruction, may prevent food from entering the stomach in adequate amounts, although the desire for food may still be present.

Malignant disease of the digestive tract, especially the stomach, is a common cause of loss of weight, and malabsorption syndromes (p. 82) are also recognized as responsible. Less frequently, impaired biliary or pancreatic function may be held to blame.

5. *Is there metabolic disorder* causing loss of weight? In diabetes there is failure to metabolize and store carbohydrates and secondarily some derangement in fat and protein metabolism. The urine should be tested in all cases of loss of weight. Conditions that speed up the metabolism have a similar effect. This is well seen in thyrotoxicosis and febrile illnesses, especially when protracted, e.g. tuberculosis and typhoid. Weight loss may occur in fevers of short duration but is quickly regained. Weight loss in diabetes and thyrotoxicosis is usually associated with a good appetite.

## ■ TABLE OF SYMPTOMS

(This table must not be regarded as complete, but it will serve as a skeleton outline to which the student can add after further reading and experience in the wards. Fuller details of the *symptoms* of disease are given in each chapter and will suggest the type of question to be asked and will explain the reason why the questions are set out here. Those symptoms which have just been dealt with more fully are not included here.)

| Symptom | Questions | Examination |
|---|---|---|
| Blood in faeces | (*See* Examination of Faeces, p. 105) | |
| Blood in urine (haematuria) | 1 Amount. Colour of urine (bright red: smoky)<br>2 Relation to micturition (before, during, or after)<br>3 Pain (renal or bladder)<br>4 Other urinary symptoms | 1 Urinary system<br>2 Microscopy of urine<br>3 Haemopoietic system<br>4 Cardiovascular system |
| Collapse | 1 Patient's description of what happened<br>2 Did he fall? Was he unconscious?<br>3 Associated symptoms (dizziness, sweating, pallor, pain, diarrhoea, fever, haemorrhage)<br>4 Food or drugs taken<br>5 Previous health. Any similar collapse before<br>6 Onlooker's observations | 1 For evidence of poisoning, infections, intestinal derangement and internal haemorrhage<br>2 Cardiovascular system<br>3 Central nervous system |

| Symptom | Questions | Examination |
|---|---|---|
| Constipation | 1 Recent or long-standing<br>2 Normal habits<br>3 Partial or absolute<br>4 If partial, is it increasing?<br>5 Associated symptoms (pain, vomiting)<br>6 Any alternation with diarrhoea | 1 Intestinal tract (abdominal and rectal examination)<br>2 Examine for general state of health, especially loss of weight<br>3 Character of stools |
| Coughing of blood (haemoptysis) | 1 Evidence that the blood was coughed (blood bright red, frothy, etc.)<br>2 Amount of blood. Was the sputum subsequently stained?<br>3 Previous symptoms of respiratory or heart disease | 1 Respiratory system<br>2 Cardiovascular system<br>3 Haemopoietic system |
| Decreased quantity of urine (oliguria, anuria) | 1 Amount passed and frequency<br>2 Fluid intake<br>3 Duration of symptom<br>4 Appearance of urine<br>5 Other symptoms of renal or heart disease<br>6 Drugs taken | 1 Cardiovascular system<br>2 Urinary system<br>3 Distinguish from retention<br><br>(*see* pp. 132, 141) |
| Diarrhoea | 1 Recent or of long duration. Intermittent or persistent<br>2 Frequency of motions and their character<br>3 Any fever or loss of weight<br>4 Food eaten. Other persons affected | 1 Intestinal tract (abdominal and rectal examination)<br>3 Examination of faeces |
| Difficulty in micturition (dysuria) | 1 Exact nature (e.g. in starting, in force of stream, in inhibition)<br>2 If accompanied by pain | 1 Urinary system<br>2 Nervous system |
| Difficulty in swallowing (dysphagia) | 1 Site—high or low<br>2 Whether for fluids or only solids<br>3 Whether increasing<br>4 History of possible trauma to oesophagus (hot liquids; corrosive poisons)<br>5 Loss of weight<br>6 Pain | 1 Neck and chest—clinically<br>2 Oesophagus—radiologically<br>3 Heart and great vessels—clinically and radiologically<br>4 Mouth, pharynx and larynx<br>5 Central nervous system<br>6 For anaemia |
| Dizziness (vertigo) | 1 Continuous or paroxysmal<br>2 Does patient tend to fall in a particular direction?<br>3 Severity (does he fall?)<br>4 Variation with posture<br>5 Associated phenomena, e.g. vomiting, deafness, tinnitus | 1 Ears, including labyrinthine function<br>2 Nervous system (especially cerebellar tests)<br>3 Cardiovascular system<br>4 Eyes<br>5 Evidence of toxaemia |

| Symptom | Questions | Examination |
|---|---|---|
| Double vision (diplopia) | 1 Is the object seen double with one eye (monocular) or with both eyes (binocular)? (Test objectively) <br> 2 Does the diplopia increase on looking to the right, left, upwards or downwards? | 1 Close each eye in turn to see if diplopia is monocular or binocular <br> 2 In monocular diplopia examine for local disease of the eye <br> 3 In binocular diplopia test integrity of cranial nerves, especially external muscles of orbit <br> 4 Examine central nervous system |
| Flatulence | 1 Relation to meals <br> 2 Whether wind belched or passed per anus <br> 3 Is the flatus offensive? | 1 Observe for air-swallowing <br> 2 Examine gastrointestinal tract and associated viscera |
| Frequency of micturition | 1 Number of times urine is passed in 24 hours <br> 2 Whether at night or in daytime or both <br> 3 Amount of urine passed each time <br> 4 If accompanied by pain | 1 Urinary system <br> 2 Nervous system |
| Inability to pass urine (retention) (Cf. Decreased quantity of urine) | 1 Sudden onset or increasing difficulty <br> 2 Any psychical trauma <br> 3 Symptoms of urological or neurological disease | 1 Abdomen for distension of bladder <br> 2 If distension, examine for surgical causes of retention (especially stricture and prostatic enlargement), and also nervous system. Catheterize if necessary <br> 3 Do not overlook retention in any severe illness, especially with clouding of consciousness |
| Incontinence of faeces | 1 Is the symptom occasional or persistent? <br> 2 Is there a call to stool? <br> 3 Is the patient conscious of defaecation? | 1 Anus, rectum and colon <br> 2 Nervous system <br> 3 General condition with special reference to mental state and consciousness |
| Incontinence of urine | 1 Does it occur only at night (in which case the term 'enuresis' is used)? <br> 2 Does the urine dribble away all the time or only periodically? | 1 Urinary system <br> 2 Nervous system <br> 3 Vaginal causes <br> 4 Mental state |
| Increased quantity of urine (polyuria) | 1 Approximate amount passed, and frequency <br> 2 Appearance of urine | 1 Urinary system, including urinalysis and specific gravity |

| Symptom | Questions | Examination |
|---|---|---|
| | 3 Whether continually or only occasionally present. Mainly day or night<br>4 Is there undue thirst? | 2 Endocrine organs (especially for diabetes mellitus and insipidus) |
| Indigestion | 1 Exact definition, e.g. pain, flatulence, anorexia<br>2 Relation to food, and bowel movement<br>3 General health; diet<br>4 Relief from antacids | 1 Digestive system<br>2 Other systems for evidence of ill health<br>3 Irritative pain arising from other systems, e.g. root irritation |
| Involuntary movements (tremors, choreiform movements, spasms, etc.) | 1 Parts of body affected<br>2 Effect of voluntary muscular action and sleep upon<br>3 Continuous or occasional | 1 Nervous system<br>2 Evidence of toxaemia, e.g. in fevers, thyrotoxicosis, renal, respiratory or hepatic failure |
| Loss of power (paresis, paralysis) | 1 Sudden or gradual<br>2 Portion of body involved and extent<br>3 Whether maximum at onset or increasing<br>4 Previous attacks<br>5 Other symptoms of nervous disease | 1 Nervous system<br>2 Other systems which may give indications of the cause, e.g. sites of embolus formation, malignant disease, etc. |
| Loss of speech (aphasia and dysarthria) | 1 Mode of onset, sudden or gradual<br>2 Does patient understand speech (e.g. execute a simple command, given without signs)?<br>3 Does he understand written words, e.g. will he execute a command given in writing?<br>4 Does the patient speak? If so, is the speech intelligible?<br>5 Can he write? | 1 Nervous system, especially:<br>a Intellectual function<br>b For evidence of paralysis of limbs<br>c For evidence of paralysis of muscles of articulation (larynx, tongue, etc.) |
| Nausea | 1 Whether related to food<br>2 Whether accompanied by vomiting<br>3 Is the patient taking any medicines? | 1 Gastrointestinal tract and associated viscera<br>2 Nervous system |
| Neuralgia | (*See* Pain, pp. 7–10) | |
| Noises in the ears or head | 1 Type of noise, e.g. singing, buzzing, voices, etc.<br>2 Are the noises persistently or occasionally present? | 1 Ears (deafness, vertigo, aural pain or discharge)<br>2 Cardiovascular system, especially arteries and blood pressure<br>3 Nervous system<br>4 Evidence of mental instability |

| Symptom | Questions | Examination |
|---|---|---|
| Numbness, tingling, pins and needles (paraesthesiae: dysaesthesiae) | 1 Extent and distribution<br>2 Sudden or gradual onset<br>3 Periodic or continuous | 1 Nervous system, especially for involvement of peripheral nerves or sensory tracts<br>2 Cardiovascular system, especially peripheral vessels |
| Obesity | 1 Family history<br>2 Sudden or gradual onset<br>3 Generalized or localized<br>4 Habits of diet and exercise<br>5 If associated with pain | 1 Distribution of fat<br>2 Endocrine organs |
| Pallor (anaemia) | 1 The patient's usual colour<br>2 Whether of sudden or gradual appearance<br>3 Has there been any haemorrhage?<br>4 Any symptoms of anaemia? (See p. 295) | 1 Haemopoietic system. Blood count in all cases<br>2 Other systems or tissues, affections of which are known to produce anaemia |
| Palpitation | 1 Whether in attacks. If so, mode of onset and offset, with particular reference to suddenness<br>2 Is the heart rate known? Does it vary?<br>3 Consciousness of irregularity<br>4 Whether the patient has been taking drugs<br>5 Association with emotion and exercise | 1 Cardiovascular system<br>2 Nervous system |
| Rashes | 1 Duration and associated symptoms<br>2 Distribution<br>3 Is there (a) pain, (b) itching?<br>4 Is the patient taking drugs?<br>5 Contact with infectious diseases or known irritants | 1 Distribution and character of rash<br>2 Presence of fever and signs of toxaemia<br>3 If the rash has disappeared, the same questions should be asked even though objective confirmation may be impossible |
| Sore tongue and mouth | 1 Duration<br>2 Patchy (e.g. ulcers) or diffuse<br>3 Whether taking any medicines<br>4 Diet<br>5 Any dysphagia | 1 Digestive system, especially tongue, teeth and buccal mucosa<br>2 Haemopoietic system |
| Swelling of abdomen | 1 Sudden or gradual onset<br>2 Total duration<br>3 Whether the swelling varies in size<br>4 Whether body-weight is changing<br>5 Menstrual cycle<br>6 Alimentary symptoms | For general obesity, tympanites, ascites, enlarged viscera, pregnancy or abdominal tumours |

| Symptom | Questions | Examination |
|---|---|---|
| *Swelling of feet (oedema)* | 1 Whether persistent or only after standing, unilateral or bilateral<br>2 Degree and duration<br>3 Other symptoms of cardiac and renal disease, anaemia, etc.<br>4 Is it limited to the legs or is the face affected? | Confirm the presence of oedema by pressure (pitting) or note 'solid' oedema which does not pit. Then examine—<br>1 Cardiovascular system, including veins<br>2 Urine<br>3 Blood<br>4 Liver<br>5 Evidence of malnutrition |
| *Thirst* | 1 Quantity of fluid taken<br>2 Is there polyuria?<br>3 Duration | 1 Examine urine (sugar and albumin and specific gravity)<br>2 Look for causes and evidence of dehydration |
| *Unsteadiness in standing or walking (ataxia)* | 1 Is it worse in the dark?<br>2 Is it paroxysmal or persistent?<br>3 Are there associated symptoms (e.g. motor or sensory disturbances, vertigo, tinnitus or deafness)?<br>4 Does the patient tend to fall to one particular side?<br>5 If of short duration, inquire as to possible poisoning, including alcohol and hypnotic drugs | 1 Nervous system<br>2 Ears (labyrinthine function) |
| *Vomiting* | 1 Frequency and forcibility<br>2 Relation to meals; time of day<br>3 Whether preceded by nausea or pain<br>4 Quantity and nature of vomitus<br>5 Drugs causing emesis<br>6 Other associated symptoms—e.g. headache, tinnitus or diarrhoea | 1 Digestive system<br>2 Nervous system<br>3 Other systems if symptoms suggest involvement, e.g. renal disease |
| *Vomiting of blood (haematemesis)* | 1 Amount and character of haemorrhage<br>2 Signs suggesting its origin (e.g. other haemorrhages, dyspeptic history)<br>3 Appearance of stools (melaena)<br>4 Is patient taking drugs, e.g. aspirin, steroids? | 1 Digestive system<br>2 Haemopoietic system<br>3 Evidence of bleeding which might have led to swallowing of blood |

*Yellow skin (jaundice)*

1 Is the skin yellow or only sallow?
2 Are the conjunctivae yellow?
3 Is the symptom associated with (*a*) pain, (*b*) gastro-intestinal disturbance, (*c*) rigors?
4 What is the colour of the urine and stools?
5 Has the patient been taking drugs or having any injections (e.g. chlorpromazine)?

1 Skin and mucosae for signs of present jaundice and anaemia. Distinguish from other types of pigmentation (*see* p. 50)
2 Abdomen (especially liver, gallbladder and spleen)
3 Urine and stools

## The case records

Accurate case records are not only essential for the continuing care of individual patients but may also be required for legal purposes, for research or for the prediction of medical service needs within a particular area. The advent of computers for the storage, retrieval and analysis of medical records has increased rather than lessened the need for precision in the recording of the case history.

The system of case recording to be followed in this chapter is set out on pp. 29–35 and consists of five 'Ds': a *Description* of the patient, the clinical *Data*, the *Diagnosis*, the *Decisions* made and the *Developments* that ensue.

### ■ DESCRIPTION OF PATIENT

To avoid any possibility of confusion, the patient's full name (and, where applicable, hospital number) should appear on every page of the case record and on all documents included in the file. Most hospitals and clinics will have a printed sheet for the recording of information needed to identify the patient, but it is the student's duty to ensure that certain basic facts are available in his own records. As a minimum, these should include full name and address, date of birth, sex, race, marital status, next of kin, occupation and the time, date and mode of presentation. This last entry should indicate whether the patient was first seen in his own home, in the surgery or in hospital and, if the latter, whether he attended a clinic or presented as an emergency.

### ■ DATA

A list should first be made of the sources from which data are available, and these sources must be stated when the case history is written up. Evidence may be obtained from relatives and from members of the hospital staff or other witnesses to the various stages of the patient's illness. Vital information about the present and previous history, including the results of investigations and surgical procedures, is often available in the family doctor's referral note or in earlier hospital records and in urgent cases should be obtained by telephone. The sifting of this documentary evidence is an important part of the student's task but should not be done until after the patient has been interviewed. These data must be incorporated in the original case sheet even if they do not come to light until long afterwards. For example, it would be wrong to leave unchanged, under the heading 'past history', a patient's statement that her hysterectomy was performed for fibroids, when later it transpires from hospital records that the operation was for carcinoma. This change must be made also in the problem list (*see* 'Problems') although it may be decided not to correct the patient's own original impression of her illness (*see* 'Explanation to patient').

The history and physical signs (*see* Chapter 3), along with any previous case documents, and the results of laboratory and other investigations constitute the basic data from which the diagnosis is made, problems identified and management planned. The history should be recorded under the traditional headings and the physical signs under the appropriate system. The date and hour at which the record is made must be clearly stated.

Although this rigid system of *recording* is necessary to permit a clear view of the patient's problems, it is equally important that the methods used for *eliciting* symptoms and signs should remain flexible. The patient's story must be allowed to flow freely with the minimum of interruption or interrogation. The student may find it helpful to write down, in the form of rough notes, what the patient has to say and later reassemble these in chronological order, excluding irrelevant matter and making clear which statements are answers to leading questions rather than volunteered. On writing out his case notes the student may find omissions which send him back to the patient's bedside for further information. He may also recognize that items recorded under past history are in fact an essential part of current illness and should therefore be transferred to the history of the present condition.

Similar principles apply to the recording of the physical examination. It may be more convenient for both patient and examiner, for example, to start with the head and finish at the feet, but the final record, compiled from rough notes made at the bedside, should present the findings according to the system affected; and again, as in the case of the history, the student must return to the patient if any gaps appear in this final systematic record. Whenever possible, diagrams should be used to illustrate abnormal findings. This applies especially to signs in the chest and abdomen, superficial sensory changes, abnormalities in the reflexes and the distribution of rashes or joint lesions. A suitable basic diagram is shown in *Fig.* 2.1.

It is of the utmost importance to record facts and observations rather than theories and inferences. This applies to the history and physical findings alike. For example, a case history may record as fact a patient's statement that he had pneumonia several years earlier. This could be an erroneous deduction on the part of the patient or his doctor from the symptoms noted at the time. If these consisted of cough, haemoptysis and pleuritic pain, which could equally well have been due to pulmonary infarction, it is these symptoms and not a 'diagnosis' which should appear under past history.

The student must also be particularly careful to record in detail the physical signs which he actually observes rather than the inferences that he draws from them. In the author's experience, a not uncommon error relates to long-standing facial palsy in which the palpebral fissure may be widened by retraction of the lower eyelid. This may be misinterpreted as narrowing of the opposite palpebral fissure, which is then wrongly attributed to ptosis. Mistakes of this kind would

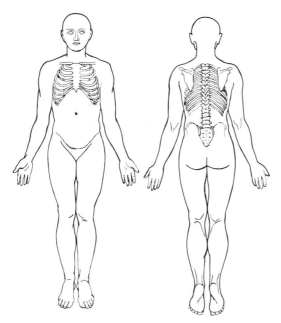

**Fig. 2.1** Basic diagram for case records to illustrate abnormal findings in physical examination.

not occur if accurate descriptions were carefully assembled before any attempt was made to interpret them.

## ■ DIAGNOSIS

When the student is satisfied that the data are as complete and accurate as possible, he should then briefly summarize the main features in the present history, in chronological order, and those items in the ancillary history which seem potentially relevant either to the chief complaints or to the abnormal signs. This should be followed by a simple list of the abnormal physical findings in each system. To facilitate this, an asterisk can be placed against all positive or relevant items in the ancillary history, the systematic questioning and the physical examination (*see* Sample Case Record, p. 30).

An attempt is then made to find a single diagnosis which will account for most or all the facts of the case. If some facts do not fit the pattern appropriate to this diagnosis, their accuracy must be checked and the original diagnosis reviewed before two or more separate diagnoses are postulated.

A complete diagnosis would describe the patient's illness in terms of the *site* (anatomy: where?), *nature* (pathophysiology: what?) and *cause* (aetiology: why?) of the disease process. In most instances, however, the physician has to be satisfied with a differential diagnosis which admits to more than a single possible answer to one or more of these three questions. The alternative diagnoses should be listed in order of probability and reasons given in support of the one which is preferred.

When considering the differential diagnosis, priority must always be given to the problems for which the patient sought medical advice. It is fair to say that in the past more emphasis has sometimes been placed upon diagnostic precision than on defining the actual problems confronting the patient and his physician. In recent years, there has been a move to construct case sheets in terms of such problems and to use the so-called 'problem-orientation' of records as the basis for management decisions.

# ■ DECISIONS

## Problems

The first decision to make is which of the patient's problems require attention (investigation, treatment or surveillance) and which, for the time being at least, can be set aside. Two lists of problems are thus compiled: 'active' and 'inactive'. These lists should appear as the front page of the case sheet as well as in the main text (*see* 'Plans' *below*), with a number or some other symbol assigned to each problem.

As time passes and more information comes to hand, 'active' problems may be redesignated as 'inactive' (or vice versa) and new problems are added to the list. Moreover, old problems are removed if they are erroneous, or amalgamated if two or more prove to be parts of the same entity. Each addition or other change to the problem list is carefully dated.

A 'problem' will only rarely be a complete diagnosis as defined in the previous section. It may consist of a symptom or sign which is not yet fully explained, a clinical syndrome of uncertain cause, a risky habit or occupation, adverse domestic or social circumstances, a predisposition to certain diseases evident in the past or family history, known allergies especially to drugs, an abnormal laboratory finding, a previous operation or a potentially dangerous form of treatment.

## Plans

A plan is devised for each 'active' problem and recorded, under the number and heading of that problem, in the section of the case sheet which follows 'Diagnosis'. The plan is set out in three parts:

*a. Investigations*: These could include ward or laboratory tests, radiographs, consultations, requests for further information about previous health or a social worker's report on the patient's home and working conditions.

*b. Treatment*: This may consist of medicinal therapy, special diets, or physical measures such as irradiation, physiotherapy or surgery. (It should be noted that the precise dosage of drugs and their route of administration are recorded also on a separate chart.)

Some indication should be given of the aims and the order of priority of the tests and treatment prescribed, the hazards that may be encountered and the action to be taken if they arise.

*c. Explanation to patient*: What is said to the patient, or even within his hearing, can determine the success or failure of management. 'They don't tell you anything' or 'They all said something different' are only too often the complaints of a patient leaving hospital. Nothing should be done to a patient nor said in his presence that has not first been explained, albeit in the simplest terms. Answers to patients' questions given by different members of the staff, whether physician, nurse or student, must be consistent.

It follows that the case records should clearly state what the patient (or, where applicable, the next of kin) is to be told or has been told about the *nature*, *treatment* and *prognosis* of his condition. The form of explanation will vary from one patient to another according to his intelligence, education and temperament. It may be decided, for example, not to reveal to a patient with an inoperable bronchial carcinoma the malignant nature of the lesion. The term used to describe his condition must be written in the case record so that he is not told by successive members of staff that he has 'an ulcer in the tubes', 'an abscess in the lung' and 'an enlarged gland in the chest' – to mention three of the commonly used euphemisms for carcinoma.

## ■ DEVELOPMENTS

After the case record has been completed and the initial plans carried out, all subsequent developments should be recorded. These may consist of new symptoms or signs, results of investigations or response to treatment. The results of investigations will usually be filed on sheets separate from the main case record but should also be included in progress notes when they either confirm or refute the original assessment of the case.

Each 'development' should be recorded under the title and number of the problem to which it is relevant and, where appropriate, changes or additions are made to the original problem list on the front sheet (*see* 'Problems' *above*, paragraph 2). The initial plans are also reviewed and further plans drawn up in the light of any new developments.

The progress or development of a case can sometimes be best displayed in the form of a graph or chart. This is done as a nursing routine in the case of pulse rate and temperature, but other examples include the haemoglobin in patients with anaemia, the blood pressure in those on hypotensive drugs, the weight as a measure of fluid balance and the serum bilirubin in patients with jaundice.

## ■ THE SYSTEM OF CASE RECORDING

| *Description* | | | | |
|---|---|---|---|---|
| | 1 | Name and address | 5 | Marital status |
| | 2 | Date of birth | 6 | Next of kin |
| | 3 | Sex | 7 | Occupation |
| | 4 | Race | 8 | Time, date and mode of presentation |

| *Data* | | | | |
|---|---|---|---|---|
| | 1 | Sources | 5 | Social history |
| | 2 | Initial complaint | 6 | Family history |
| | 3 | History of present condition | 7 | Physical signs |
| | 4 | Past history | | |

| *Diagnosis* | | |
|---|---|---|
| | 1 | Summary of relevant data |
| | 2 | Differential diagnosis |

| *Decisions* | 1 | Problems: Active or inactive |
| | 2 | Plans: Investigations, treatment, explanation to patient |

| *Developments* | 1 | New symptoms or signs |
| | 2 | Results of investigations |
| | 3 | Response to treatment |
| | 4 | Changes in problems or plans |

## SAMPLE CASE RECORD

### DESCRIPTION OF PATIENT

John Smith, 15 Castle Road, Chester
Born: 21.9.47
Male, Caucasian
Married. Next of kin: Mrs Catherine Smith (wife): same address
Occupation: Builder's labourer

Arrived in Emergency Dept. by ambulance at 15·00 hours on 10 Jan., 1987.

### DATA

*Sources*

Family doctor's letter, Emergency Dept. records, previous hospital case sheet, patient's wife.

*Initial Complaint:*
*10.1.87 15·50 hours*

Headaches and confusion: 1 hour (from patient and wife)

*Past History*

*Rheumatic fever: 1957
Appendicectomy: 1958
*Gastric ulcer diagnosed by barium meal: 1976
(check previous hospital records). No symptoms in last 8 years
*Jaundice: anorexia, nausea, dark urine; cleared in 3 weeks; treated at home; no records available: 1979
*Bronchitis: cough, sputum and wheezing dyspnoea; off work for 4 weeks: February, 1986.

*Family History*

*Wife has rheumatoid arthritis – cannot manage stairs unaided
2 sons well, aged 10 and 6
Mother well, aged 78
*Father died aged 62: stroke
*1 brother died aged 49: heart attack
2 sisters well, aged 36 and 42 years.

*Social History*

*Home: lives with wife and two sons in 3-bedroom, 2-storey flat
Work: builder's labourer
Meals: regular and adequate
*Habits: smokes 30 cigarettes per day. No alcohol or drugs
Hobbies: gardening
Abroad: to France in 1985. Never in tropics
*Worries: About his ability to continue work and pay mortgage on flat; also about wife's illness preventing her from looking after the children.

*History of Present Condition:*
*4 months*

Tires easily. Short of breath, first noticed when digging in the garden and subsequently when playing with the children.

*6 weeks ago*

Sudden palpitations when gardening. Have recurred at irregular intervals since then, sometimes at rest.

*Today*

*History from wife.* Came home for lunch. Slumped over the table. Called out but could not say what was wrong. Wife noticed that his face was twisted and his speech strange. Tried to get up but fell to the floor. Doctor sent for.

*Doctor's letter.* Found patient stuporose on floor, stertorous breathing, fast irregular pulse, right facial weakness, resisted attempts to undress him. Last seen with bronchitis in 1986. Ambulance sent for.

*Emergency Dept. records.* Patient conscious but apparently aphasic. Had a predominantly right-sided convulsive attack with urinary incontinence shortly after arrival. Admitted direct to ward.

*Patient.* Since admission, has complained of frontal headache and a confused feeling. Knows where he is and understands what is said but has difficulty in finding the right words.

*Systematic questioning:*

Appetite: good
No indigestion or vomiting
Bowels and micturition: normal
*Cough: in mornings; no sputum
Dyspnoea: as above; no orthopnoea
No chest or abdominal pain
No ankle swelling
Vision and hearing: good
No dysphagia
*Paraesthesiae: numb feeling in right hand
No previous fits or faints
Weight: steady.

*Physical examination:*

Well-nourished man of thin build. Seems apprehensive. Colour, skin, hair, lymph nodes, nails: normal.

*RS*

Equal expansion
Trachea central
Percussion note, breath sounds, voice sounds: normal
*Basal inspiratory crepitations; no wheeze.

*CVS*

No jugular venous engorgement or oedema
Pulse: normal volume and rhythm. Rate: 80/min.
BP: 130/85
Apex: 5th interspace; 9 cm from midline
*Apical 1st sound: increased
No opening snap or 3rd heart sound
*Apical pan-systolic murmur→axilla (gr.2)
*Apical mid-diastolic murmur (gr.3)
No aortic murmurs.

*DS*

Mouth: healthy
Abdo: no abnormal masses
Genitalia and rectum: normal.

CNS   Cerebral function: co-operative
      Orientated in time and place
      Understands and obeys the spoken and written word
      *Slight delay in finding the right word, e.g. in identifying objects
      *Cranial nerves: R. homonymous hemianopia; slight drooping of R.
      mouth angle
      *Trunk: R. adbominal reflexes absent
      Limbs: Normal power and tone
            *Reflexes: *See* diagram
            Normal sensation and co-ordination
            Gait: uncertain on legs but can walk unaided and without a
            limp.

| Reflexes | R | L |
|---|---|---|
| | – | + |
| Abdos | – | + |
| Bic. | + + | + |
| Tric. | + + | + |
| Sup. | + | + |
| KJ | + + | + |
| AJ | + + | + |
| PLS | ↕ | ↓ |

## DIAGNOSIS

### Summary

A 39-year-old man presenting with sudden right-sided weakness and difficulty in speech accompanied by a fast irregular pulse and followed by right-sided convulsions. He had complained of effort dyspnoea for 4 months and bouts of palpitation for 6 weeks. Past illnesses include rheumatic fever, gastric ulcer, jaundice and bronchitis. He smokes cigarettes and has a morning cough. There is a family history of premature vascular disease. On examination, there are mitral systolic and diastolic murmurs, basal lung crepitations, a right homonymous hemianopia with right corticospinal tract signs and motor dysphasia.

### Differential diagnosis

The physical signs in the heart indicate mitral stenosis and regurgitation, probably rheumatic in origin. Paroxysmal atrial fibrillation could account for the palpitations and the irregular pulse noted by the family doctor. The neurological features point to a lesion in the left cerebral hemisphere, probably vascular in view of the sudden onset. Embolism from the left atrium is the most likely cause, but in this heavy smoker with a family history of vascular disease atheroma is an alternative possibility. The effort dyspnoea and bronchitis could result from heavy smoking, from pulmonary congestion due to mitral disease or from a combination of the two.

## DECISIONS
*(to go on front page of Case Records)*

### Problem list

| Active | Noted | Resolved | Inactive |
|---|---|---|---|
| 1 Mitral stenosis and regurgitation | 10.1.87 | | |
| 2 History of cardiac dysrhythmia<br>→ Atrial fibrillation | 10.1.87<br>12.1.87 | | |
| 3 R. hemiparesis with dysphasia and convulsions | 10.1.87 | | |
| 4 Cigarette smoking | 10.1.87 | 14.1.87 | → Stopped smoking |
| 5 History of bronchitis<br>→ Problem 1 | Feb. 1986<br>13.1.87 | | |
| 6 History of jaundice | 1979 | 14.1.87 | → SH antigen negative |
| 7 | 1958 | 1958 | Appendicectomy |
| 8 Gastric ulcer | 1970 | 12.1.87 | → Ba. meal and gastroscopy negative |
| 9 Crippled wife – ? care of children | 10.1.87 | 12.1.87 | → Help obtained at home |
| 10 | 1957 | 1957 | Rheumatic fever |

## Decisions list: plans for active problems

| Problems | Plans Investigations | Treatment |
|---|---|---|
| 1 Mitral stenosis and regurgitation | ECG. Cardiac screening with Ba swallow. Blood count. Electrolytes. Cardiologist's opinion – ? catheter studies or echocardiography. | Heparin 10 000 units i.v. 6-hourly |
| | *Explanation* (to patient and wife). Scarred mitral valve in the heart. Probably caused a small clot to break off and lodge in a brain blood vessel. Treatment being given to prevent future clots and tests to decide whether a valve operation is needed and also whether the old gastric ulcer is still active. | |
| 2 Cardiac dysrhythmia | ECG monitor | |
| 3 R. hemiparesis with dysphasia and convulsions | Fasting serum lipids EEG Prothrombin time – ? anti-coagulants | Physiotherapy Speech therapy Phenytoin sodium 200 mg orally t.d.s. |
| 4 Cigarette smoking | | Stop smoking |
| 5 History of bronchitis | Lung function tests | |
| 6 History of jaundice | Liver function tests SH antigen | Warn laboratory |
| 8 Gastric ulcer | Hourly pulse (?bleeding from heparin). Faeces for occult blood. Urgent gastroscopy and Ba meal (? anticoagulants). Obtain 1976 hospital records | Gastric diet 2-hourly milk |
| 9 Crippled wife – ? care of children | Social worker | |

## DEVELOPMENTS

| | | | |
|---|---|---|---|
| *11.1.87* | *10·15 hours* | (1) | No signs of cardiac failure<br>ECG: bifid P waves. Otherwise normal<br>Sinus rhythm<br>Blood count and electrolytes normal. |
| | | (3) | No further convulsions. |
| | | (4) | Still smoking – riot act read! |
| | | (8) | No gastric symptoms or signs of bleeding. |
| *12.1.87* | *11·30 hours* | (1) and 2) | Complains of palpitations and dyspnoea; basal creps +. Atrial fibrillation confirmed in ECG. Heart rate 130/min.<br>*Start* Lanoxin 250 µg 6-hourly<br>Frusemide 40 mg each morning<br>Slow-K 1200 mg b.d. |
| | | (3) | Prothrombin time: 13 s (normal). |
| | | (8) | Gastroscopy and Ba meal: no evidence of gastric ulcer<br>Faeces negative for occult blood<br>*Start* Warfarin (details)<br>*Stop* Heparin (details). |
| *13.1.87* | *11·00 hours* | (1) and (5) | Lung function tests: no evidence of airways obstruction; mild restrictive pattern only.<br>Cardiologist opinion: Mitral stenosis and regurgitation with fixed calcified valve. Respiratory symptoms probably due to mitral disease not bronchitis. Will arrange catheter studies with view to mitral valve replacement. Patient and wife notified of arrangements. |
| *14.1.87* | *10·20 hours* | (2) | Atrial fibrillation controlled. Heart rate: 84/min.<br>Lung bases clear. |
| | | (3) | Neurological signs unchanged<br>Serum lipids: normal. |
| | | (4) | Has stopped smoking. |
| | | (6) | SH antigen negative: laboratory notified. |
| | | (8) | No gastric symptoms or signs of bleeding. |
| | | (9) | Social worker: home help obtained for wife.<br>Wife's sister coming to look after children. |

# External manifestations of disease

■ ## INSPECTION OF EXTERIOR OF BODY

While talking to a patient and taking the history outlined in the last chapter, the student should be noting any special characteristics which suggest disease. Such preliminary inspection of the patient as a whole may give clues to diagnosis which could be missed during a detailed examination of the systems. For example, a general slowing of the body's physical or mental activity may be unaccompanied by any focal signs in the early stages of Parkinsonism and hypothyroidism. An impression may also be formed about the general health of the patient and whether he is suffering from any physical discomfort such as pain or dyspnoea. The patient's emotional state and attitude to his illness should also be noted at this stage.

The following observations should then be made: (1) Facial characteristics; (2) Abnormalities in the head and neck; (3) Examination of the mouth (*see* Chapter 4); (4) Character and distribution of hair; (5) Height and weight; (6) Posture and gait; (7) Skin; (8) Genitalia; (9) Extremities.

### FACIAL CHARACTERISTICS

Abnormalities of colour may be most evident in the face but can be reliably detected only in natural light. Screens should, therefore, not be drawn around the bed until colour changes have been excluded. The yellow tint of jaundice is confirmed by inspection of the sclera and the pallor of anaemia by examining the conjunctival lining of the lower eyelid. Cyanosis, the blue colour imparted by hypoxic blood, is usually best seen in the lips, nose and ears; blueness of the tongue (*see* p.164) indicates that the cyanosis has a central origin. A deep dusky red colour suggests polycythaemia. The brown pigmentation of Addison's disease may show in the face, especially over areas of friction (e.g. the nasal bridge in those who wear glasses) but, unlike sunburn, it may also occur in the buccal mucosa.

Thickening of the subcutaneous tissues may be seen in acromegaly and myxoedema, and the puffiness of the eyelids in the latter condition may simulate the true subcutaneous oedema of renal disease (*Fig.* 3.1) or superior vena caval

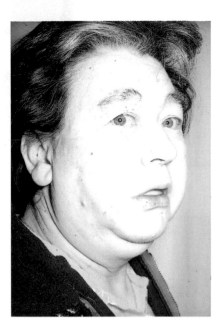

**Fig. 3.1** Hypothyroidism.

obstruction. A puffy swollen face with closure of the eyelids may also occur as an allergic reaction to certain drugs, foods or insect bites. In old age and dehydration (e.g. in diabetes and severe diarrhoea) the skin may be parched and wrinkled.

The condition of the blood vessels should be recorded. Dilated vessels are often seen in mitral disease and in alcoholics: in the former especially on the cheeks, in the latter on the nose but similar changes occur in those who work out of doors. The butterfly rash occurs in rosacea and lupus erythematosus (*see* p. 41 and *Fig.* 3.10, p. 42). Spider naevi are common in cirrhosis of the liver. All changes in the skin of the face must be compared with those of other parts of the body.

The individual's personality and mood may affect the facial characteristics. This is partly due to the alteration in facial lines and wrinkles which may become modified by pain, fear, anxiety and apathy. Grosser changes may occur in *mental disease* when there may be a stupid expression or a fatuous grin. Changes in character due to alcohol, heroin, morphine, cocaine and other forms of drug addiction may be suspected from the facies. The expression of the drugtaker is often shifty, though when deprived he may show agitation and terror. The alcoholic often looks self-satisfied and is plausible in manner.

It is none the less important not to jump to conclusions about alterations in expression because they may merely indicate nervousness, shyness, or be evidence of some other psychological imbalance.

Wasting and plumpness may be noticed first in the face, though they should be looked for elsewhere. A notable rounding of the facial contours is not uncommon in patients on corticosteroid therapy ('moon face'). Many nervous diseases such as Parkinsonism and myopathies, which will be described later, have typical facies.

### The eyes

Local diseases of the eyes are beyond the scope of this book and will be considered only in so far as they have a bearing on general medical diagnosis.

*Ptosis, squint, irregularity in the pupils and other evidence of oculomotor pareses* are of particular importance in the diagnosis of nervous diseases and are considered more fully in Chapter 10, p. 357 (*see also* p. 352 *for examination of the optic nerve*).

*Exophthalmos or proptosis* (*Fig. 3.2, see also* p. 358) is a notable feature of primary hyperthyroidism and may also result, though more rarely, from tumours affecting the orbit or from thrombosis of the cavernous sinus (generally unilateral) (*Fig.* 3.3).

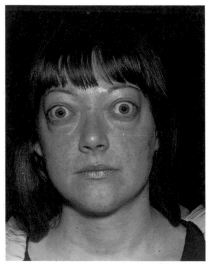 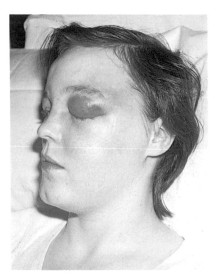

**Fig. 3.2**
Exophthalmos. Note staring expression with abnormal exposure of the sclera between the iris and the eyelids.

**Fig. 3.3**
Cavernous sinus thrombosis. Shows redness and oedema of eyelid, obscuring proptosis. Requires differential diagnosis from erysipelas and insect bites.

*Enophthalmos* (recession of the eyes) may occur in serious wasting diseases and dehydration; in the latter, gentle pressure over the closed eye will reveal an abnormal softness and inelasticity of the eyeball. Abnormal hardness on palpation of the closed eye indicates raised intraocular tension (glaucoma) which is an important cause of ocular pain and visual impairment in the elderly.

Inspection of the eyeball itself should take into account abnormalities of the conjunctiva, sclera, cornea, iris and lens.

*Conjunctival* changes of general medical import include the pallor of anaemia; oedema ('chemosis') due to hypoproteinaemia or impaired venous drainage (*Fig.*

3.4; *see also Fig.* 11.10, p. 469); abnormal dryness ('conjunctivitis sicca') in lacrimal gland disease, e.g. Sjögren's syndrome; inflammation in certain infective and allergic disorders such as measles, hay fever or the Stevens–Johnson syndrome (*Fig.* 3.5); increased vascularity imparting a glistening appearance to the eyes in respiratory failure and polycythaemia; haemorrhage resulting from blood diseases, fractured skull or violent cough (e.g. whooping-cough).

*The sclera* is yellow in jaundice and may show inflammatory changes ('episcleritis') in rheumatoid arthritis (*see Fig.* 9.13). Rarely, the blue sclerotics of fragilitas ossium are seen (*Fig.* 3.6).

The commonest abnormality of the *cornea* is arcus senilis which appears as an opalescent ring of lipoid material obscuring the periphery of the iris in elderly

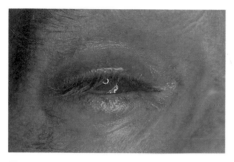

**Fig. 3.4**
Chemosis and oedema
of eyelid due to metastasis in
orbit from bronchial carcinoma.

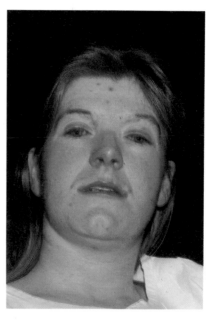

**Fig. 3.5**
Acute conjunctivitis in
Stevens–Johnson syndrome
(*see also Fig.* 3.21).

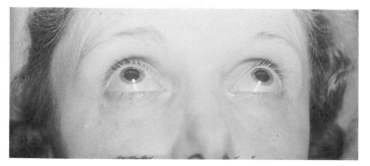

**Fig. 3.6** Fragilitas ossium. The patient, aged 40, had suffered numerous fractures since childhood—spontaneously or from minor injuries. Her son, aged 16, had the same complaint.

subjects. A premature arcus senilis sometimes results from hyperlipidaemia, which may be associated with arterial atheroma.

The cornea may be rendered opaque by the interstitial keratitis of congenital or acquired syphilis. In hepato-lenticular degeneration, a golden-brown deposition of copper (Kayser-Fleischer ring) can sometimes be seen at the periphery of the cornea with the aid of a slit lamp.

**The iris** Iritis occurs in rheumatoid arthritis, ulcerative colitis and sarcoidosis, and may be recognized by the discoloration and distortion of the iris and irregularity of the pupil. A rim of iris atrophy also surrounds the Argyll Robertson pupil of neurosyphilis. In albinism, there is lack of pigmentation of the iris, and also of the skin and hair, associated with impaired vision and nystagmus. The eye thus has a pink appearance and the eyelashes are white.

**The lens** Diabetes and prolonged hypocalcaemia both predispose to cataract which can sometimes be seen with the naked eye as a grey opacity behind the pupil. A rare abnormality is the curious shimmering movement of the iris caused by the ectopic lens in Marfan's syndrome.

### The lips

Indications of ill health may be given by the lips. They are dry and cracked in most illnesses, even of a trivial nature, but *sordes*, a collection of epithelial debris, food and bacteria, are present in the more serious diseases such as uraemia and prolonged fevers. Angular stomatitis, especially with a sore magenta-coloured tongue, may indicate ariboflavinosis (*Fig.* 3.7) but can occur in other deficiency states. Angular stomatitis may also result from ill-fitting dentures and from fungal infections such as candidiasis (thrush).

*Herpes simplex*, a virus infection of the skin, is recognized as an eruption of

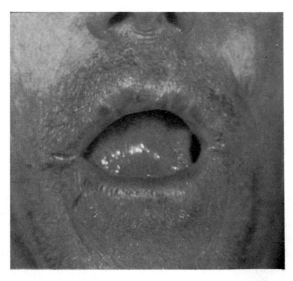

**Fig. 3.7** Ariboflavinosis. Smooth magenta-coloured tongue and angular stomatitis.

vesicles which soon burst and form scabs. It appears not only on the lips but occasionally on other parts of the face (*Fig.* 3.8). The lesions are often described by the patient as 'cold sores' and are a common accompaniment of both upper and lower respiratory tract infections. Herpes simplex is therefore a useful physical sign in the differential diagnosis of pulmonary infection, in which it is commonly present, from pulmonary infarction.

Anaemia and cyanosis are particularly well seen in the lips, but are considered elsewhere. The lips are thick in myxoedema and acromegaly. In the myopathic facies the lower lip is pendulous, exhibiting part of the mucous membrane (*see Fig.* 10.73, p. 412). in scleroderma the lips are puckered (*see Fig.* 3.29, p. 56) while in Addison's disease they may be pigmented.

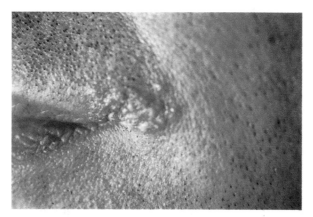

**Fig. 3.8** Herpes simplex.

### The nose

The nose is large in acromegaly, due partly to thickening of the subcutaneous tissues, and partly to bony overgrowth. In hypothyroidism it tends to broaden.

The skin and underlying tissues of the nose may be damaged and destroyed by tuberculous infection (*lupus vulgaris*) or by the granulomatous lesion of sarcoid (*lupus pernio*) or Wegener's granuloma (*Fig.* 3.9). The resulting exposure of the nostrils gives rise to a wolf-like appearance (L. *lupus*, a wolf).

In congenital syphilis the bridge of the nose is depressed, giving a saddle-back appearance.

Rosacea is characterized by a reddening of the nose and cheeks, giving the 'butterfly-wings' appearance. It is seen in alcoholics and, in exaggerated form, occurs as the 'strawberry nose'. An appearance similar to rosacea occurs in lupus erythematosus which may have manifestations in other organs (*Fig.* 3.10).

Perhaps the commonest abnormality of the nose is obstruction to the airway leading to mouth-breathing and a 'nasal' voice; this may be accompanied by discharge (rhinorrhoea) or signs of inflammation over the paranasal sinuses. These changes may reflect allergic or infective conditions of the respiratory tract as a whole and, in particular, can be associated with asthma or bronchiectasis.

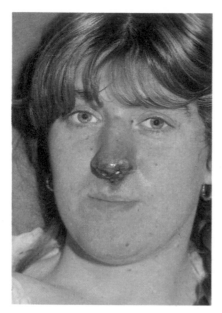
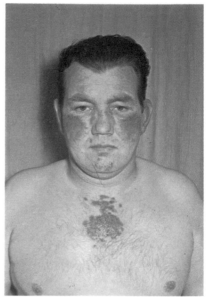

**Fig. 3.9**
Wegener's granuloma of the nose.

**Fig. 3.10**
Systemic lupus erythematosus: typical distribution of rash, including the butterfly-wing appearance on the face.

Examination of the interior of the nose with a speculum may reveal mucosal changes relevant to systemic disease, e.g. the source of epistaxes in patients with vascular or haematological disorders and nasal polyps in asthmatic subjects.

### The ears

The ears may be deformed. The usual malformation is an absence of well-defined lobes and a fusion of the ear to the face where the lobe should normally be freely dependent. Ears of this type are common in mental defectives and in epileptics. In Down's syndrome (mongolism) the ears are usually large.

Note should be taken of any cyanosis of the periphery of the ear, which may occur in all conditions causing cyanosis. A herpetic eruption may be seen on the ear in the Ramsay–Hunt syndrome (*Fig.* 10.30. p. 364). Any discharge from the meatus should be recorded, as it may indicate middle-ear infection and have an important bearing in suspected intracranial abscess. In such cases, the mastoid area should be examined for tenderness and other signs of inflammation. The external auditory meatus and eardrum can be inspected by means of an auroscope (*Fig.* 3.11).

*Tophi* ('chalk-stones') are collections of uric acid salts which occur in gout. They appear as whitish masses stretching the skin of the ears and sometimes protruding through it (*Fig.* 3.12). They may be seen in other parts of the body.

*Abnormalities of hearing*: See p. 364 *et seq.*

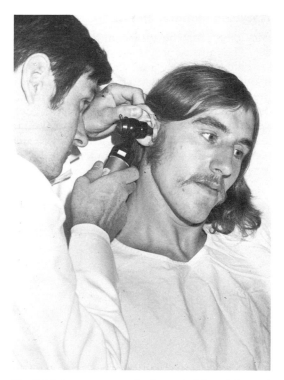

**Fig. 3.11** Auroscopy: to obtain good vision of the eardrum, the auricle is drawn upwards and backwards while the speculum is directed slightly forwards.

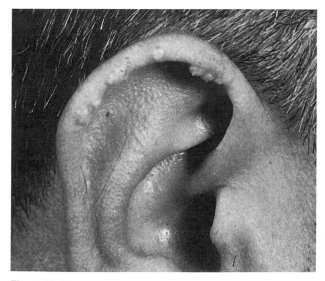

**Fig. 3.12** Gouty tophi in the ear.

### The salivary and lacrimal glands

The salivary glands may be enlarged. Parotid swellings are situated chiefly in front of the ear. The most important from the physician's point of view is the bilateral painful swelling of these glands caused by *mumps*. In this disease there is pyrexia and it is sometimes complicated by orchitis, parotitis or a meningo-encephalopathy. Unilateral parotitis is more often due to sepsis, usually associated with a salivary calculus, but may be a feature of typhoid. Swellings beneath the chin may be due to enlargement of the submaxillary or sublingual glands, but their diagnosis falls more within the scope of surgical practice. Rarely, involvement of salivary and lacrimal glands may be seen in leukaemias, sarcoidosis and Sjögren's syndrome (*see Fig.* 3.13).

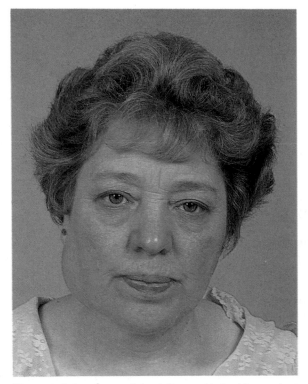

**Fig. 3.13** Enlargement of the right parotid gland in a patient with Sjögren's syndrome.

### Facial movements

These are considered under the nervous system. They give indications of lesions of the facial nerve, of hypertonicity or hypotonicity of the facial muscles, choreiform movements and other signs of neurological importance.

## ABNORMALITIES IN THE HEAD AND NECK*

The shape and size of the head is sometimes of diagnostic importance. In *hydrocephalus* it is often immense in proportion to the rest of the body, and the forehead appears to overhang the orbits, giving a sunken effect to the eyes, which are directed downwards. In such cases the sutures are unduly separated and the fontanelles enlarged and bulging (*Fig.* 3.14).

*Frontal bossing* occurs in rickets and in congenital syphilis, both rare now.

Generalized gradual enlargement of the head in adults, noticeable to the patient by the increase in the size of his hats, is almost a pathognomonic sign of osteitis deformans (Paget's disease) (*see Fig.* 9.1).

The great thickening and prominence of the superciliary arches with the receding forehead above contribute much to the simian appearance of the acromegalic (*Fig.* 3.15).

Lastly, *nodular irregularities* should suggest the possibility of secondary growths or primary tumours of bone or underlying structures such as myeloma or meningioma. (*Fig.* 3.16).

Enlargement of the thyroid gland is known as a *goitre* (*Fig.* 3.17). Note should be taken of the size, regularity or irregularity, consistency and movements of the gland on swallowing. Free movement distinguishes the goitre from enlargement of lymph nodes. When the latter are present, their extent and physical character (pp. 460, 465) should be observed. In particular, local malignant disease, e.g. of the bronchus, lips or tongue, may produce hard irregular lumps in the neck which contrast with the soft, tender, breaking down masses of septic nodes. Soft or 'rubbery' enlargement of lymph nodes without tenderness suggests a granulomatous lesion such as tuberculosis or sarcoid, a lymphoma (e.g. Hodgkin's disease) or a haematogenous disorder as in leukaemia and glandular fever. (*See also* The Haemopoietic System, p. 295.)

The position of the trachea (p. 167) and the activity of the accessory muscles of respiration are of importance in respiratory diseases.

Arterial pulsation or lack of it and prominence of the jugular veins may be observed. Their significance is dealt with under The Cardiovascular System (pp. 220, 292).

Examination of the musculoskeletal structures in the neck includes the noting of any abnormal posture such as torticollis, the compensatory hyperextension of ankylosing spondylitis (*see Fig.* 9.18, p. 333), and the short 'webbed neck' of Turner's syndrome (*see Fig.* 11.22, p. 477). The range of movement of the cervical and temporomandibular joints should be measured (*see also* Skeletal System, p. 324) and the function of the 11th (accessory) cranial nerve examined by testing the power of the sternomastoid muscles (*see also* Central Nervous System, p. 368).

## EXAMINATION OF THE MOUTH

(*See* p. 65.)

---

* *See also* The Examination of Children, Chapter 13.

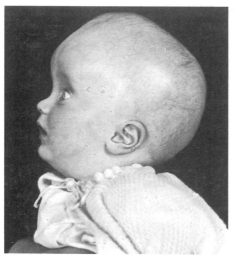

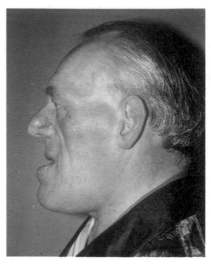

**Fig. 3.14**
Hydrocephalus. Great
enlargement of head, making
the face look
disproportionately small.

**Fig. 3.15**
Acromegaly: prognathism;
enlarged nose and ears;
prominent superciliary arches.

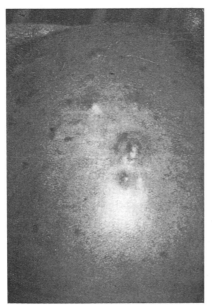

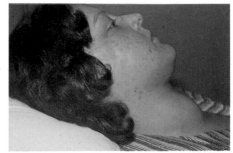

**Fig. 3.16**
Bronchial carcinoma:
secondary deposits in the
scalp.

**Fig. 3.17 Goitre.**
Goitre.

## CHARACTER AND DISTRIBUTION OF HAIR

Serious illness can result in dryness and temporary hair fall. In hypothyroidism these characters are especially noticeable, and the hair is thick, coarse and scanty, falling out particularly over the frontal region. The outer third of the eyebrows is also sometimes lost in hypothyroidism. A more complete loss of hair, axillary, pubic and facial, is a feature of anterior hypopituitarism (p. 470), Addison's disease in women and chronic hepatic failure (p. 119). In mongolism the hair is silky. Patchy loss of hair occurs in alopecia areata, a condition of unknown cause (but sometimes related to psychogenic illness) and also in secondary syphilis. Loss of hair from the legs in men may be a sign of arterial insufficiency. Excessive hairiness (hirsutism) (*Fig.* 3.18) in the female, especially over the moustache area and limbs, is not necessarily pathological and is common after the menopause. Grosser distribution over the trunk and limbs with moustache and beard formation requiring shaving call attention to the various types of virilism, especially adrenal.

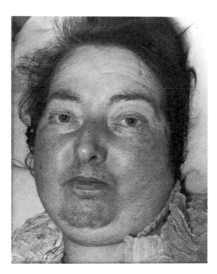

**Fig. 3.18**
Cushing's syndrome.
Hirsutism and moonface.

## HEIGHT AND WEIGHT

### Height

The height should be taken into consideration with the age and build of the patient (*see also* Examination of Children, Chapter 13), but although tables of height and weight give a rough indication of the correct proportion between these, they must be interpreted with considerable latitude. Height may be determined by ethnic or genetic factors, and the average height of other members of the patient's race and family must therefore be taken into account.

Excessive height, *gigantism*, suggests overactivity of the anterior lobe of the pituitary gland (excess of growth hormone) occurring before puberty, i.e. before the long bones have attained their full length. Other features of pituitary hyperfunction may also be present (*see* pp. 470–73). A tall, thin build with relatively long limbs is characteristic of *eunuchoidism* (*Fig.* 11.4, p. 464) and of Marfan's syndrome (*see Fig.* 7.55, p. 263).

Small stature, *dwarfism*, may be due to: (1) inherited skeletal anomalies such as achondroplasia or (2) to certain diseases acquired in early life before growth is complete. The acquired causes include: (*a*) impaired nutrition from faulty diet or malabsorption (e.g. coeliac disease; cystic fibrosis of pancreas); (*b*) conditions associated with chronic hypoxia such as asthma and congenital heart disease; (*c*) in tropical and developing countries especially, chronic infections and infestations; (*d*) endocrine disorders which include hypopituitarism (deficient growth hormone), untreated hypothyroidism (cretinism) and prolonged corticosteroid therapy for asthma or other childhood ailments; (*e*) chronic renal disease with calcium depletion ('renal rickets').

### Weight

The weight may be permanently below or above the average, but more significance attaches to a rapid change in weight.

Great *increase in weight* may be a familial characteristic, often occurring at the same age in different members. Although common in middle age, it may even occur in youth. This familial obesity may be aggravated by over-eating and lack of exercise. Obesity of this kind is of great importance in favouring the development of many diseases, especially those associated with disordered lipid metabolism (diabetes, atheroma, gallstones) and those due to muscular deficiency or gravitational stresses (inguinal and hiatal hernia, diverticulitis, uterine prolapse, varicose veins, osteoarthrosis). Obesity also increases the work and impedes the action of the heart and lungs and will thus aggravate dyspnoea, whatever its cause.

Obesity is seen in childhood as a temporary phenomenon which rectifies itself soon after puberty. More rarely in children or adults it is due to endocrine disturbance as in pituitary–hypothalamic syndromes, certain adrenal diseases, and sometimes in eunuchoidism. Weight increase in hypothyroidism is not due to fat.

Irregular distribution of fat occurs in the rarer lipodystrophies, in some of which the lower part of the body is obese and the upper part emaciated (descending lipodystrophy). In Dercum's disease, adiposis dolorosa, the masses of fat are painful to touch. A special form of localized accumulation of fatty tissue is the *lipoma*, which is often multiple. This is a very common but harmless condition which can be distinguished from other subcutaneous tumours by its soft consistency, lobulated surface and free movement in relation to deeper structures (*Fig.* 3.19).

*Decrease of weight* is described on p. 17.

The term *cachexia* usually implies serious wasting, a greyish or 'earthy' pallor and, frequently, an altered texture of the skin (dry and wrinkled). It is commonly reserved for cases of malignant disease, of which wasting is an essential symptom. Anorexia nervosa gives a similar appearance (p. 80). Occasionally, the word is applied to the general condition in grave diseases such as leukaemia, chronic renal disease, chronic tuberculosis and so forth.

### POSTURE AND GAIT

The posture of a patient sitting in a chair or lying in bed, or the gait as he walks into the consulting room, may provide the first clue to the nature

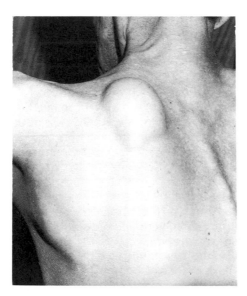
**Fig. 3.19**
Lipoma.

of his disease. Abnormalities are due most often to skeletal or neuromuscular disorders and these are dealt with in Chapters 9 and 10 (*see especially* pp. 384 *et seq.*).

### Posture

Skeletal and neurological lesions usually give rise to chronic and persistent disorders of posture such as kyphoscoliosis, ulnar deviation of the fingers, wrist drop and the rigidity of Parkinsonism. Abnormalities of posture arising in other systems are often more acute and transient and result from discomfort, pain or impairment of consciousness rather than from deformity. Patients in respiratory distress, especially of cardiac origin, tend to sit upright clasping their knees or hanging their legs over the edge of the bed. During a severe febrile illness with clouding of consciousness, the patient will lie flat and log-like. In anxiety states and hyperthyroidism, the patient will often sit bolt upright or perched on the edge of the chair, while in cases of depression or thyroid deficiency, a slumped slouching attitude is adopted. Pain may give rise to characteristic postures, as when the patient clutches or supports the affected part or avoids lying on tender areas of the body. In severe abdominal pain, the knees are often drawn up and the body as a whole is 'doubled up'. When the posterior parietal peritoneum is involved, as in carcinoma of the pancreas, relief may be obtained by leaning forwards over the edge of the bed or chair.

### Gait

As in the case of posture, abnormalities of gait due to causes other than skeletal or neuromuscular (*see* p. 384) usually result from discomfort or pain. For example, a limp may be due to painful infective, ulcerative or ischaemic lesions of the skin and subcutaneous tissues of the leg or, more rarely, inflammatory processes involving the psoas muscle in the abdomen. Severe varicose veins, thrombophlebitis and gross oedema of the legs can also cause discomfort on walking, with disturbance of gait. When walking causes dyspnoea, angina or ischaemic pain in the legs, the gait may be slow and cautious with frequent pauses.

## SKIN

Some of the points to be observed have been mentioned in describing the skin of the face, but it is necessary to inspect the skin of the whole body.

Undue *sweating* is common in certain infections, and is also usual during the subsidence of any pyrexia. The sweating of pulmonary tuberculosis occurs characteristically during sleep. Sweating is also common in hyperthyroidism and psychoneuroses and in many illnesses which cause exhaustion or severe pain. In most forms of shock there is a cold clammy skin. This may also occur in hypoglycaemia.

*Dryness* of the skin is also common in fevers in their earlier phases. It is a characteristic of hypothyroidism (*see* p. 466) and of some skin diseases (e.g. ichthyosis), and also results from dehydration.

The degree of *pigmentation* of the skin should next be noted. Increased pigmentation varying from light to dark shades of brown is a classic sign of Addison's disease (*see* pp. 473, 474) (adrenal insufficiency), but should be sought also in the mucous membrane of the mouth. Similar pigmentation may be caused by arsenical poisoning, chronic liver disease, intestinal malabsorption, malignant cachexia and pellagra, but the mucous membranes are rarely affected. The appearance of dirty patients may imitate some of these conditions. *Café au lait* spots may be seen in von Recklinghausen's disease. Pigmentation may also result from chronic venous congestion and is commonly seen in the lower parts of the legs in patients with varicose veins (*see Fig.* 3·43, p. 62). Therapeutic irradiation is another cause of localized pigmentation. The possibility that pigmentation is due to sunburn or to racial origin should be ruled out before it is attributed to disease. Patchy loss of pigment ('vitiligo') may occur as a congenital anomaly in healthy people or in association with hyperpigmentation and it is an occasional feature of autoimmune disorders (*Fig.* 3.20*a*). Pallor, cyanosis and jaundice are dealt with elsewhere, but note should be made of the rare yellow of carotinaemia (*Fig.* 3.20*b*), the grey of haemochromatosis and the yellowish raised patches of xanthomatosis. (*See* Xanthelasma, *Fig.* 7.2.)

Blackness of the skin may occur in gangrene, commonly the result of arterial obstruction (*see Fig.* 3.37, p. 60).

*Excoriation* due to scratching may result from irritation of the skin ('pruritus'). This accompanies certain rashes (*see below*) but can also provide important evidence of systemic disease, such as obstructive jaundice, lymphoma (e.g. Hodgkin's disease) and polycythaemia vera. Pruritus around the vulva is a common early manifestation of diabetes.

*Flushing* of the skin from transient capillary dilatation most often affects the head and neck, when it is usually due to emotional causes ('blushing') or to hormonal imbalance at the menopause ('hot flushes'). Generalized flushing occurs in fever, hyperthyroidism and hypercarbia. Rarer causes include Hodgkin's disease (in which flushing may be provoked by alcohol) and a carcinoid tumour secreting a vasodilatory substance (5-hydroxytryptamine) from hepatic metastases. Polycythaemia and chronic vasodilatation due to corticosteroid ther-

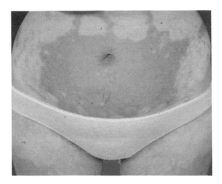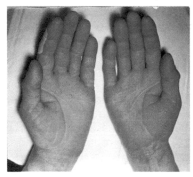

**Fig. 3.20** *a*, Vitiligo. *b*, Yellowish coloration of hands (also affecting the feet) in a patient consuming large quantities of raw carrots. This may also occur in hypothyroidism.

apy or alcoholism may give rise to a more persistent cutaneous flush often with telangiectases.

The texture of the skin may change. Apart from skin diseases, reference has already been made, in describing facial characteristics, to the increased thickness and coarse texture in myxoedema. This may affect the skin of other parts of the body.

### Rashes

Rashes are of great clinical importance. Sometimes the rash is the principal physical sign, as in the exanthemata—for example, measles and chickenpox; sometimes it is only subsidiary—for example, the purpura of haemorrhagic fevers and certain blood diseases. Drug reaction, whether due to overdose or undue susceptibility, is today among the commonest causes of an unusual rash; barbiturates, antibiotics (e.g. penicillin) and diuretics are specially liable to upset the skin. Drugs may also induce the Stevens–Johnson syndrome in which characteristic 'target' lesions in the skin (*Fig.* 3.21) are accompanied by conjunctivitis (*see Fig.* 3.5) and mucosal ulceration. A rash is a prominent feature of some vitamin-deficiency diseases, e.g. scurvy and pellagra. The extent and distribution of the rash and how it spreads (centrifugally or centripetally) should be noted; also the site of onset and whether or not there is irritation.

The commoner types of skin eruption are:

1. *Macular*, consisting of coloured spots, not raised above the surrounding skin. Examples are the rashes of measles and glandular fever and less commonly of syphilis and typhoid fever, and the more diffuse and densely distributed spots of scarlet fever. Haemorrhagic rashes, *purpura*, also fall into this category (*see Fig.* 8.2, p. 297).

2. *Papular*, or rashes in which the elements are raised into tiny nodes. This type of rash occurs in certain stages of the exanthemas, e.g. chickenpox and in essential diseases of the skin with which this book has no concern.

3. *Vesicular*, comprised of small blisters or papules, the tops of which are filled with a clear fluid. Good examples are seen in herpes simplex (*see* The Lips, p. 40 and *Fig*. 3.8), and herpes zoster, a vesicular rash due to an infection of the posterior root ganglia, and usually distributed in a girdle-like manner around one-half of the trunk (to which the disease owes its popular name of 'shingles' (Lat. *cingulum*, a girdle). (*Fig*.3.22.) Chickenpox is a related disease, and the rash presents somewhat similar characteristics.

4. *Bullous*, consisting of larger blisters generally containing clear fluid. They are well seen in burns and scalds and occasionally in erysipelas. Sometimes they occur in severe nervous lesions and drug intoxication (*Fig*. 3.23). The various forms of pemphigus, of which bullae are the essential features, cannot be considered here.

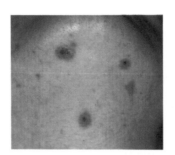

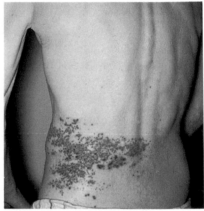

**Fig. 3.21**
Target lesions in Stevens–Johnson syndrome (*see also Fig*. 3.5).

**Fig. 3.22**
Herpes zoster ('shingles').
The vesicles in this case are haemorrhagic.

5. *Pustular*, in many ways resembling a vesicular rash, but in which the little nodules are filled with turbid or purulent instead of clear fluid. Pustules are familiarly seen in acne vulgaris, in which they are non-infective in origin, and to a lesser extent in chickenpox. The malignant pustule of anthrax shows a black centre with surrounding redness.

6. *Nodular* rashes consist of swellings in the skin generally of greater size than the average vesicle or pustule. They are also firmer to touch. An important example of a nodular rash is found in *erythema nodosum* (*Fig*. 3.24). This occurs on the legs, especially the shins, as painful reddish-blue nodules varying in size from a millimetre to several centimetres in diameter. This is commonly due to sarcoidosis, but it may be a response to various infections, especially streptococcal and tuberculous, and also to drugs and other allergens; it may also accompany inflammatory bowel disease. Other examples of a nodular rash are the secondary deposits in the skin of carcinoma or leukaemia, and the deposition of syphilitic, tuberculous and leprous granulation tissue in the form of gummas, tuberculomas

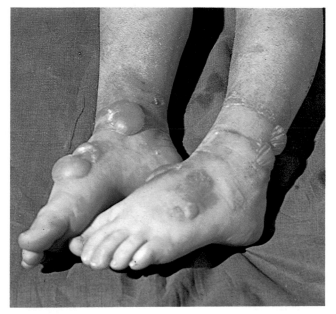

**Fig. 3.23** Bullous eruption on the feet due to a reaction to nalidixic acid (Negram) used to treat a urinary infection.

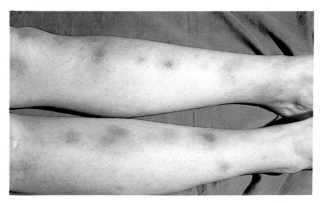

**Fig. 3.24** Erythema nodosum.

and lepromas. Except in the developing countries, these infective forms of granulomas are now relatively less common as a cause of skin nodules than vasculitic granulomas resulting from immune reactions and the purple lesions of Kaposi sarcoma in patients with AIDS. A gross form of nodular change in the skin is neurofibromatosis (*Fig.* 3.25) in which the lesions may be pedunculated (on stalks). Patches of pigmentation (*café au lait* spots) are also found in this condition.

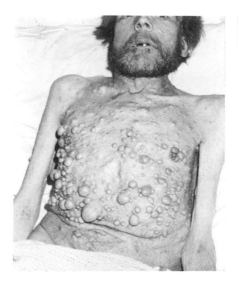

**Fig. 3.25**
Neurofibromatosis (von
Recklinghausen's disease).

7. *Weals* These are raised areas, sometimes pale, sometimes red, which are often seen in sensitive skins even after slight trauma or exposure to irritants (e.g. nettle stings, insect bites). They may appear as 'writing' on the skin (dermographia, *Fig.* 3.26). They also occur spontaneously in various forms of urticaria and are often an expression of hypersensitivity to foreign proteins either ingested (e.g. shell-fish) or injected (e.g. antitetanic serum). Thus they may have a connection with allergic diseases such as asthma, hay fever and angioneurotic oedema. Other features of a weal are its transient nature and irritable characteristics (itching, burning).

These essential elements of a rash may be accompanied by secondary changes. The area around pustules is usually reddened and swollen from inflammatory

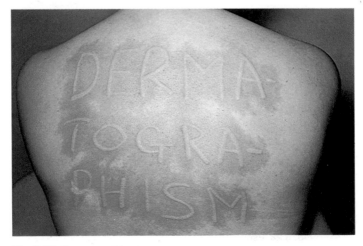

**Fig. 3.26** Dermographia.

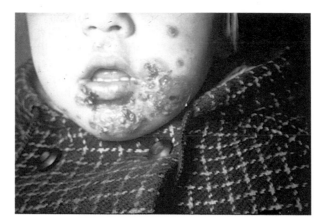

**Fig. 3.27** Impetigo.

reaction. When the pustules burst, *crusts* may form, e.g. in impetigo (*see Fig.* 3.27). *Desquamation* is the name given to shedding of the superficial layers of the epidermis which occurs after many fevers, but is particularly characteristic of scarlet fever and of some drug eruptions. More localized scaling or desquamative rashes include flexural eczema, which, with asthma and hay fever, is a common manifestation of an 'atopic' or allergic state, and also psoriasis which may be associated with a rheumatoid form of arthritis (*Fig.* 3.28). Erosion of the deeper layers of the skin and loss of tissue result in *ulcers*; these may follow infections or injuries, especially when the circulation is abnormal due to varicose veins or arterial atheroma, or when the nerve-supply is interrupted. In these cases, the distal parts of the limbs are most often affected. Skin ulcers more rarely result from the breakdown of malignant or granulomatous nodules. *Scars* may be

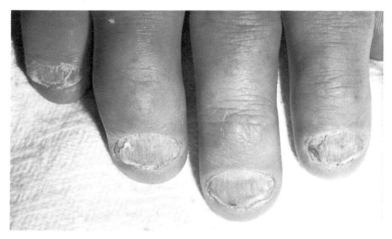

**Fig. 3.28** Psoriasis: arthritis of the terminal interphalangeal joints with deformity and discoloration of the nails.

significant of old skin lesions, especially of acne, smallpox, herpes zoster and healed varicose ulcers (*see Fig*. 3.43, p. 62). The scars of operations and injuries must not be overlooked, as they may bear upon the present illness.

In many rashes several elements are combined. Thus in smallpox, macules, papules, vesicles and pustules are seen on the skin successively. In allergic purpura, the essential haemorrhagic rash is frequently combined with the weals of urticaria.

Pathological changes in the skin, such as *telangiectases*, may be associated with similar lesions in other organs. For example, hereditary haemorrhagic telangiectasia, in which there is multiple localized dilatation of the venules and capillaries in the skin and mucosae, may explain haemorrhages from the nose, lungs, gastrointestinal tract and kidneys. Telangiectasia may also accompany systemic sclerosis (scleroderma) (*Fig*. 3.29) and hepatic disease (spider naevi) and may be seen after irradiation of the skin (*Fig*. 3.30).

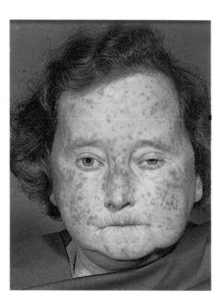

**Fig. 3.29**
Systemic sclerosis, showing puckering of the mouth due to scleroderma, and telangiectasia.

In recent years, many cutaneous 'markers' of internal malignant disease have been recognized, especially certain persistent erythematous rashes (*see Fig*. 3.31).

### GENITALIA

The size and form of the genitalia are of especial importance in endocrine disorders (*see* Chapter 11).

The penis and testes fail to reach adult proportions in several types of infantilism: hypopituitarism, hypothyroidism and eunuchoidism are notable causes. In these cases the normal sexual functions are also in abeyance, and the secondary sex characters (in boys, deepening of the voice, growth of hair on the pubes and in masculine sites) do not develop at puberty. In females the main sign of genital infantilism is the failure to menstruate; the pubic hair may be delayed in

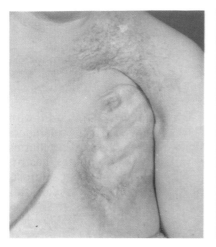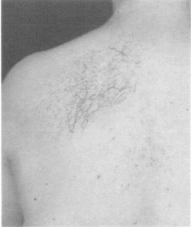

**Fig. 3.30** Post-radiation telangiectasia. Note also skin scarring.

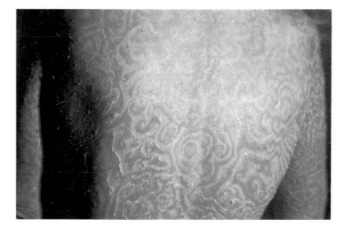

**Fig. 3.31** Erythema gyratum repens in a patient with bronchial carcinoma.

appearance, and the general bodily configuration remains sexless without breast development.

By contrast, sexual precocity may be found in adrenal cortical hyperplasia or tumours and in certain rare diseases of the endocrines or brain. Male children may develop a penis of adult proportions at an early age (erection and ejaculation of spermatozoa may occur). Precocious puberty in females may develop along masculine or feminine lines; if the former (premature heterosexual maturation), the clitoris may enlarge and hirsutism appear as in the adrenogenital syndrome; if the latter, the normal sex characteristics, e.g. breast formation and menstruation, are unduly early (*Fig.* 3.32).

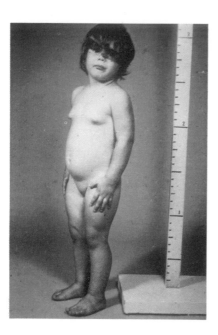

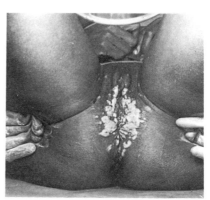

**Fig. 3.32**
Precocious puberty in a four-year-old.

**Fig. 3.33**
Condylomas from a case of secondary syphilis.

The external genital organs may also exhibit evidence of local disease, particularly venereal manifestations such as syphilitic chancre on the penis or vulva, the presence of secondary manifestations of the disease, e.g. condylomas (*Fig.* 3.33), or the presence of urethral or vaginal discharge in gonorrhoea and other local infections and in non-specific urethritis (*see* Reiter's syndrome, p. 332). Herpes simplex may also affect the genitalia as a sexually transmitted disease.

### EXTREMITIES

In certain diseases the shape of the hands may be modified. In myxoedema they are broad and the fingers appear short and stubby from thickening of the subcutaneous tissues. In acromegaly they are large, broad and paw-like (*Fig.* 3.34), but in hypogonadism they are often slender and feminine. Long spidery fingers—arachnodactyly—occur in Marfan's syndrome and are sometimes associated with atrial septal defect or other congenital cardiac anomalies (*Fig.* 3.35).

The joint affections of the hands are described in Chapter 9. It remains to add that many types of crippling deformity may result from arthritis. Two are worthy of mention here: first, *ulnar deviation* in rheumatoid arthritis, in which the whole hand, but especially the fingers from the metacarpophalangeal joints, is deflected to the ulnar side; secondly, *Heberden's nodes* (*Fig.* 9.21, p. 334), bony prominences at the distal interphalangeal joints which occur in osteoarthrosis. Another common deformity of the hand results from fibrous thickening of palmar tissues with flexion of the fingers: Dupuytren's contracture (*Fig.* 3.36). This is usually inherited but may accompany alcoholic cirrhosis of the liver.

Gangrene, causing blackness of the skin, is usually the result of serious and permanent arterial obstruction due to thrombosis complicating atheroma or

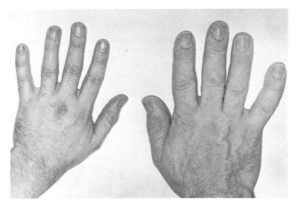

**Fig. 3.34** Acromegaly: spade-shaped hand compared with the normal hand on the left.

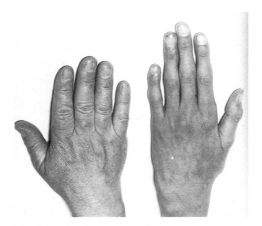

**Fig. 3.35** Arachnodactyly. The spidery fingers are compared with those of a normal hand on the left. (*See also Fig.* 7.55, p. 263.)

vasculitis, or to embolism. (*See also* p. 289.) The toes are most often affected in atheroma (e.g. diabetic gangrene, *Fig.* 3.37) and the fingers in inflammatory vascular conditions associated with a Raynaud phenomenon (e.g. systemic sclerosis, *see Fig.* 7.81, p. 287). In this latter condition, the skin of the fingers is taut and shiny, sometimes with telangiectases, and the ends of the fingers may be tapered due to ischaemic resorption of bone.

In respiratory and cardiac disease, clubbing of the fingers and toes should be sought, but this and the abnormalities of the hands due to nervous diseases will be considered in later chapters.

Traumatic and infective lesions of the hands and feet are common and the latter may be complicated by lymphangitis (*Fig.* 3.38).

Finally, the *nails* should be inspected. Pitting, ribbing and brittleness are often

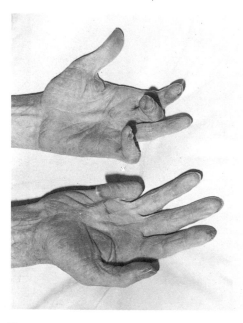

**Fig. 3.36** Bilateral Dupuytren contractures in a patient with alcoholic cirrhosis of the liver.

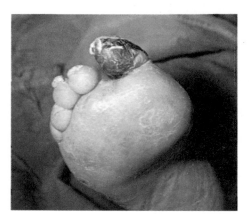 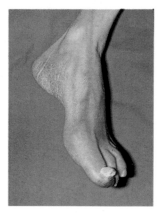

**Fig. 3.37**
Diabetic gangrene.

**Fig. 3.38**
Lymphangitis spreading
from an infected
gangrenous toe.

seen after severe illness and in malabsorption syndromes (*Fig.* 3.39). The short irregular nails of the nail-biter may suggest some instability of personality. Koilonychia (spoon-shaped nails) is seen in iron-deficiency anaemias (*Fig.* 3.40, and *Fig.* 8.8, p. 308). In psoriasis, the nails may be deformed, pitted and yellow

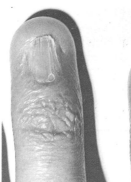
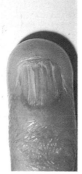
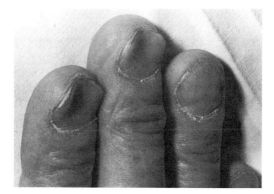

**Fig. 3.39**
Ribbing of the nails associated with the malabsorption syndrome.

**Fig. 3.40**
Koilonychia.

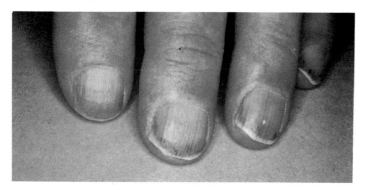

**Fig. 3.41** Splinter haemorrhages seen best in the 5th finger. There are also fading lesions in the middle finger.

in colour (*see Fig.* 3.35). A rare cause of yellow nails is lymphatic obstruction, usually accompanied by pleural effusion (*see Fig.* 6.37). Leukonychia, abnormal whiteness at the base of the nails, sometimes occurs in chronic liver failure (*see Fig.* 8.8, p. 308) and other conditions associated with hypoalbuminaemia. Splinter haemorrhages may appear beneath the nails in blood diseases and as the result of emboli in bacterial endocarditis (*see Fig.* 3.41). A similar appearance in the nailbed may be caused by small digital infarcts in patients with a vasculitis, e.g. systemic lupus erythematosus.

*Tremors* are generally seen best in the hands. Apart from neurological causes dealt with on p. 377, they may be present in senility, thyrotoxicosis, alcoholism, carbon dioxide retention and in renal and hepatic failure.

The *legs* should be specially inspected for evidence of circulatory disorders, both venous and arterial. Examination of the legs for evidence of deep vein thrombosis is especially important when pulmonary embolism is suspected. This evidence may include tenderness in the thigh or calf, pain in the calf on dorsi-flexion of the foot (Homans' sign), pitting oedema or an increase in the girth of one leg when compared with the other (*see Fig.* 3.42). Venous congestion or obstruction causes pitting oedema which can best be elicited over the tibiae and ankles. Chronic impairment of venous return may lead to varicose veins associated with eczema, pigmentation and ulceration over the lower part of the legs (*Fig.* 3.43). Evidence of arterial ischaemia includes pallor, cyanosis, coldness, loss of hair, anaesthesia and trophic changes such as gangrene (*see Fig.* 3.37).

Because of gravity, haemorrhagic rashes associated with increased capillary fragility as in scurvy and other forms of purpura may be seen best in the lower

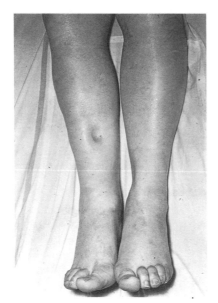

**Fig. 3.42**
Pitting pretibial oedema due to deep vein thrombosis.

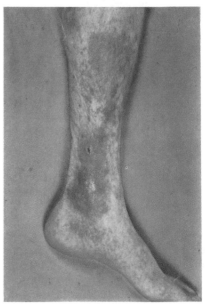

**Fig. 3.43**
Eczema, pigmentation and ulcer scars associated with varicose veins.

limbs (*see Fig*. 3.44). Erythema nodosum (*see Fig*. 3.24, p. 53) also favours the legs.

*Bone deformities* such as bow-legs (*Fig*. 3.45), knock-knees and sabre tibiae must also be noted, although these are now relatively uncommon. Deformity of the feet, especially pes cavus, may occur with congenital neurological disorders including syringomyelia and the hereditary ataxias.

The toe nails may be clubbed and may also show evidence of neglect (*Fig*. 3.46).

The *joints* of the lower limb are particularly prone to disease. Osteoarthrosis

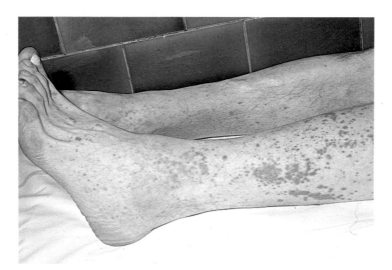

**Fig. 3.44** Purpuric rash on the legs.

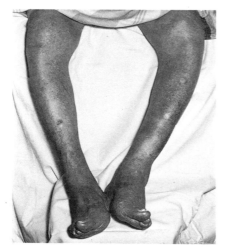
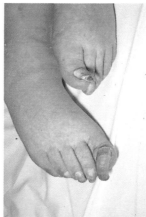

**Fig. 3.45**
Paget's disease: bow-legs.

**Fig. 3.46**
Onychogryphosis.

affects the weight-bearing joints of the hip, knee and ankle; rheumatoid arthritis commonly involves the small joints of the feet, and gout favours the metatarso-phalangeal joint of the big toe (*see also* Chapter 9).

*Neurological abnormalities* of the legs are described in Chapter 10.

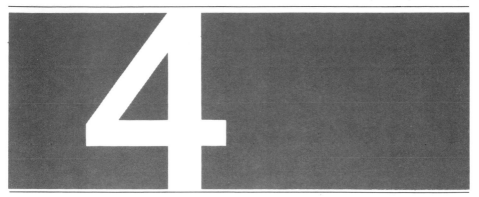

## The digestive system

The digestive system comprises the alimentary tract and the accessory organs and tissues concerned in the digestion of food. It will be convenient to describe the symptoms and objective examination of each part separately, though certain general descriptions of symptoms common to all parts and the method of examining the abdomen as a whole will be necessary.

### ■ THE MOUTH*

#### Symptoms

Symptoms arising in the mouth include thirst and dryness, increased salivation, loss or disorder of taste, difficulty in speech, chewing or swallowing, soreness and pain.

#### Thirst and dryness

Thirst usually reflects the degree of cellular dehydration and can thus result from diminished intake or excessive loss of water, or from increased consumption of salt. Severe diarrhoea, polyuria in diabetes mellitus and renal failure and profuse sweating, especially in fevers, are notable causes, aggravated sometimes because the patient is too weak to drink. Dryness of the mouth from decreased salivation is a familiar transient feature in fear, but it may be more persistent in mouth breathers from nasal obstruction. It may also result from diseases of the salivary glands, e.g. mumps, Sjögren's disease and salivary calculi, and is usual in the states of dehydration causing thirst. In acute illness such dryness may be a useful indication of the necessity for fluids. Drugs such as anticholinergics and anti-depressants may produce a dry mouth as may depression even without medication.

#### Increased salivation

This occurs in irritant lesions of the buccal mucosa (e.g. stomatitis, teething in infants), in Parkinsonism (*see* p. 412) and as an accompaniment of

---

* *See also* The Respiratory System (Chapter 6) and Haemopoietic System (Chapter 8).

nausea. Salivation is often a distressing symptom of oesophageal obstruction because the normal secretions cannot be swallowed. Anxiety states may produce an increase in saliva, which patients find difficult to swallow.

### Loss or disorder of taste (*see also* Central Nervous System, Chapter 10)

The sensory nerve endings in the tongue can only distinguish the primary sensations of taste: sweet, bitter, sour, salt. Loss of these sensations usually indicates a lesion of the 7th or 9th or more rarely the mandibular division of the 5th cranial nerves. More often, a patient complaining of loss of 'taste' cannot distinguish those more subtle flavours of food which depend upon the sense of smell. This symptom, which commonly results in anorexia, is rarely due to lesions of the olfactory nerves and more commonly to disease of the nasal mucosa or obstruction of the nasal airway. The presence of an unpleasant taste in the mouth or a distortion in the flavour of food sometimes occurs in cerebral lesions or as an aura in epilepsy (*see* p. 440), but is also a frequent psychogenic symptom associated with the fear that the breath is offensive to others. An unpleasant taste is in fact only rarely associated with an offensive breath (*see* p. 70).

### Difficulty in speech, chewing or swallowing

These symptoms can result from diminished salivary secretion, inadequate teeth or an ill-fitting denture and painful conditions of the mouth or throat. The neuromuscular causes are dealt with in Chapter 10.

### Soreness and pain

Soreness of the mucous membrane covering the mouth or tongue is found in the various forms of stomatitis, and inflammation of the buccal mucosa due to local or systemic causes (*see below*). The soreness is felt especially when very hot or acid foods are taken and during speech, chewing or swallowing. The commonest form of pain arising in the mouth is toothache due to dental caries or periodontal abscess. The pain is constant, aching in character, aggravated by chewing or by cold foods, and it may radiate to the ear, the temple or the orbit.

## PHYSICAL SIGNS: EXAMINATION OF THE MOUTH

The examination of the mouth requires a good light, and preferably the use of an electric torch if bright daylight is not available.

### The teeth

The teeth should be inspected and their number and condition noted. Deficient or carious teeth and ill-fitting false teeth which prevent adequate chewing, or discourage the patient from wearing the denture at meal times, may be contributory causes of dyspepsia. Abnormal formation of the teeth is important in the diagnosis of congenital syphilis in which the incisors may be notched (Hutchinsonian teeth, *Fig.* 4.1). Discoloration may be due to poor dental hygiene, but is sometimes seen when the fluorine content of water is unduly high. The teeth then show a mottled brownish appearance. This may also be produced by

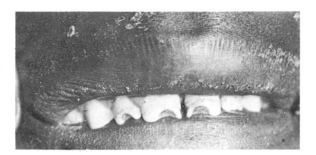

**Fig. 4.1** Photograph of an African boy, aged 14, with congenital syphilis. Note the notched character of the teeth, especially the central incisors. (Hutchinsonian teeth.)

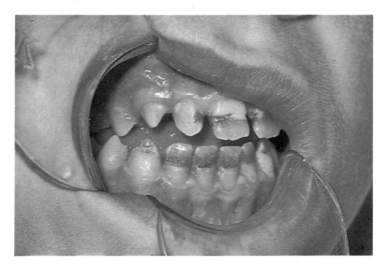

**Fig. 4.2** Staining of the teeth due to tetracyclines given during childhood for fibrocystic disease of the lung.

tetracyclines (*Fig.* 4.2). A rare phenomenon is the pink fluorescence of the teeth in congenital porphyria.

### The gums

The state of the gums should next be noted. A deep-red congestion with easy bleeding is present when the gums are inflamed (*gingivitis*), and in *pyorrhoea* pus can be squeezed from the gum margins. Both in gingivitis and pyorrhoea the teeth are generally affected and are often loose and covered with a greenish-yellow exudate. The gum margins retract. Oral sepsis of this kind may in certain circumstances give rise to bacterial endocarditis or to lung abscess; it can also be an aggravating factor in gastric disorders. The gums are pale in anaemia, and in lead poisoning a blue line may be seen at the gum margin. The blue line is due to a deposit of lead sulphide in the gum tissues; thus it cannot be cleaned away with a pledget of cotton-wool, and it is seen even better if the gum margins between the teeth are transilluminated from behind by a small electric torch. This does not occur in edentulous patients and has become rare. A yellow line may similarly be caused by cadmium sulphide. (*See also* Haemopoietic System, p. 295.) In scurvy the gums are soft and spongy and bleed easily (*see also* p. 316). Vincent's angina may cause ulceration and sloughing of the gingiva as well as faucial manifestations. Hypertrophy of the gums may occur in epileptics taking phenytoin over a long period of time (*see Fig.* 10.89, p. 442) and also in certain leukaemias (*see Fig.* 8.5, p. 301).

## The tongue and buccal mucous membrane

The normal papillae of the tongue give rise to a furred appearance best seen in the posterior part. Dryness of the tongue is an important sign of dehydration (*see* p. 65) and may be accompanied by thickening, discoloration and 'caking' of the fur.

Anaemia, cyanosis and jaundice may be evident in the tongue. In certain anaemias (pernicious anaemia and iron-deficiency anaemias particularly) the tongue is depapillated, i.e. smooth and shiny and sometimes sore (*see* p. 300). Cyanosis of the tongue is always central in origin (*see* p. 164). The ventral aspect of the tongue must be inspected as haemorrhages, neoplastic ulcer and leucoplakia (*Fig.* 4.3) may only be seen from below.

The tongue is large in acromegaly and in cretins and mongols, and in the latter often fissured. Macroglossia for which no other obvious cause is found may be due to amyloidosis (*Fig.* 4.4).

Paralysis, atrophy, tremors and abnormalties of movement of the tongue and soft palate will be noted incidentally but are referred to under the nervous system.

Small ulcers indicate the presence of stomatitis (*see* p. 70). The more serious ulcers of syphilis and malignant disease should not be overlooked; the former

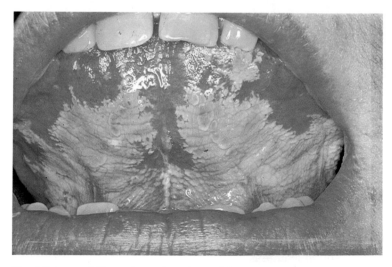

**Fig. 4.3** Leucoplakia on the undersurface of the tongue.

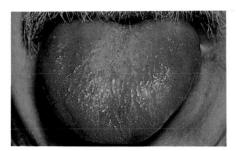

**Fig. 4.4**
Macroglossia due to amyloid.

tend to be central and the latter marginal. Leucoplakia may be syphilitic and sometimes precancerous. It is characterized by white and sometimes thickened patches in the mucosa (*Fig.* 4.3). Tuberculous ulceration is associated with pulmonary infection and commonly involves the tip of the tongue. With the decline in syphilis and tuberculosis, Crohn's disease has become a relatively more common cause of mouth ulcers. Swabs or sections from the ulcer may help to identify such conditons as Crohn's disease, syphilis, tuberculosis and malignant disease. In Addison's disease, brownish areas of pigmentation may be seen in the buccal mucous membrane, a useful confirmatory sign in doubtful cases (*Fig.* 4.5). Buccal pigmentation can also occur in normal people, especially Negroes, and rarely in haemochromatosis. Telangiectasia are seen on the lips in hereditary haemorrhagic telangiectasia, systemic sclerosis and scleroderma (*Fig.* 4.6). Pigmentation of the lips and mouth is a cutaneous marker for the Peutz–Jegher's syndrome in

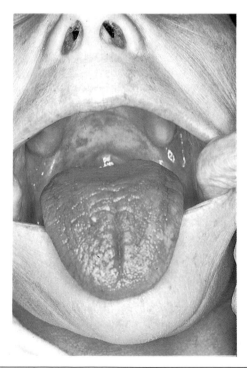

**Fig. 4.5**
Buccal pigmentation. Patches of brown pigment on the palate in a patient with Addison's disease.

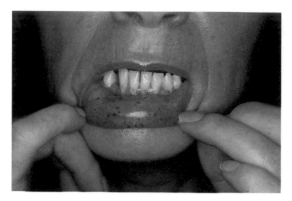

**Fig. 4.6** Telangiectasia of the lips in systemic sclerosis.

which gastrointestinal polyps may cause intussusception or bleeding. Haemorrhages are occasionally found in purpura and if accompanied by thrush may suggest leukaemia. Note will be made of the movements of the soft palate and uvula.

(*See also* Koplik's Spots, p. 531.)

### The breath

An offensive faecal odour to the breath sometimes occurs in symptomless people due to putrefaction of food fragments retained around the teeth or the proliferation of organisms in the gums or tonsils. More rarely, a foul smell can arise from the stomach contents, as in gastric carcinoma and intestinal obstruction, or from chronic suppuration in the lung (bronchiectasis; lung abscess). A sweet smell may be imparted to the breath by acetone in cases of diabetic coma and in acidosis, especially in children. The breath in uraemia sometimes has a urinose smell, while that in hepatic coma is musty. The smell of alcohol on the breath does not always mean that it has been consumed to excess, or that it is responsible for any symptoms, but chronic alcoholism should be suspected if the smell is evident before about 11.00 a.m. (*see* Coma, p. 17).

## DIAGNOSIS OF DISEASES OF THE MOUTH

Many diseases of the mouth are within the province of surgical diagnosis and will not be described here. One which deserves mention is stomatitis.

### Stomatitis

The term embraces a number of conditions of varying aetiology, characterized by signs of inflammation, exudate and ulceration usually with increased salivation. Sometimes these are due to mechanical traumatic causes such as jagged teeth, ill-fitting dentures or burns. They may be due to local infections such as moniliasis ('thrush') which is characterized by a patchy white exudate scattered throughout the mouth but especially on the soft palate (*Fig.* 4.7). Today this is one of the commonest forms of mouth infection and appears especially in

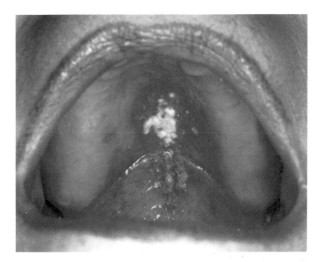

**Fig. 4.7** White patches on the soft palate due to moniliasis.

those receiving broad-spectrum antibiotics or corticosteroid inhalers. Systemic causes of an ulcerative stomatitis include leukaemia, uraemia, metallic poisons such as mercury and, in tropical areas, kala-azar.

The term *aphthous stomatitis* is applied to a fairly common condition in which small vesicles may change to ulcers of superficial but painful nature (*Figs.* 4.8). The cause is obscure, but it may be associated with Crohn's disease in a few cases.

Nutritional causes should be looked for, especially in tropical zones where deficiency in vitamin-B complexes are common. (*See also* Scurvy and Agranulocytosis, pp. 316, 306.)

*Angular Stomatitis* (cheilosis) is a characteristic feature of nutritional deficiency (*see Fig.* 4.8 *and also* Chapter 8).

A number of skin conditions also have buccal mucous membrane manifestations, e.g. erythema multiforme.

## ■ THE OESOPHAGUS

### SYMPTOMS

#### Dysphagia

Dysphagia or difficulty in swallowing is the principal symptom of oesophageal disease. Dysphagia may consist of a difficulty in emptying the mouth because of poor salivation, paresis of the tongue or painful conditions of the mouth or pharynx. In oesophageal dysphagia, the food is felt to lodge in the throat or behind the sternum. The obstruction can sometimes be accurately localized by the patient, but a lower oesophageal obstruction can sometimes give rise to dysphagia at a higher level. The commoner causes of dysphagia are listed in *Table* 4.1. Of these, carcinoma and peptic stricture are the commonest. At first, the

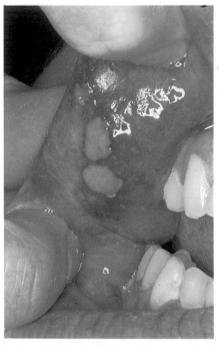

*a*

*b*

**Fig. 4.8** *a*, Aphthous ulcers; *b*, angular stomatitis.

patient has difficulty only with solid foods and for a time this can be overcome by chewing food until it is of fluid consistency; later, as obstruction increases, fluids and even saliva cannot be swallowed. Dysphagia due to other causes is rarely complete and, in a the case of achalasia, may be intermittent over a period of many years and affects solids and fluids equally, Dysphagia of neuromuscular origin may be accompanied by a bout of coughing due to food entering the larynx.

| Table 4.1 | **Causes of dysphagia** |
|-----------|------------------------|
| *High* | Carcinoma (pharynx or oesophagus)<br>Cervical tumours (lymph nodes; goitre)<br>Neuromuscular (bulbar palsy; myasthenia; psychogenic)<br>Iron deficiency (*see* Chapter 8)<br>Diverticulum (pharynx or oesophagus) |
| *Middle* | Carcinoma of oesophagus<br>Mediastinal tumours (lymph nodes; aneurysm) |
| *Low* | Carcinoma (stomach or oesophagus)<br>Peptic stricture (usually with hiatus hernia)<br>Achalasia<br>Systemic sclerosis |

### Pain

Pain which accompanies dysphagia is probably due to muscle contractions in the oesophagus above the obstruction. This pain is retrosternal and maximal at the site of the obstruction, but it can spread across the chest and radiate into the neck and through to the back. It may thus simulate cardiac pain, but it usually occurs immediately after swallowing and can be eased by regurgitation of food. A more persistent pain of this nature can result from rupture or perforation of the oesophagus. A lower sternal burning pain provoked by stooping and relieved by antacids suggests an oesophagitis due to reflux of acid from the stomach. This occurs particularly in hiatus hernia (*see also* Heartburn, p. 81). Painful swallowing without obstruction (odynophagia) occurs in oesophagitis secondary to peptic reflux or infections such as candidiasis or herpes simplex.

### Regurgitation

Food and secretions may be retained behind an obstruction of the oesophagus or within a diverticulum and subsequently regurgitated. Regurgitation, as distinct from vomiting (i.e. evacuation of the gastric contents) is rarely preceded by nausea and is often effortless. The regurgitated food is undigested but it may undergo bacterial putrefaction and become foul-smelling. The inhalation of regurgitated matter during sleep is an occasional cause of nocturnal bouts of coughing and can lead to serious pulmonary infections.

### Haemorrhage

Oesophageal haemorrhage presents as haematemesis or melaena (*see* p. 104) or, more insidiously, as anaemia. The bleeding may come from peptic oesophagitis or from oesophageal varices, secondary to portal hypertension. A massive haemorrhage from ruptured varices can present as an effortless regurgitation of dark venous blood unaltered by gastric acid. Fresh blood at the conclusion of forceful vomiting suggests a traumatic tear at the gastro-oesophageal junction—a Mallory–Weiss tear.

## ■ PHYSICAL SIGNS: EXAMINATION OF THE OESOPHAGUS

The examination of the oesophagus is largely dependent on X-rays, oesophagoscopy and biopsy. The clinician relies chiefly upon the history, but observes difficulties in swallowing and notes any glandular enlargement in the neck or evidence of mediastinal obstruction.

## DIAGNOSIS OF DISEASES OF THE OESOPHAGUS

### Carcinoma of oesophagus

This tumour causes pain, progressive dysphagia and regurgitation of food which may be foul and bloodstained. The exclusion of solid food and, later, of fluids from the stomach leads to thirst, wasting, dehydration, anaemia and other signs of malnutrition. Inability to swallow saliva can be a particularly distressing symptom. Rarely, the symptoms appear suddenly. The structures adjacent to the oesophagus may be invaded at a relatively early stage of the disease (*see* Mediastinal Obstruction, p. 167). If the obstruction cannot be relieved, the patient will die of starvation or from pneumonia due to the inhalation of regurgitated food.

### Achalasia of the cardia

Achalasia is due to the failure of the lower oesophagus to relax before the oncoming bolus of food. This has been attributed to an incoordinated peristaltic wave rather than to spasm of the cardia and results from degeneration of Auerbach's plexus. Achalasia tends to affect younger people than does carcinoma but may persist throughout life if untreated; the dysphagia is usually more variable and less relentless in its progression, and it can be temporarily relieved by drugs which relax smooth muscle. Nutrition is often well maintained.

### Perforation and rupture

Although these are surgical emergencies, they are mentioned here because they so often present to the physician in the guise of myocardial infarction with severe retrosternal pain and signs of 'shock'. When symptoms of this kind come on after a meal containing sharp bones (e.g. fish, chicken, chop), oesophageal perforation should always be considered. Forceful vomiting after a heavy meal with a lot of alcohol can result in spontaneous rupture of the oesophagus. In either case, the diagnosis is supported by the finding of palpable crepitus in the neck (surgical emphysema) due to air tracking up from the mediastinum and, later, by the signs of a pleural effusion usually on the left side. The breach in the wall of the oesophagus is confirmed by radiographs taken after the patient has swallowed a radio-opaque material.

### Reflux oesophagitis

Reflux of the gastric contents into the lower oesophagus is particularly likely in the presence of pregnancy, obesity, raised intra-abdominal pressure or herniation of the stomach through the oesophageal hiatus (hiatus hernia). The resulting symptoms are heartburn on stooping or lying and regurgitation of bitter fluid. If severe peptic oesophagitis ensues, then pain, dysphagia and bleeding may occur. After long-standing reflux oesophagitis, there may be columnar metaplasia of the epithelium (Barrett's oesophagus) and this is a premalignant condition.

### Special investigations

Abnormalities in the outline of the oesophageal lumen can be demonstrated by radiological screening while the patient swallows barium sulphate, a substance opaque to X-rays. Lesions of the oesophageal mucosa can also be identified by direct vision through a flexible endoscope (*fibreoptic endoscopy*), by cytological examination of aspirated contents and, if indicated, a biopsy of the mucosa can be taken for histological examination.

Considerable increase in understanding of oesophageal abnormalities has been made possible by the more scientific measurements of pressure and motility, namely manometric studies. These have been particularly valuable in showing lack of co-ordination in the contraction of different segments, as in achalasia and the rarer cork-screw oesophagus of elderly persons.

Acid perfusion of the oesophagus may induce the pain of oesophageal regurgitation and may thus be helpful in the differential diagnosis of retrosternal pain.

## ■ GENERAL SYMPTOMS OF ABDOMINAL DISEASE

### ABDOMINAL PAIN

Pain has been considered on p. 7, and special characteristics in relation to individual abdominal viscera will be described later. Abdominal pain of organic origin falls into two classes:

1. *Visceral pain*, due to increased tension on the splanchnic nerve endings in the muscular wall of the affected viscus. This pain is deeply situated, sometimes colicky in type, and is found most commonly in obstructive lesions of the intestines and bile ducts. A similar pain is found in obstruction of other tubes, particularly the ureter in cases of renal colic. When an organ is inflamed, the threshold to visceral pain is lowered, and it may then be induced by a variety of stimuli (e.g. acid secretion or local pressure in the case of peptic ulceration).

2. *Referred pain*, probably due in many cases to the irritative effects of inflammatory, haemorrhage or neoplastic diseases of the abdominal viscera upon the parietal peritoneum. The parietal peritoneum in contact with the viscus receives its nerve supply from the same segments of the spinal cord as the overlying parts of the abdominal wall. This explains why the pain and tenderness are experienced in many cases over the viscus, although the pain is referred. In other cases, as in the instance of shouldertip pain, the area of skin is situated remotely from the irritated peritoneum. Here irritation of the peritoneum (or pleura) covering the central portions of the diaphragm, which receives its nerve supply from the phrenic nerve (3rd, 4th and 5th cervical segments), causes the pain to be felt in an area supplied by other somatic nerves arising at the same level, namely over the tip of the shoulder. The pain of peritoneal irritation is usually associated with deep tenderness and often with muscular rigidity. It is more constant than visceral pain and is generally stabbing, cutting or burning in character.

## Special features to be noted (*Table* 4.2)

An accurate description by the patient of his pain is of the greatest value in the diagnosis of digestive diseases. The following points should be ascertained in every case:

1. *The Situation*. From the preceding sections it follows that when pain is due to peritoneal irritation it is usually experienced over the affected viscus, but when truly visceral it may be more vaguely situated, and in the case of gastrointestinal pain it is usually central. Visceral pain, as already pointed out, depends for its position on the embryological origin of the viscus. Fuller details are given in dealing with individual viscera.

2. *The Character*. This includes the severity, which varies from the slight discomfort of gastric flatulence to the agonizing pain of a perforated ulcer. The description of the type of pain—'griping', 'gnawing', 'stabbing', 'cutting' and so forth—depends a good deal upon the intelligence and descriptive ability of the

| Table 4.2 | **Analysis of severe abdominal pain** | | |
|---|---|---|---|
| | *Perforation* | *Appendicitis* | *Acute haemorrhagic pancreatitis* |
| Site | Epigastric | Umbilical | Epigastrium or right hypochondrium |
| Radiation | Whole abdomen and left shoulder | Right iliac fossa later | Back and whole abdomen |
| Type | Sharp | Colicky, becoming constant | Constant |
| Severity | Very severe | Severe | Very severe |
| Onset and duration | Instantaneous and persistent | Fairly rapid onset, many hours | Sudden and persistent |
| Aggravating factors | Movement | Walking causing movement of the iliopsoas behind inflamed viscus | Nil |
| Relieving factors | Nil | Nil | Nil |
| Associated symptoms | Shock and vomiting | Vomiting, fever | Vomiting and shock |
| Physical signs | Board-like rigidity | Tenderness and guarding in right iliac fossa | Abdomen rigid after initial softness |
| Investigations | Air under diaphragm seen on radiograph | Nil | Increased serum and urinary amylase |

patient, and too much stress, therefore, cannot be laid upon it as a point in diagnosis. The distinction between visceral and somatic pain may be recognized from the patient's description.

3. *Conditions Aggravating the Pain.* Abdominal pain so frequently arises from the stomach, intestines or organs which modify the function of these that it naturally bears a close relationship to meals. Inquiry should be made whether the pain occurs after meals; if so, for how long and whether relief is afforded by taking more food. The patient should also be asked whether any particular kind of food disagrees with him and precipitates pain.

4. *Conditions Relieving the Pain.* The effect of starvation should be ascertained, or whether abstention from particular articles of diet gives relief. Relief given by medicines, particularly antacids, may also be a valuable diagnostic point. Comfort produced by evacuation of the bladder or rectum may suggest these organs as the seat of pain.

| *Gallbladder colic* | *Renal colic* | *Large-bowel obstruction (complete)* | *Small-bowel obstruction* |
|---|---|---|---|
| Right hypochondrium and epigastrium | Loin | Hypogastric | Umbilical |
| Right scapula | Towards groin | Flanks | Nil |
| Colicky or continuous | Colicky | Colicky | Colicky |
| Very severe | Very severe | Severe | Severe |
| Sudden, lasting hours | Sudden, minutes to hours | Slow onset, lasting days | Fairly rapid onset, hours to days |
| Nil | Jolting | Nil | Nil |
| Nil | Nil | Nil | Nil |
| Vomiting and sometimes fever with rigors | Vomiting, frequency, haematuria | Constipation. Vomiting at a late stage | Vomiting |
| Tenderness in right hypochondrium. Transient jaundice | Nil | Flank distension, increased bowel sounds. Rectum ballooned and empty | Central distension. Bowel sounds increased. Rectum ballooned and empty |
| Cholecystogram may show calculus | Radiograph may show calculus | Intestinal fluid levels on radiograph | Intestinal fluid levels on radiograph |

5. *Duration.* If the pain comes on after meals, the patient should be asked whether it disappears before the next meal or whether it is continuous. In apparently continuous pain there are often spells in which the patient is comparatively comfortable. Intervals of freedom from the attacks of pain should also be noted. It is characteristic, for example, in gastric and duodenal ulcer to find periods of some weeks in which the patient is entirely free from discomfort. On the contrary, pain due to gastric and other visceral carcinomas often starts gradually and becomes more severe and continuous as time goes on. Pain of short duration is more likely to be due to obstructive causes such as renal or biliary colic than to inflammation or neoplasm.

6. *Associated Phenomena.* Indications of the severity of the pain and its reflex effects are often seen in the association of vomiting, sweating and collapse. Severe pain, especially due to peptic ulcer, may wake the patient at night. It should be particularly noted whether vomiting gives relief from the pain, a common history in cases of gastric disease. The association of constipation or diarrhoea with abdominal pain should focus attention on the intestinal tract. Fever suggests an inflammatory lesion such as appendicitis, cholecystitis or cholangitis complicating bile duct obstruction by stone. The combination of fever with rigors, jaundice and abdominal pain is characteristic of ascending cholangitis (Charcot's triad) usually caused by a bile duct stone.

## VOMITING

Vomiting is another symptom common to so many diseases of the digestive and other systems that it is convenient to describe it before proceeding further. It is a reflex act induced through the vomiting centre of the medulla and may be caused by central or peripheral stimulation. Central stimulation of the vomiting centre may occur from external causes such as disgusting smells or sights or from increased intracranial pressure as in cerebral tumour. It may arise reflexly from labyrinthine disturbances, e.g. in seasickness and Menière's disease. It is also a fairly constant symptom in the early months of pregnancy and may arise from metabolic causes such as uraemia and hypercalcaemia. However, in this chapter we are concerned with vomiting arising from irritation of the gastric mucosa. It is common as a result of indiscretions in diet, it may occur in organic disease of the stomach such as ulcer or cancer, in reflex disturbance of the stomach from disease of the gallbladder, appendix or other viscera, and when the pylorus or small intestine is obstructed. In pyloric stenosis there may be food remnants recongizable as several days old and in intestinal obstruction the vomitus may be faeculent due to bacterial invasion.

Vomiting must be distinguished from the regurgitation of food into the mouth (*see* Regurgitation, p. 73). True vomiting implies the ejection of appreciable quantities of the stomach contents, sometimes consisting of undigested food, sometimes of partially digested food to which the gastric secretions have been added.

### Special features to be noted

A careful note should be made of the following points:

1. *The relationship of the vomiting to any pain.* Note whether the pain precedes or follows the vomiting and at what interval.

2. *The time of day at which vomiting occurs.* In cases of pyloric stenosis, each meal adds to the gastric contents, and vomiting may not occur until the latter part of the day when a large quantity has accumulated. The vomiting of pregnancy and alcoholic gastritis occur characteristically in the mornings.

3. *The presence or absence of nausea.* Nausea generally precedes vomiting due to diseases of the digestive system, but in cases of increased intracranial pressure is often absent.

For details of the character of the vomitus, *see* p. 104.

## ■ SYMPTOMS ASSOCIATED WITH INDIVIDUAL VISCERA

### THE STOMACH AND DUODENUM

Both pain and vomiting are common in gastric and duodenal disease.

### Pain

In peptic ulceration pain is generally of the visceral type, localized in the epigastrium and confined to a small area irrespective of whether the ulcer is duodenal or gastric. The pain pathway is via the splanchnic nerves, but when the ulcer penetrates the mucosa and involves the peritoneum, cerebrospinal pathways may be implicated.

Muscle spasm and powerful peristaltic contractions are secondary rather than primary causes of the pain.

Tenderness on deep pressure over the ulcer may also be of direct visceral origin, but where tenderness is extreme and associated with muscular rigidity, then involvement of the parietal peritoneum should be suspected.

In cancer of the stomach, the pain is often more constant because of partial penetration of the stomach wall and involvement of the peritoneum.

Disease of other viscera, e.g. appendicitis and cholecystitis, may cause pain imitating that of a peptic ulcer (*see also* p. 107).

### Vomiting

This is a common but not invariable feature of organic disease of the stomach such as ulcer or neoplasm. Vomiting generally occurs after digestion has been in process for some time, often, also, when gastric pain is at its height. By relieving the tension of the hypertonic stomach wall it may diminish or abolish pain, and an intragastric cause may reasonably be suspected when abdominal pain is relieved by vomiting. Vomiting occurs especially when the pylorus is obstructed (*see* p. 109), in which case the vomitus may be large in amount and, particularly in infants, projectile in character.

### Haematemesis (vomiting of blood)

This is most frequent in cases of peptic ulcer and is less commonly found in neoplasm of the stomach, where anaemia from chronic blood loss into the stool is more usual. A serious complication of hepatic cirrhosis is rupture of the oesophageal and gastric veins engorged as a result of portal hypertension. The amount of blood vomited varies from a mouthful to several litres. The exact amount is difficult to estimate as the blood is usually mixed with the gastric contents, which alter its colour and sometimes give the vomit a 'coffee-grounds' appearance. If the loss of blood is great, the general signs of haemorrhage will also be present. Substantial haematemesis can occur, even in patients without a chronic peptic ulcer, as a result of violent vomiting causing a breach in the gastric mucosa (Mallory–Weiss syndrome) or from superficial erosions induced by a gastric irritant such as aspirin.

These three symptoms, pain, vomiting and haematemesis, are found usually in organic disease of the stomach, but pain and vomiting, like the symptoms now to be described, may also be found in reflex disturbances of the stomach function due to disease of other viscera, to faulty habits of life, especially diet, and to psychological causes.

### Nausea

This is a sensation of sickness without actual vomiting, and is frequently accompanied by salivation, sweating and a feeling of faintness. It often results from psychic causes such as unpleasant sights or smells but also occurs in organic disease of the digestive system, notably carcinoma of the stomach. The possibility of drug-induced nausea should always be considered in patients receiving medicinal treatment. Vomiting of gastric origin is generally preceded by nausea.

### Flatulence

The stomach or intestines may be distended with gas, and the patient then complains of 'wind' or 'flatulence' or in America 'gas'. The wind may be belched through the mouth or passed per rectum; the former is gastric flatulence, the latter intestinal. Flatulence is common in many types of digestive disorder, but even more in functional than in organic disease. The gas in the great majority of cases of gastric flatulence is swallowed air (aerophagy). This may follow attempts to relieve epigastric discomfort from any cause, but frequent belching of large amounts of gas usually indicates compulsive air swallowing of psychogenic origin.

### Disturbance of appetite

Loss of appetite or *anorexia* must be distinguished from a fear of eating because of peptic ulceration or painful conditions of the mouth or gullet. True anorexia is common as a temporary phenomenon and of little significance, but when it is persistent it is of great importance. It may then be caused by serious disease in many parts of the body, but is particularly common in local diseases of the stomach such as gastritis and carcinoma. General debilitating diseases such as tuberculosis and severe aneamias have a similar effect. Profound loss of appetite may be of psychogenic origin as in anorexia nervosa and in certain mental disorders. An aversion to particular kinds of food sometimes occurs, as in diseases of the liver and biliary system when fats are not tolerated.

Excessive appetite with compulsive eating between meals is common in certain anxiety states, especially in women, and can lead to considerable obesity. Increased appetite of more moderate grade may be a feature of diseases where tissue waste is accelerated as in thyrotoxicosis and diabetes.

### Heartburn, waterbrash and eructations

These symptoms are often confused by the patient, who should therefore be asked to define clearly what he means by the terms.

*Heartburn* is a scalding or burning sensation experienced behind the sternum usually a little while after a meal or on stooping. In most cases, it is due to reflux of acid into the oesophagus especially when the pain threshold is lowered by oesophagitis (e.g. in hiatus hernia). However, it may also occur with reflux by duodenal juices containing bile and pancreatic enzymes.

*Waterbrash* consists in the filling of the mouth with a watery fluid composed of saliva. It is not necessarily a symptom of organic disease, but it may accompany the pain of duodenal ulcer or be due to reflex stimulation of saliva from gastrointestinal tract lesions.

*Eructations* of small amounts of the acid gastric contents along with flatus are common both in functional and organic disease of the stomach.

### ■ THE INTESTINES

*Pain, constipation and diarrhoea* are the most important symptoms caused by intestinal disease. Constipation and diarrhoea are even more common in temporary disturbances of health than in serious organic disease. As in the case of most gastrointestinal symptoms, persistence is a most significant point, for temporary constipation or diarrhoea rarely causes alarm except in acute abdominal disease.

### Pain

Pain is usually of the visceral type, vaguely localized and colicky in nature. It is almost certainly caused by increased tension on the intestinal musculature and exaggerated peristalsis, i.e. mechanical in origin. In gross intestinal obstruction where peristalsis is visible through the abdominal wall, the pain may be seen to coincide with the waves of peristalsis. Pain arising from the small intestine is generally situated in the centre of the abdomen. When the upper parts of the small intestine (jejunum) are affected, the pain is generally higher in the abdomen then when the lower parts are involved (ileum). Pain from the large intestine may also be experienced in the centre of the abdomen and left iliac fossa, but appears also to be common in the loins. Possibly the latter pain is not truly visceral but due to irritant effects or dragging upon the neighbouring parietal peritoneum.

### Constipation

In the average person evacution of the bowels takes place once daily, but the event may occur twice daily or only once in 2 days in persons in quite good health. It is therefore of importance to inquire as to the normal habits of the individual over a period of some years. Most persons regard themselves as constipated if they do not have one action of the bowels in 24 hours. A sudden change in habit is significant.

The degree of constipation should be ascertained and precisely what the patient means by the term, e.g. less frequent evacuation or dry stools or small amounts, often pellets. In all forms of intestinal obstruction absolute constipation may take place, that is there is passage neither of faeces nor of gas. In partial intestinal obstruction incomplete constipation may occur. The patient finds he needs increasing quantities of purgatives, but the stools when passed are usually soft or liquid and may be modified in shape—e.g. the ribbon-shaped stool—if the constricted area is in the rectum. There is as a rule no difficulty in the passage of flatus in partial intestinal obstruction.

Intestinal obstruction is the most serious cause of constipation but by no means the commonest. Constipation may arise from a great variety of factors, such as improper or temporarily reduced diet, insufficient exercise, carelessness in habits and general ill health from disease in other parts of the body. It is important to distinguish between delay in the passage of faeces through the large bowel into the rectum due to a hold-up at or above the sigmoid (colonic 'spastic' constipation) and delay in emptying of the rectum itself. In persons of careless habits the faeces frequently pass normally through the colon into the rectum, but, owing to neglect of the call to defaecation, they accumulate and cause distension of the rectum with loss of tone in its walls. This condition is called *dyschezia*, rectal constipation, and as a result of it a greater and greater amount of faeces is required to give the necessary sense of fullness which provokes the desire for defaecation. When faeces are retained in the bowel, water is absorbed so that the stool becomes hard and nodular and thus more difficult to evacuate. Rectal constipation, sometimes with impaction of faeces needing manual evacuation, is common in the elderly because of weakness of the pelvic musculature and, in some cases, difficulty in visiting the lavatory. Such patients often present with faecal incontinence due to pseudo-diarrhoea (*see below*).

### Diarrhoea

As in the case of constipation, the patient's definition of diarrhoea should be checked against the accepted idea that this symptom implies an increased frequency in evacuation of stools of liquid or semi-liquid character, not the discharge of mucus, blood or other abnormal constituents, though these may also be present. In most cases the stools are paler than normal, especially so in steatorrhoea, in which condition the stool also tends to float in the pan and is difficult to flush away.

Diarrhoea due to organic causes commonly occurs during the night and early morning as well as during the day. When diarrhoea is severe and persistent, the passage of frequent fluid stools may lead to physical exhaustion, dehydration with peripheral circulatory failure, the symptoms of potassium deficiency and protein loss (muscle weakness, oedema, etc.) and painful excoriation of the perianal skin.

The causes of diarrhoea include:

1. Those of temporary duration (a few hours to a few days), such as nervousness, allergic responses to food and drugs and acute infections of short duration, e.g. by Salmonella and other organisms.

2. More severe and prolonged infections such as bacillary and amoebic dysentery which with intestinal tuberculosis are more commonly seen in tropical zones. An acute form is exemplified by cholera with 'rice-water' stools containing enormous numbers of the vibrio.

3. Colonic diseases such as neoplasm, ulcerative colitis and irritable colon (p. 115).

4. Toxic states such as poisoning with heavy metals, e.g. arsenic, or toxaemias such as uraemia.

5. The excessive use of purgatives or 'pseudo-diarrhoea' due to the liquefaction of impacted or obstructed faeces.

6. Endocrine causes including hyperthyroidism and gastrin-secreting tumours of the pancreas (Zollinger–Ellison syndrome).

7. Malabsorption syndromes such as coeliac disease and chronic pancreatitis.

8. Crohn's disease of the small or large intestine.

In separating these various causes several points must be considered, e.g. the position and character of any pain; the character of the stools; evidence of gastric, thyroid, pancreatic and malabsorption syndromes; pyrexia and exposure to infections. The presence of blood in the faeces may be noted by the patient and signifies organic rather than functional disease of the lower bowel.

### Tenesmus

Tenesmus often accompanies diarrhoea and consists in straining with a desire to empty the lower bowel without evacuation taking place.

## ■ THE BILIARY TRACT

The special symptoms which need consideration in connection with the bilary tract are *pain* and *jaundice*, though many of the symptoms which have been described under The Stomach may also be reflexly produced by disease in the gallbladder or bile ducts.

### Pain

A stone in the cystic duct affords the best example of the type of pain which results from obstruction in the biliary system. The pain is due to the violent peristaltic movements of the wall of the duct attempting to force onwards a hard foreign body. It is not strictly a colicky pain as it is continuous rather than intermittent. It is felt in the epigastrium and right hypochondrium and is of such great intensity that the patient rolls about in agony, sweats and frequently vomits. In some cases the pain radiates to the angle of the right scapula. It is essentially visceral and lasts a few hours, but may be followed by a more localized pain in the right hypochondrium lasting several days. The latter is due to secondary cholecystitis and peritoneal involvement. This pain is associated with tenderness and rigidity on pressure (*Fig.* 4.9) and sometimes with fever or rigors. Similar pain occurs if the stone is impacted at the ampulla, and jaundice may then occur.

### Jaundice

Jaundice is a yellow pigmentation of the skin and mucous membranes caused by the presence in the blood of an excess of bile pigments. It is best seen in daylight. Jaundice may be due to increased production of bile pigments, defective transport or conjugation of bilirubin within the liver cell or obstruction to the outflow of bile from the liver to the duodenum. Some knowledge of the

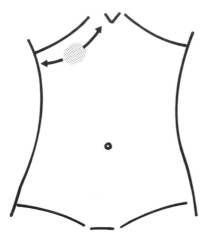

**Fig. 4.9**
Area of pain in biliary colic.
Often spreads to epigastrium
and inferior angle of right
scapula.

biochemistry of bile pigments is essential for the proper understanding of jaundice.

In health *unconjugated bilirubin* (haemobilirubin) is water-insoluble and derived from the breakdown of red cells by the reticuloendothelial system. It passes, attached to plasma albumin, to the liver where it is conjugated with glucuronide and possibly other substances.

Conjugated bilirubin glucuronide (hepatobilirubin) is water-soluble and is the major constituent of bile, which passes into the intestine. There it is changed by bacterial action into urobilinogen, the major part excreted in the faeces but some is reabsorbed to enter the liver and a small part absorbed into the general circulation to appear in the urine (*Fig.* 4.10).

**Prehepatic (Haemolytic) Jaundice** This form of jaundice is due to the presence in the blood of an excess of unconjugated bilirubin. Although haemolysis is the most important cause of prehepatic jaundice, it is now recognized that about 1 per cent of the population have a mild unconjugated hyperbilirubinaemia of an entirely benign nature—Gilbert's syndrome. The jaundice is often not clinically detectable, but may deepen during fasting or intercurrent illness, resulting in a mistaken diagnosis of hepatitis.

Haemolytic jaundice may result from an inherited abnormality in the red cells or from acquired causes. Since these forms of haemolysis are usually accompanied by anaemia, they are dealt with in Chapter 8 (p. 295). Sometimes a breakdown of red cells, as in gross pulmonary infarction or incompatible blood transfusion, causes prehepatic jaundice without anaemia.

When the red cells themselves are abnormal, as in hereditary spherocytosis, thalassaemia and to a lesser extent in pernicious anaemia, a genetic factor is at work and the cells may become osmotically and mechanically more fragile and are thus destroyed by the reticuloendothelial system. The history of previous attacks of jaundice or a family history of this complaint is of diagnostic importance.

Auto-antibodies, neoplasia and certain virus infections may similarly cause acquired haemolytic jaundice.

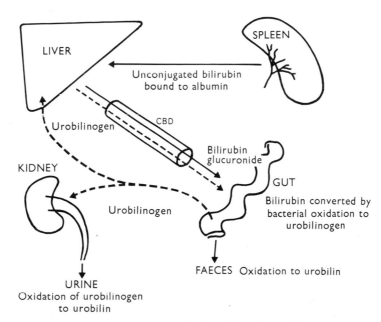

**Fig. 4.10** Physiological phases in bile formation and excretion.
CBD = common bile duct.

In most forms of prehepatic jaundice, the skin and mucosae are delicately jaundiced (a lemon-yellow tint), but the urine and faeces remain normal in colour, though the urine may darken on standing due to oxidation of the excess urobilinogen.

**Hepatocellular jaundice** This results from damage to the liver parenchyma interfering with the transport or conjugation of bilirubin and sometimes with its excretion through the canaliculi. The commonest cause of hepatocellular jaundice is a virus hepatitis (*see* p. 119), so that a history of transfusion, contact with another case or, in hospital workers, contact with the blood of a carrier may be obtained. Rarer infective causes include Weil's disease and yellow fever. The possibility of exposure to a medicinal liver toxin, such as chlorpromazine, testosterone, halothane or rifampicin, or an industrial one such as carbon tetrachloride, should always be considered. Hepatocellular jaundice also occurs in congestive cardiac failure and in the later stages of cirrhosis. When hepatic damage is accompanied by obstruction to the bile canaliculi (*cholestatic jaundice*), the characteristics of the jaundice itself are similar to those described under posthepatic obstruction (*see below*). The history of events preceding the jaundice, notably the prodromal period of anorexia and nausea in virus hepatitis, is of particular importance in differentiating the hepatocellular and posthepatic varieties (*see Table* 4.3). Liver function tests may also be helpful (*see* p. 124).

**Posthepatic (obstructive) jaundice** This form of jaundice results from obstruction to the bile ducts outside the liver. The common causes include gallstones, primary carcinoma of the head of pancreas or bile ducts, and secondary carcinomatous masses in the porta hepatis. When the obstruction is due to gallstones

**Table 4.3   The differential diagnosis of jaundice**

| | *Prehepatic (haemolytic)* | *Hepatocellular* | *Posthepatic (obstructive)* |
|---|---|---|---|
| *Mechanism* | Increased bilirubin formation | Hepatocellular failure | Bile duct obstruction |
| *Common causes* | Haemolysis. Gilbert's syndrome | Virus hepatitis. Drugs, e.g. chlorpromazine. Chronic liver disease. Cirrhosis | Gallstones. Carcinoma of pancreas |
| *Past history* | May be previous attacks or a family history | History of contact, of injections, or of taking hepatotoxic drugs | May be previous attacks (stone) |
| *Mode of development* | Rapid, with anaemia and sometimes fever and rigors. Periodic attacks | After a period of anorexia and nausea; gradual onset and recovery | After an attack of pain. Rapid and sometimes intermittent (stone). Insidious and progressive (carcinoma) |
| *Pruritus (bile salt retention)* | Absent | Occasional (if cholestasis). Primary biliary cirrhosis | Present |
| *Skin colour* | Faint lemon-yellow | Yellow | Brilliant or dark yellow |
| *Urine* | Colourless at first. Urobilinogen present; later by oxidation urobilin occurs and urine darkens slightly | Dark. (Bilirubin and urobilinogen) | Very dark. (Bilirubin; no urobilinogen) |
| *Faeces* | Normal | Pale (if cholestasis) | Pale |
| *Gallbladder* | Nil | Nil | May be palpable in carcinoma; not with stone |
| *Enlarged spleen* | Usually | Sometimes | Nil |
| *Bilirubin* | Unconjugated | Mixed | Conjugated |
| *Serum alkaline phosphatase* | Normal | Raised (if cholestasis) | Markedly raised |
| *Tests for hepatocellular function* | Normal | Grossly abnormal | Slightly abnormal |
| *Tests for haemolysis* | Positive | Negative | Negative |

the jaundice is usually preceded by biliary colic and may be intermittent. Jaundice due to carcinoma tends to be insidious in onset and progressive in its course, and the gallbladder is sometimes palpable (*see Fig.* 4.19, p. 99). Obstructive jaundice varies in intensity from a slight yellowish tinge in the skin and mucous membranes to a pronounced canary yellow, or, in long-standing cases, a dark greenish-yellow discoloration. It affects the skin of the whole body (*Fig.* 4.11), but is most marked on the trunk and proximal parts of the limbs. Even before the skin is affected, the yellowing is seen in the mucous membranes and should be sought in the conjunctivae and soft palate. Intolerable itching is common and is probably due to bile salts, as it may precede the actual pigmentation of the skin and mucosae. The excess of bile pigments (conjugated bilirubin) in the blood leads to their appearance in the urine, which may be visibly bile-stained or in which bile may be detected by special tests (*see* p. 116, *et seq.*). The lack of the normal flow of bile into the duodenum deprives the faeces of one of their colouring constituents and further interferes with the digestion and absorption of fats because of the lack of bile salts. As a result, the faeces have a lighter colour than normal and are often clay-coloured. In complete obstruction, urobilinogen is absent from the urine.

In conclusion, it must be stressed that more than one of the three types of jaundice can exist in the same patient. It has already been said that intrahepatic obstruction is common in hepatocellular jaundice, and obstruction due to pigment stones may also occur in haemolytic jaundice. Moreover, liver-cell dysfunction can result from the damming back of bile and ascending infection in obstructive jaundice. Special laboratory investigations are therefore needed for the precise diagnosis of jaundice and for the differentiation of the three types.

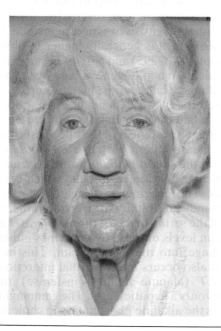

**Fig. 4.11**
Yellow pigmentation of the skin and greenish yellow sclerae due to carcinoma of the bile ducts.

## Biochemical tests

Biochemical tests of the blood and urine differentiate between the three types of jaundice (*Table* 4.4).

In prehepatic or haemolytic jaundice an excess of unconjugated bilirubin is formed in the blood but cannot pass into the urine as, unlike bilirubin glucuronide, it is unable to cross the glomerular membrane. However, the urine does contain an excess of urobilinogen derived from the increased quantity of bile pigments entering the bowel (*see Table* 4.3, p. 86).

In posthepatic and hepatocellular jaundice bilirubin glucuronide is formed normally in the liver but seeps back into the blood because it cannot generally reach the bowel. It is then excreted in the urine, while the faeces are deprived of bile pigments.

| Table 4.4 | Urine testing in normal and jaundiced patients | | | |
|---|---|---|---|---|
| | *Normal* | *Prehepatic* | *Posthepatic* | *Hepatocellular* |
| Bilirubin | − | − | + + | + + |
| Urobilin | + | + + + | − | + + |

In hepatocellular jaundice, *some* bile pigment will reach the intestine and be absorbed into the bloodstream, but the damaged liver cells cannot cope with it all and urobilinogen may then appear to excess in the urine which must be examined fresh.

The presence of jaundice, especially when doubtful or in subclinical forms, can be confirmed by the finding of a raised *total serum bilirubin*, i.e. bilirubin and bilirubin glucuronide (*see* p. 144). The relative proportions of these two forms of bilirubin may help to distinguish haemolytic from obstructive forms of jaundice.

Other tests used in the differential diagnosis of jaundice include measurement of the *serum alkaline phosphatase* which is generally higher in obstructive than hepatocellular jaundice (*see* Chapter 8, p. 295) and *tests for hepatocellular function* (*see below*) may be abnormal chiefly in hepatogenous jaundice. They are therefore useful in detection of liver damage in hepatitis, hepatic necrosis or cirrhosis.

The tests most commonly used today are dependent upon a derangement in those functions of the liver that relate to the metabolism of protein, the cellular enzymes and the excretion of foreign substances in the bile. Tests based upon the metabolism of proteins include measurement of the *serum albumin*, which may be decreased in liver disease, and the *serum globulin*, which is usually increased in active liver disease; the particular fraction of globulin which is increased can be identified by *electrophoresis*. The enzyme tests include the *serum alkaline phosphatase* (elevation of which indicates biliary obstruction rather than hepatocellular damage, *see below*), and the serum levels of the *transferases* and *dehydrogenases*. An increase in the serum levels of these two enzymes indicates that cell damage is permitting their leakage into the bloodstream. This increase is not specific to liver damage, since it also occurs in myocardial infarction, but a relatively greater increase in *ALT* (alanine-amino transferase) than in *AST* (aspartate-amino transferase) favours a hepatic cause. The gammaglutamyl transpeptidase ($\gamma GT$) enzyme mirrors the alkaline phosphatase in cholestasis but does not rise in bone disease; it is therefore useful in distinguishing an elevated alkaline phosphatase of liver and bone origin. The γGT is also elevated by enzyme-inducing agents, particularly by alcohol, and is a useful guide to alcohol abuse even in the absence of hepatic damage. In this context the average size of circulating red cells (MCV) is valuable, being commonly elevated in alcoholism quite independent of folate or $B_{12}$ deficiency.

## ■ ANATOMICAL CONSIDERATIONS

Before proceeding to the detailed examination of the abdomen, certain anatomical facts may be recalled. It is customary for purposes of clinical description to divide the abdomen into nine regions by two vertical and two horizontal lines. Each vertical line may be taken from the midclavicle to the midinguinal region. The upper horizontal line passes across the abdomen at the lowest point of the 10th costal arches. The lower horizontal line joins the two anterior superior spines of the illia.* The 'regions' thus marked out (*Fig.* 4.12) are:

*In the upper abdomen*—the right hypochondrium, epigastrium and left hypochondrium.

*In the middle*—the right lumbar, umbilical and left lumbar.

*In the lower abdomen*—the right iliac fossa, hypogastrium and left iliac fossa.

It must be emphasized that the main value of the regions is to describe the position of pain, tenderness, rigidity, tumours, etc. Lists of viscera contained in these regions are fallacious. The stomach, intestines and kidneys (and other viscera to a lesser extent) are so mobile that they are not constantly found in the same regions, even in the same individual, and in different normal individuals differ widely in position.

Some organs, however, are more or less fixed. The gallbladder is generally

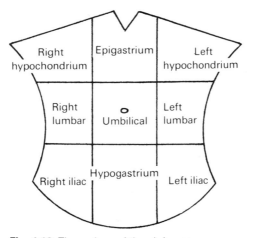

**Fig. 4.12** The regions of the abdomen.

* Other lines are also in use, and it matters little which the student employs, as the division of the abdomen into regions is purely arbitrary and is of more clinical than anatomical value.

found in the right hypochondrium, the liver in the right hypochondrium and epigastrium, the spleen in the left hypochondrium. The hypogastrium contains the full bladder or pregnant uterus. Posture and respiration have a profound effect on the position of the viscera.

■ PHYSICAL SIGNS: EXAMINATION OF THE ABDOMEN

A careful history is most important in the diagnosis of diseases of the digestive system, and it is often disappointing that the symptoms are not corroborated by abnormal physical signs and that for a diagnosis the physician must frequently resort to special methods of investigation, such as radiology and endoscopy. This admission, however, forms no excuse for the omission of the well-recognized clinical methods of examination. The examination of the mouth and oesophagus has already been considered. The examination of the abdominal viscera requires a knowledge of the method of examination of the abdomen in general, and certain special details concerning the individual viscera.

Examination of the abdomen should follow the routine described under the respiratory and cardiovascular systems – inspection, palpation, percussion and auscultation—though inspection and palpation are by far the most important methods of approach.

*Inspection* shows the condition of the abdominal wall, the size of the abdomen and any irregularity in its contour caused by enlargement of viscera or the presence of abnormal swellings in the abdominal cavity. It also shows certain motile phenomena such as the movement of the abdominal wall with respiration, the presence of visible peristalsis in the stomach or intestines and the pulsations of the aorta or an engorged liver. The external genitalia may be inspected at the same time (*see* p. 56).

*Palpation* determines the presence of superficial or deep tenderness and of undue rigidity or laxity of the abdominal wall. It is the principal method by which the enlargement of viscera such as the liver, spleen and kidneys, and the presence of tumours and herniae, are detected.

*Percussion* may add confirmatory information in the case of enlarged viscera or tumours, and may help in recognizing the presence of free fluid in the peritoneal cavity. In cases of tympanites (gastrointestinal distension) the note on percussion is drum-like.

*Auscultation* is of special value in distinguishing between paralytic ileus, in which the abdomen is silent, and intestinal obstruction, in which the bowel sounds are increased.

### INSPECTION

Inspection of the abdomen must be carried out in a good light and if possible with the patient both in the erect and recumbent postures.

#### Condition of the abdominal wall

The *skin* of the abdomen should first be observed. When abdominal distension is present from any cause, the skin is stretched, smooth and shiny, and the umbilicus may be flattened or even everted. In obese subjects the abdomen may appear distended, but the umbilical cleft is deeper than normal. Undue laxity of the abdominal wall, causing wrinkling of the skin, is found when intra-abdominal pressure is suddenly decreased, as after childbirth (especially in multi-parae), and after removal of fluid from the peritoneal cavity. After repeated pregnancies or loss of weight in a previously obese subject, broad silvery lines or 'stretch marks' appear on the abdominal wall. Similar marks, often purple in colour, are also seen in Cushing's syndrome (*see* Chapter 11).

*Enlarged veins* are useful evidence of obstruction in the inferior vena caval or portal systems. The greater the distension and the more numerous the veins, the greater the obstruction is likely to be.

Obstruction in the inferior vena cava or common iliac veins usually causes veins to appear at the sides of the abdomen (*Fig.* 4.13), and when the veins are emptied by pressure with the fingers, they will be seen to fill again from below. The blood bypasses the inferior vena cava, travelling from the lower limbs (and certain viscera) to the thorax via the veins of the abdominal wall. These superficial veins are arranged longitudinally. Thrombosis of the inferior vena cava, owing to its completeness in obstructing the circulation, will cause the most pronounced collateral circulation to become apparent on the abdominal wall, but any increase in the intra-abdominal pressure (e.g. ascites) will have a similar though less striking result.

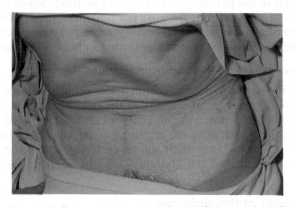

**Fig. 4.13** Enlarged abdominal veins in inferior venal caval obstruction.

If the obstruction is in the portal system (cirrhosis of the liver, or more rarely thrombosis of the portal vein), the engorged veins are centrally placed and may form a little cluster around the umbilicus (caput medusae). The blood in these veins flows in all directions away from the umbilicus. The direction of the blood flow should always be tested.

A section of vein can be emptied by 'milking' it with the fingers, and each end of the emptied part is sealed with the pressure of a finger. One finger can then be removed and the rate at which the vein fills is noted. The performance is repeated, removing the finger at the other end. The blood enters more rapidly from the direction of the blood flow.

Secondary nodules may be found in the skin in certain types of malignant disease (*Fig.* 4.14). Oedema of the abdominal wall may be demonstrated by the

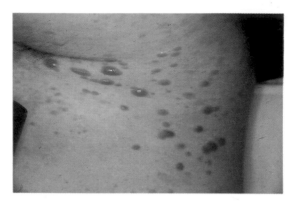

**Fig. 4.14** Secondary nodules in abdominal skin due to carcinoma of the gallbladder.

usual phenomenon of pitting (best elicited by pinching a fold of the abdominal wall), and has the same origin as oedema elsewhere. It is not to be confused with the presence of fluid in the peritoneal cavity itself (ascites). Small herniae due to extrusion of pieces of extraperitoneal fat are not uncommonly seen in the midline of the upper abdomen. They are usually symptomless. Larger herniae may be seen at or near the umbilicus or protruding through abdominal scars.

### Movements of the abdominal wall

The movements of the abdominal wall should be carefully watched. In men with the abdominal type of respiration the movement should be free and equal on the two sides. In women the movement is often restricted owing to the costal type of breathing. An absolute fixation of the whole or greater part of the abdominal wall is a most important sign of generalized peritonitis. Unequal movement of the two sides of the abdomen may be seen in cases of phrenic paralysis.

### Contour of the abdomen

The contour of the abdomen should next be noted. When abnormal swelling is present it is important to observe whether it is uniform or asymmetrical. Uniform swelling may be caused by obesity, by distension of the abdomen by gas in the gastrointestinal tract or by fluid in the peritoneal cavity. Large abdominal tumours such as an overfilled bladder, pregnant uterus or large ovarian cyst (*Fig.* 4.15) cause swelling of the abdomen which at first glance may appear uniform, but which closer inspection shows to be limited to the contour of the enlarged viscus or tumour.

*Irregularities in the contour* of the abdomen may be caused by enlargement of viscera such as the liver (*Fig.* 4.16), spleen, kidneys, or gallbladder, or by tumours arising from these and other organs, e.g. the stomach, intestines, pancreas or peritoneum (*Fig.* 4.17). Distension of one portion of the alimentary tract may also produce irregularity in the abdominal contour, e.g. gastric distension producing a bulge in the epigastrium or colonic distension causing a fullness in the flanks. The

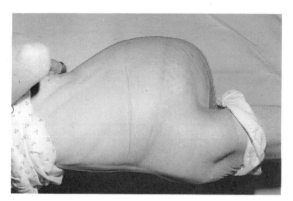

**Fig. 4.15** Ovarian cyst. Note generalized distension, apparently arising from the pelvis.

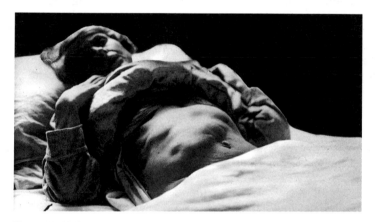

**Fig. 4.16** Malignant disease of the liver. Enormous liver enlargement due to secondary growths from neoplasm of ovary. Note especially the nodular irregularity.

type and degree of irregularity in the contour of the abdominal wall will depend upon the size, shape and irregularity of the underlying swelling.

## Movements beneath the abdominal wall

Care should be taken to observe any movements occurring beneath the abdominal wall or communicated through it. Visible pulsation of the abdominal aorta is frequent in nervous individuals, especially in those with a thin abdominal wall, and must be distinguished from aneurysm of the abdominal aorta. In this condition the pulsation is usually more marked, and it is generally possible

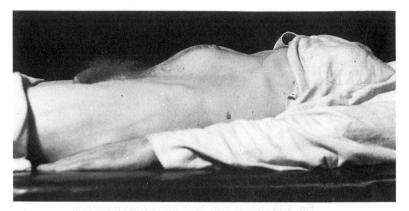

**Fig. 4.17** Abdominal swelling due to mesenteric cyst. The curve of the swelling has a fairly steep rise at the pubis and in the epigastrium, and obviously occupies chiefly the central abdomen. (*See* for comparison *Fig.* 5.4, p. 138, Distended bladder.)

by palpation to define the outline of an enlarged expansile arterial swelling. Often aortic pulsation is transmitted through an overlying viscus or tumour. For example, the aorta may cause pulsation of a carcinoma of the stomach, which must then be differentiated from aneurysm. In these cases of transmitted pulsation the pulsating tumour is usually irregular, and its pulsations may cease if the patient is examined in the knee–elbow position, so that the tumour falls away from the underlying aorta. The enlargement of mobile organs such as the liver and spleen or a tumour in the stomach may be revealed as a downward-moving ripple beneath the skin when the patient breathes in.

*Peristalsis* may be visible in cases of obstruction in the gastrointestinal tract. Obstruction at the pylorus causes increased peristaltic movements of the stomach, seen through the abdominal wall as a slow wave moving from left to right across the upper abdomen. Obstruction in the large intestine may also be accompanied by peristaltic waves in the upper abdomen, in this case moving from right to left. In obstruction of the small intestine the peristaltic waves may be seen in a ladder pattern down the centre of the abdomen. Such movements can be induced by gentle kneading of the abdomen, by applying a cold stimulus to the skin or by giving the patient soda-water to drink.

Intestinal peristalsis may be observed especially in elderly women with a lax abdominal wall but no organic disease.

## PALPATION

Successful palpation needs much practice. The most favourable posture for the patient is lying flat on his back with the head slightly raised (one pillow), the arms to the side, and the knees extended. When the abdominal muscles are held tense it may be helpful to draw up the patient's knees. The blankets should be folded well out of the way and the edge of the sheet drawn across the groins to cover the genitalia until they are examined. The patient should be asked to breathe quietly and rather more deeply than normal, keeping the mouth open to encourage the abdominal type of respiration. When the examiner is satisfied that the abdomen is moving freely, palpation may begin, using the flat hand but exerting pressure with the fingers. The fingertips should be used only after the flat hand has first been employed, and then only under special circumstances, as the discomfort caused by their use leads to reflex spasm of the abdominal wall, which prevents satisfactory examination. Each region of the abdomen is examined in turn, very light palpation being used first to locate areas of tenderness or guarding. The following points should be systematically observed:

### 1 Tenderness

Tenderness means pain on pressure. *Deep tenderness* is most commonly found in inflammatory lesions of the viscera and their surrounding peritoneum. Tenderness, for example, in the right iliac fossa is frequently found in appendicitis, tenderness in the right hypochondrium in cholecystitis, and epigastric tenderness in peptic ulceration with peritoneal involvement, while purely visceral pain such as gastric or intestinal colic is not associated with any tenderness. Occasionally pressure in one region of the abdomen may cause pain in another. For example, pressure in the left iliac fossa sometimes causes pain in the right, in cases of appendicitis. This is the exception rather than the rule and is probably explained by transmission of the pressure to the right iliac fossa, e.g. through the colon. Tenderness is usually found over the region where the inflamed viscus is lying. If an area of tenderness is expected, the palpating hand should first be placed on the abdomen in some region distant from the suspected area. In appendicitis, for example, palpation should begin in the left iliac fossa, which, being normal, will form a contrast to the tenderness in the right iliac fossa.

Closely allied to deep tenderness are *cutaneous hyperaesthesia* and *tenderness in the superficial tissues* of the abdominal wall.

All forms of tenderness may be found in neurotic individuals who have no local abdominal disease. As a temporary phenomen *tympanites* (distension of the gastrointestinal tract with gas) may also give rise to tenderness.

### 2 Guarding and rigidity

Abdominal guarding is due to muscular contraction, which often occurs reflexly as a part of a defence mechanism over an inflamed organ. This has already been discussed.

Some patients hold the abdominal wall so tightly that examination is difficult or impossible, but in the majority, if the patient is put in a comfortable position and his mind set at rest by explaining that no undue pain will be caused by the examination, the abdominal muscles gradually relax. Nervous guarding of this type generally affects the whole abdominal wall. So also does the contraction of the abdominal muscles if the patient raises his head to satisfy his curiosity about the examination. Localized guarding is therefore more suggestive of disease. The notable exception to this is the case of acute generalized peritonitis in which there occurs a true generalized rigidity of the abdominal wall which cannot be relaxed ('board-like' rigidity).

As in the examination for tenderness, the palpating hand should first test the abdominal muscles in some part away from the suspected lesion. For example, if cholecystitis is suspected, palpation should begin in the left hypochondrium, which then forms a standard of control to the rigidity in the right hypochondrium. The bellies of the rectus muscles sometimes cause difficulty in the examination of the abdomen. Portions of them may be so prominent as to simulate a lump beneath the abdominal wall, and it is important to compare carefully the two recti. If the rectus muscles are brought into use, such a 'tumour' becomes more pronounced. In some patients, on the other hand, the rectus muscles are so poorly developed and toneless that the hand can palpate through them with the same ease as through other portions of the abdominal wall. In perfectly healthy individuals it is not uncommon to find separation of the rectus muscles producing a wide gap in which the abdominal wall is so thin that the viscera beneath can be palpated more distinctly than normal (divarication of the recti).

### 3 Enlargement of viscera

**The liver** Palpation of the liver is made by resting the flat of one or both hands on the abdomen with the tips of the fingers gently inserted beneath the costal margin. To avoid overlooking gross enlargement it is advisable to move the hand from the right iliac fossa gradually upwards until any increased sense of resistance is noted. At this point the fingertips may be used to locate the liver edge accurately (*Fig.* 4.18a). The liver in a healthy subject may sometimes be felt 1–2 cm below the costal margin during inspiration but in certain diseases can extend well into the right iliac fossa. For this method of palpation, the examiner has to sit on the edge of the bed and the patient's knees cannot be fully flexed. An alternative method is to place the right hand across the abdomen and to seek the liver edge with the radial border of the index finger (*Fig.* 4.18b).

The *character of the edge* should be recorded. When palpable in health it is sharp, firm and regular, gradually passing upwards as it crosses the epigastrium into the left hypochondrium. Deformities of the chest (e.g. in kyphoscoliosis emphysema) are sometimes responsible for displacing the liver downwards so that it appears to be enlarged. In infants also the liver is relatively large and may be palpable in health.

An unusual tongue of liver substance, Riedel's lobe, may occasionally give rise to difficulty. It is sometimes freely mobile and may be mistaken for a movable kidney, or, if situated nearer the middle line, for a gallbladder swelling. It is almost invariably in the right upper quadrant of the abdomen.

When the liver is enlarged from fatty changes, its edge is soft and difficult to feel, especially in an obese person. Fortunately, this type of enlargement, though common, is rarely an important point in the diagnosis. In most other forms of liver enlargement the edge is firm or even harder than normal. Thus in passive congestion of the liver due to cardiac failure the edge is firmer than normal, while in malignant disease it may be very hard and irregular.

The *surface of the liver* should next be palpated. In cancerous infiltration it may be grossly irregular owing to the presence of large nodules. The nodularity is clinically less obvious, however, in micronodular cirrhosis. Gross nodularity of the liver in a patient with cirrhosis suggests hepatoma. In most other forms of liver enlargement (*see Table* 4.5) the surface of the organ is quite smooth.

The *degree of enlargement* also gives useful information. In the congestion of heart failure, for example, the size of the liver is often roughly proportionate to the

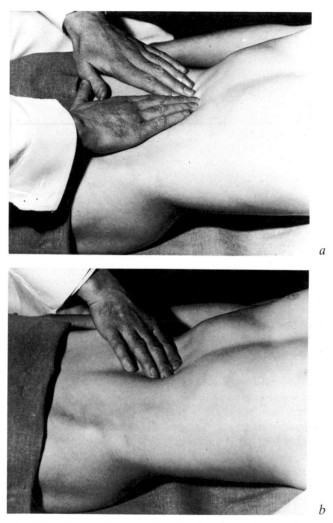

*a*

*b*

**Fig. 4.18** Palpation of liver. *a*, Both hands are placed flat on the abdomen with the fingers directed towards the costal margin and gradually moved upwards until resistance is encountered. The patient then takes a deep breath and the edge of the liver rides over the fingers. *b*, An alternative method.

degree of cardiac failure, and its shrinkage is a useful indication of the response to treatment. In moderate degrees of heart failure the liver edge extends 5–8 cm below the costal margin, but in tricuspid incompetence it may reach the level of the umbilicus or lower. Such gross enlargement of the liver is also common in cancer, amyloidosis, amoebic abscess and certain blood diseases. Moderate enlargement of the liver occurs in obstruction of the common bile duct (e.g. with gallstones) and in infective hepatitis. In cirrhosis, the liver is usually enlarged but later shrinks in advanced cirrhosis, especially in the macronodular variety.

| Table 4.5 | **Causes of hepatic enlargement** |
|---|---|
| *Tender enlargement* | *Painless enlargement* |
| Rapid distension from any cause (e.g. venous congestion in cardiac failure) | Biliary obstruction (e.g. stone, carcinoma, cholestatic hepatitis) |
| Acute inflammation (e.g. virus and amoebic hepatitis) | Cirrhosis (e.g. posthepatitis, biliary, cardiac) |
| Hepatic abscess (e.g. portal pyaemia and amoebic abscess) | Malignant disease (e.g. secondary carcinoma, primary hepatoma) |
| | Haemopoietic disease (e.g. Hodgkin's disease, leukaemia) |
| | Chronic infections (e.g. malaria) |
| | Amyloidosis (e.g. chronic suppuration, rheumatoid arthritis) |
| | Infiltrations (e.g. fatty liver, lipoidoses, sarcoidosis) |

It should be noted whether the liver is tender or painless on palpation. Tenderness is often found in the congested liver of heart failure and in inflammatory lesions, e.g. hepatitis and liver abscess, while the gross enlargements of cancer and other diseases may remain quite painless. (*See Table* 4.5.)

Finally, the presence of pulsation should be sought, especially in patients with signs of congestive cardiac failure. Pulsation of the liver suggests incompetence of the tricuspid valve (*see* p. 221).

**The gallbladder** In obstruction of the cystic duct, commonly by stone, or of the common bile duct, particularly by growth of the head of the pancreas, enlargement of the gallbladder may be found. The organ is felt as a smooth tense swelling projecting beneath the right costal margin in the direction of the umbilicus. If the enlargement is great, the swelling may be mistaken for another viscus—for example an enlarged right kidney. Moderate degrees of enlargement may be obscured if the gallbladder is covered by the liver. A distended gallbladder in the presence of jaundice is due to some cause other than gallstones (generally to carcinoma of the head of the pancreas). This is known as *Courvoisier's Law* (*Fig.* 4.19), but, as with all 'laws' in medicine, exceptions do occur. It is explained by the fact that gallstones, if present for a considerable time, cause fibrosis of the gallbladder. Thus when a stone is later impacted in the common bile duct, jaundice results, but the gallbladder is less likely to expand than in the case of a healthy gallbladder proximal to a malignant obstruction.

**The colon** The colon may be palpable as a sausage-shaped tumour when distended with gas or faeces. In normal subjects the descending colon can often be felt as a firm tube in the left iliac fossa and sometimes the caecum can also be palpated. (The characteristics of colonic tumour are described below.)

The palpation of other enlarged abdominal viscera, e.g. the kidneys and spleen, not directly connected with the digestive tract, will be dealt with under the appropriate system.

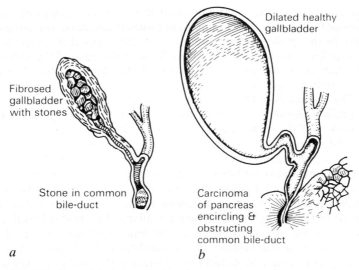

Dilated healthy
gallbladder

Fibrosed
gallbladder
with stones

Stone in common
bile-duct

Carcinoma
of pancreas
encircling &
obstructing
common bile-duct

*a*                                    *b*

**Fig. 4.19** Courvoisier's Law. *a*, Jaundice caused by a gallstone
in the common duct. The gallbladder cannot dilate as it is
fibrosed from cholecystitis due to stones within it. *b*, Jaundice
due to obstruction of the common bile duct by carcinoma of the
head of the pancreas. The gallbladder is dilated owing to the
back-pressure of the bile.

### 4 Abdominal tumour

On detection of a tumour in the abdomen the following points
should be observed.

**Position** An accurate description of the position often helps to decide the organ
from which the tumour is growing, and when its outline has been defined, the
observer should consider what organs and tissues lie in this region of the abdomen.
The localization of tumours is sometimes difficult owing to the fact that only a
small portion may present at the abdominal wall, and the bulk of the tumour may
be impalpable because of its deep situation. When a tumour does not lie in the
region of a particular viscus, the possibility of a peritoneal origin should be considered. Malignant or inflammatory masses may, for example, be distributed
irregularly in the omentum or mesentery, and in the latter cysts also occur. Care
should be taken also to exclude the possibility of the tumour arising from the
abdominal wall. In this case modifications of the shape and size of the tumour
can be produced by making the patient move the abdominal muscles.

**Size** The larger the tumour, the more difficult it is to determine the tissue from
which it is growing, but certain tumours by their very size (e.g. an ovarian cyst,
which forms a large round swelling in the lower abdomen) give a valuable clue
to their nature (*see Fig.* 4.15, p. 93).

**Consistency** Some organs and tissues, e.g. the stomach, intestines and bladder,
are normally impalpable unless they are distended respectively by gas, intestinal
contents or urine. The consistency of organs such as the liver and spleen may help

to distinguish a simple enlargement of these viscera from enlargement due to neoplastic infiltration. Most malignant tumours are hard and irregular.

**Shape** In the early stages a tumour may correspond in shape with the viscus from which it is arising. This is especially so in the case of the kidney and spleen. As the tumour grows larger, the characteristic shape is often lost and therefore gives no information as to its origin.

**Mobility** Tumours of the stomach, transverse colon, liver, gallbladder, kidneys and spleen generally move downwards with the diaphragm during inspiration, but tumours of the pancreas, the para-aortic lymph nodes and the viscera in the lower abdomen (bladder, uterus, descending colon, caecum, etc.), upon which respiratory movements have little effect, are usually immobile.

**Ability to get above or below the tumour** It is sometimes possible to define the upper border of an enlarged kidney or a pyloric tumour, but not in the case of an enlarged liver or spleen. Likewise in the pelvis, the hand may reach below a tumour of the colon but not below an enlarged uterus or bladder.

Masses in the upper abdomen are at times partially obscured by the costal margins and lie in the hollows of the diaphragmatic domes. They may be more accurately delineated by putting the patient (after suitable explanation) over a 'bridge' made by placing a pillow in the concavity of the lumbar spine. This manoeuvre may enable one 'to get above' a tumour.

### 5  Fluid in the peritoneal cavity

When free fluid is present in the peritoneal cavity (*Fig.* 4.20), palpation of enlarged viscera is difficult, but the edge of the enlarged organ, e.g. the liver or spleen, may be felt by *dipping* or *ballotting*. This method of palpation is performed by a quick pressure of the tips of the fingers over the region where the edge of the viscus is expected. The pressure displaces the fluid temporarily and allows the fingers to come in contact with the enlarged viscus (*Fig.* 4.21).

The *fluid thrill* is also used to detect the presence of free fluid. The observer places one hand flat on one flank and with the fingers of the other hand gives a sharp tap on the opposite flank. This produces a wave in the fluid which is detectable by the palpating hand. A similar sensation may be obtained if the abdominal

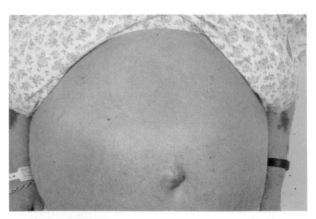

**Fig. 4.20** Malignant ascites.

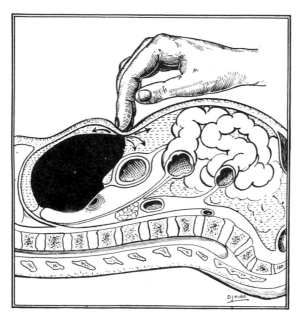

**Fig. 4.21** 'Dipping' for enlarged liver. The palpating fingers prod sharply over the expected enlarged viscus, the fluid is displaced as shown by the arrows, and the fingers strike the surface or edge of the organ. Note also the gas-containing intestines which float to the surface and give a central area of resonance on percussion.

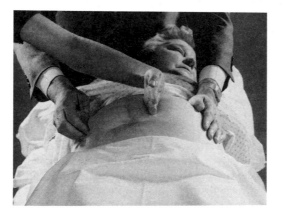

**Fig. 4.22** The fluid thrill. The nurse's hand is placed firmly along the linea alba. The observer places one hand flat on the flank, while the fingers of the other percuss on the opposite flank.

wall is very fat, and to avoid this a second person should place the edge of his hand along the linea alba, exerting firm pressure so as to damp out any vibrations in the abdominal wall itself (*Fig.* 4.22). (*See also* Percussion, p. 102.)

### 6 The hernial rings

The superficial inguinal rings should be carefully examined in every case and evidence of herniation should also be sought in the epigastric and umbilical areas. This is particularly necessary in any case that suggests intestinal obstruction, of which strangulation of an inguinal or femoral hernia is quite a common cause. In the male, when no hernia is visible on standing, a finger should be inserted through the invaginated scrotum into the external abdominal ring and the patient asked to cough. Small herniae can be detected in this way as they give a forcible impulse to the palpating finger.

### RECTAL EXAMINATION AND PROCTOSCOPY

Examination of the rectum is employed for many purposes and is mentioned more fully in Chapter 5. In the examination of the digestive tract it is used to determine the tone of the anal sphincter, the presence of any haemorrhoids, the condition of emptiness or fullness of the rectum, and, above all, the presence of any new growth in the rectum itself or any tumour of the surrounding tissues which may press on or obstruct the rectum. 'Ballooning' of the rectum suggests obstruction at the junction of the sigmoid colon and rectum.

The small amount of faeces obtained on the glove or fingerstall after rectal examination may be enough to provide for certain quick observations. The colour may confirm pale stools in steatorrhoea, bright blood in rectal haemorrhage or melaena from higher intestinal bleeding. Tests for occult blood, microscopy for ova, and examination under ultraviolet light in cases of porphyria variegata are examples.

Fuller details of faecal characteristics are given later (pp. 105–107).

### PERCUSSION

Percussion has only a limited use in the examination of the alimentary system. However, it is important in delineating the upper border of the liver, usually at the level of the fifth or sixth right intercostal spaces in the midclavicular line, thus distinguishing an enlarged liver from one that is merely displaced downwards by overinflated lungs. Light percussion as a rule gives more information than heavy and is of most value in helping to elucidate the cause of abdominal enlargement. Uniform enlargement caused by gastrointestinal distension with gas yields a tympanitic note, whilst a similar enlargement caused by fluid yields a dull note, which may be present all over the abdomen if the fluid is large in amount, or only in the flanks if the fluid is insufficient to cover the centrally placed coils of intestine (*Fig.* 4.21). When fluid is suspected, percussion should be performed first with the patient lying on his back and then lying alternately on each side. This movement will lead to a displacement of the fluid into the flank nearest the bed, over which a dull note will be obtained, whilst the empty upper flank will yield a tympanitic note. This phenomenon is known as *shifting dullness*. Care must be taken to percuss a strictly comparable site on each side of the abdomen: with the patient recumbent the percussion may start centrally and continue laterally until dullness appears. Percussion must take place with the finger running the length of the abdomen parallel to the level present in the flank (*Fig.* 4.23).

Percussion may be used as an accessory method to palpation in defining the

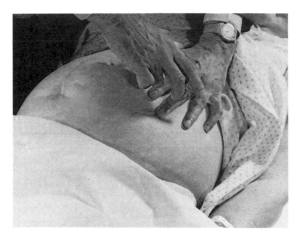

**Fig. 4.23** Ascites demonstrated by shifting dullness. Note how the struck finger is parallel to the long axis of the abdomen and hence the fluid level.

outline of enlarged viscera or abdominal tumours. The nearer the viscus or tumour lies to the abdominal wall, the more definite will be the results of percussion. An enlarged spleen, over which the percussion note is dull, can thus be distinguished from an enlarged left kidney over which the percussion note is resonant because of intervening colon. The lower edge of the liver can also be detected by percussing the abdomen from the right iliac fossa up towards the costal margin. When the liver is either enlarged or displaced downwards, a dull note is elicited at some point below the costal margin. In the case of downward displacement, the upper border of liver dullness will be lower than normal.

## AUSCULTATION

In cases of paralytic ileus due to peritonitis or other causes, the absence of the normal sounds due to peristaltic activity may be a suggestive sign, but it may be necessary to listen for several minutes. In peritonitis, the sounds disappear first in the neighbourhood of the lesion. On the other hand, in obstructive lesions of the gastrointestinal tract the sounds may be greatly exaggerated (*borborygmi*) and sometimes have a high-pitched tinkling note. Their intensity corresponds with waves of pain.

When the pylorus is obstructed gastric contents are retained for longer than 3 or 4 h after a meal. A 'succussion splash' can then be elicited by palpation over the stomach or by gently rolling the patient from side to side.

Auscultation of the abdomen may also reveal sounds of vascular origin. A systolic murmur suggests narrowing of an artery by atheroma or, more rarely, by tumour (e.g. pancreatic carcinoma invading the splenic artery to give a systolic murmur radiating towards the left side). Systolic murmurs in the lower abdomen or groins usually originate in the aorta or iliac arteries; those in the upper abdomen may indicate narrowing of superior mesenteric vessels but can be referred from the heart. More continuous murmurs are sometimes heard, especially in the upper abdomen. These can arise from vascular tumours such as hepatoma or hypernephroma. They may also occur in the form of a venous hum, increasing on inspiration, over porto-systemic anatomoses in patients with portal obstruction.

## ■ EXAMINATION OF THE GASTROINTESTINAL CONTENTS

The naked-eye inspection of vomited material or of the gastric contents removed by the stomach tube, and of the stools, often gives invaluable help in the diagnosis of gastrointestinal diseases. The more detailed analyses of the gastric contents and of the faeces by microscopical and chemical tests are mentioned later, under Special Investigations.

### VOMITUS

Instruction should be given to the nurse or whoever is in charge of the patient to save any vomited material. This should be examined for its quantity, odour, colour and reaction, and for the presence of normal and abnormal constituents.

#### Quantity

The vomit may be large in quantity if there is delay in the passage of the food through the pylorus, especially when this is due to pyloric carcinoma, and the gastric contents increase throughout the day to be vomited in the afternoon or evening. In organic lesions causing pyloric obstruction the food is frequently undigested, and the nature of the last meal should always be ascertained so that undigested articles of diet may be recognized.

#### Odour

Most vomit possesses a sour odour due to the acid present, but offensiveness usually indicates serious disease, e.g. malignant disease of the pylorus due to excessive fermentation in the retained gastric contents. It occurs late in intestinal obstruction, when the vomit may have a faeculent odour.

#### Colour and constituents

The colour of the vomit varies considerably with the length of time the food has been in the stomach, with the amount of duodenal regurgitation, and with the presence of abnormal constituents. *Blood* may give it a bright-red appearance if vomiting occurs soon after the haemorrhage, but usually the blood remains in the stomach sufficiently long to be altered to a dark brown colour—'coffee-grounds' due to acid haematin (*see* Haematemesis, p. 79). *Bile* is a normal constituent, giving a yellowish or greenish appearance to the vomit, but it may be excessive in disease such as intestinal obstruction and absent in pyloric stenosis. In certain phases of intestinal obstruction the vomit may consist very largely of bile, later being replaced by a thin brownish fluid derived from the small intestine and recognized only by a faeculent odour. *Mucus* is identified by its jelly-like appearance and is present in small amounts in most vomit. In large amounts it suggests inflammation of the gastric mucosa—chronic gastritis. Rarer constituents of vomit are *pus*, which may be swallowed or derived from some extrinsic abscess, pieces of new growth, and various parasites and ova. These constituents usually require microscopy for their recognition. The presence of food items ingested days earlier is diagnostic of pyloric stenosis.

## THE FAECES

A simple examination of the stools should never be omitted when the patient has symptoms of alimentary disease.

The faeces are made up of voluminous soap gels, residues of intestinal secretions, excretions and innumerable bacteria, many of them dead. Normally the only food residues are remnants of muscle fibre and the rough debris of vegetables, for practically all the food is digested and absorbed by the time it reaches the ileocaecal valve.

The *quantity, odour, colour, consistency and presence or absence of abnormal constituents* should be systematically noted.

### Quantity

This varies considerably in different individuals and according to the type of diet, but is usually about 100–200 g daily in one or two motions. It may be considerably increased by undigested food, as in the bulky stools of certain types of pancreatic disease and malabsorption syndromes as well as a high residue diet (*see Table* 4.6).

### Odour

A certain degree of offensiveness is normal, due to the presence of indol and skatol, constituents which are more plentiful when the diet contains much meat. When offensiveness is excessive some derangement of digestion or absorption should be suspected, though it may only be temporary and have no serious significance. Putrefaction of protein, such as may occur in pancreatic disease, gives a musty smell; carbohydrate fermentation produces 'acids of fermentation' and the rancid smell of butyric acid.

### Colour

The colour also varies with the type of diet. In persons on a milk diet the stools are canary yellow in colour; in those taking much meat they are dark. In an average mixed diet the stools are usually of a light brown colour. Certain articles of diet, such as wines, fruit and stout, may cause darkening of the stools, as may medicinal preparations, especially those containing iron or bismuth. These points should be borne in mind before attributing any pathological significance to an alteration in the colour of the stools. When peristalsis is excessive and the intestinal contents are hurried downwards, bile gives a yellowish-green or greenish appearance to the faeces. When bile pigments do not reach the intestine, the stools become clay coloured. In steatorrhoea the stools are pale and yellow owing to increased fat content. Blood is found in the stools in two forms: first, bright-red blood in small or large amounts derived from the large intestine, especially in its lower parts (e.g. haemorrhoids, cancer and polyps of the lower bowel); secondly, altered blood originating from the stomach or small intestine and partially digested on its way down, so that it gives the stool a dark tarry appearance—melaena (e.g. from gastric and duodenal ulcer). Small amounts of blood may not be visible on inspection but can be shown by tests for occult blood.

The combination of melaena and steatorrhoea, as caused by a bleeding carcinoma of the ampulla of Vater, produces a characteristic 'silver stool' known as a 'flash in the pan!'

## Consistency

The normal stool has a pultaceous consistency. It should be sufficiently soft for it to be moulded by the intestinal tube, the shape of which it retains. If too soft it may have the liquid or semi-liquid consistency of a diarrhoeic stool (see Diarrhoea, p. 82). If the stool is unusually hard it may form rounded masses called *scybala*. In extreme cases of constipation these scybalous masses may be very dry owing to the great absorption of water from them during their prolonged stay in the large intestine.

## Abnormal constituents

Many of these are more easily recognized by microscopical examination and may cause considerable difficulty to the inexperienced observer.

Faeces may be abnormal either because normal constituents are absent (e.g. stercobilin, derived from bile pigments) or because abnormal constituents are present (e.g. undigested food constituents, blood, serum, pus, mucus, parasites). *Mucus* occurs in two forms: as small flakes, intimately mixed with the faeces (usually due to inflammation), and as jelly-like masses either coating the surface of a hard faecal mass, or appearing separately as a cast or membrane (irritable colon). The recognition of *blood* has already been mentioned in describing colour of the stools, but unaltered blood may be passed without any faecal material. Excess of translucent *starch granules*, which stain blue with iodine, suggests failure of carbohydrate digestion. Excess of *fats* is recognized by the light, greasy nature of the stool and generally indicates failure of fat digestion through insufficiency of bile or pancreatic secretion or impaired absorption from the small intestine. This type of stool may be associated with visible grease or fat floating in the lavatory. However, it should be noted that 20 per cent of normal people have colonic bacterial flora producing sufficient hydrogen and methane to cause the stool to float. Failure of protein digestion may lead to the presence of undigested *meat fibres*, which, though generally recognized through the microscope, may appear as light brown threads in the stool (see also Table 4.6). *Pus* may appear in masses separate from the faeces, especially when it is derived from an extrinsic abscess bursting into the intestine. It is more intimately mixed with the stool in ulcerative conditions of the bowel such as malignant disease and ulcerative colitis.

*Foreign constituents* such as gallstones, rarely enteroliths, but many types of worms and ova may establish or give valuable clues to the diagnosis.

In Europe and North America the commonest types of worm to infest the bowel are tape-worms, round-worms and thread-worms. Tape-worms (*Taenia saginata or solium*) can be recognized by their great length, segmented body and a head surmounted by hooks and suckers. Round-worms (*Ascaris lumbricoides*) are usually several centimetres in length and resemble the common earth-worm. Thread-worms (*Enterobius vermicularis*) appear like minute strands of white cotton. In tropical countries many other helminths are causative of disease. Among those seen in the faeces examples are hook-worms (*Ancylostoma duodenale*), both worms and their ova, *Schistosoma mansoni* and numerous others, which affect many people, but with a light infestation may cause little or no ill health. An example of the last group is giardiasis, although this has now become quite a common cause of mild but persistent diarrhoea in European countries. (*See also* Chapter 12.) Stool porphyrin analysis will help to characterize a particular type of porphyria but cannot be used as a screening test.

# ■ DIAGNOSIS OF DISEASES OF INDIVIDUAL VISCERA

## THE STOMACH

When the symptoms suggest a lesion of the stomach it is to be remembered that the organic lesions of this organ are few. The more important are described below.

### Gastritis

Acute gastritis is most commonly the result of alcohol or anti-inflammatory agents such as aspirin, and presents with gastrointestinal bleeding. Very rarely, acute phlegmonous gastritis may occur as a result of intramural infection with alpha-haemolytic streptococci or gas-forming organisms. Chronic gastritis is either related to an immunological disturbance (when pernicious anaemia frequently ensues) or is part of the spectrum of peptic ulceration and is related to damage by agents such as bile and alcohol. In this condition morning vomiting, pain and sometimes fever with epigastric tenderness are found. The diagnosis is confirmed at endoscopy.

### Ulcer

Peptic ulcer may arise in the stomach or duodenum, and more rarely in the oesophagus or jejunum. The cause is not known, but the ulcers are often grouped together and called 'acid peptic disease' or 'peptic ulcer' because of the part played by hyperchlorhydria in their development. It has become increasingly evident that genetic factors are at work, especially in duodenal ulcer. It is known that there is a liability for first-degree relatives of propositi to develop the same type of ulcer. One of the factors contributory to the duodenal diathesis is the genetic phenotype, salivary ABH non-secretor. The possession of blood group O tends to make the consequences of a duodenal ulcer more serious, with a greater tendency to bleed or perforate than in the other ABO phenotypes. Because of these genetic and other considerations opinion has now swung much in favour of regarding primary gastric and duodenal ulcer as separate entities.

Possibly a hormonal factor is suggested by the higher incidence of peptic ulcer in men than in women (especially before the menopause).

Both gastric (*Fig.* 4.24, *see also Fig.* 4.29) and duodenal ulcers (*Fig.*4.25, *see also Fig.* 4.30) are characterized by periodic attacks of epigastric pain, often in the spring or autumn months, separated by symptom-free intervals. The pain usually occurs in a steady fashion from 30 min to 3 h after meals and is relieved by antacids and by certain foods, milk especially.

Duodenal ulcer is more common and has a more easily recognizable clinical pattern. The pain tends to occur some hours after a meal or shortly before the next; hence the term 'hunger pains', which are generally relieved by food. A

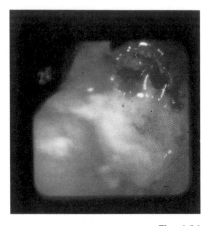 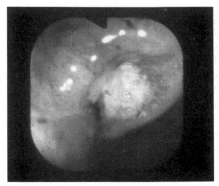

**Fig. 4.24**   **Fig. 4.25**
Benign gastric ulcer.   Duodenal ulcer.

similar picture may occur in gastric and other forms of peptic ulceration, and sometimes in oesophagitis. Associated symptoms include heartburn, waterbrash, vomiting (which may relieve the pain), and in gastric ulcer there may be loss of appetite and weight confusing the diagnosis with carcinoma. Tenderness in the epigastrium during exacerbations is the only constant physical sign. In differential diagnosis neoplasm must always be considered, but in tropical areas and sometimes in the immigrant population hook-worm diseae (*Ancylostoma duodenale*) may cause a very similar syndrome to that of duodenal ulcer.

Inquiry should be made as to whether the patient is taking drugs which may favour or exacerbate ulceration, e.g. aspirin or steroids.

Peptic ulcer may be complicated by haemorrhage (*Fig.* 4.26), pyloric stenosis or perforation. Pain in the back may be due to penetration of posterior abdominal structures, sometimes the pancreas, but may be ill-explained or may possibly be merely radiation from the main site.

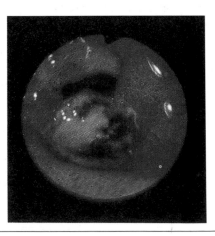

**Fig. 4.26**
Bleeding duodenal ulcer
showing vessel.

### Neoplasm

Carcinoma of the stomach causes symptoms similar to those of gastric ulcer but as the tumour progresses the pain is less regular, remissions do not occur, the appetite disappears, and there is progressive loss of weight. The diagnosis should be suspected in any patient complaining of persistent indigestion for the first time in middle or later life. Physical examination may reveal evidence of weight-loss, a lump in the epigastrium or signs of spread to other parts (e.g. a hard nodular enlargement of the liver or malignant nodes in the left supraclavicular fossa—Virchow's node, *Fig.* 4.27). Early diagnosis depends upon a careful history and radiological studies followed, if ulcer or neoplasm is suspected, by endoscopic inspection and biopsy of the gastric mucosa (*Fig.* 4.28, *see also Fig.* 4.31).

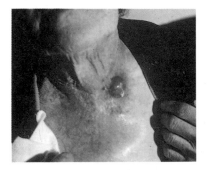

**Fig. 4.27**
Virchow's node. Malignant lymph node in the left supraclavicular fossa due to carcinoma of the stomach.

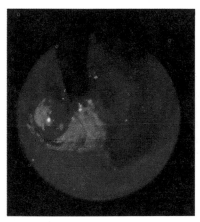

**Fig. 4.28**
Polypoid gastric carcinoma.

### Mechanical deformities

These often result from ulcer or neoplasm. The most important is *pyloric stenosis*, an obstruction at the pylorus intefering with the normal onward passage of the gastric contents. The digesting food is retained in the stomach and periodically vomited in large quantities in which food eaten many hours previously may be recognized. Pyloric stenosis may also be congenital, manifesting itself early in infancy, when the vomiting is often projectile in character.

The chief physical signs of pyloric stenosis are visible peristalsis and succussion splash. The loss of gastric contents by vomiting may lead to alkalosis and disturbance of electrolytes.

Other deformities of the stomach may be demonstrated in radiographs but are not necessarily associated with symptoms. These include herniation of the stomach into the thorax (hiatus hernia, *see* p. 74), 'hour-glass' stomach and other deformities consequent upon the healing by fibrosis of a gastric ulcer, and displacement or distortion of the stomach from extrinsic masses such as a pancreatic cyst or enlarged spleen.

## Miscellaneous disorders

The symptoms and signs may take such definite shape as to make diagnosis easy, but radiography and endoscopy along with appropriate laboratory techniques are usually needed to establish the diagnosis. If these organic diseases can be excluded, attention is next directed to certain dyspepsias in which an organic lesion of some other tissue is responsible for derangement of the stomach function. Appendicitis, cholecystitis and pancreatic disease are examples of diseases in this category, but the cause is not always to be found in a lesion of the abdominal viscera. Familiar examples of remote causes are bronchial carcinoma, pulmonary tuberculosis, uraemia and cerebral tumour.

Lastly, there remain many cases of indigestion or dyspepsia of a functional nature, that is in which no organic lesion is to be found in the stomach or other related organ. For these some cause will usually be found if the general health and habits of the patient are carefully considered. Examples of such causes are anxiety states, dietary indiscretion, and excessive smoking.

## SPECIAL INVESTIGATIONS

Diseases of the stomach which alter the internal outline or peristaltic activity of the viscus (e.g. ulcer, carcinoma) can be demonstrated by radiological examination using a radio-opaque meal such as barium (*see Figs.* 4.29–4.31).

The development of the flexible fibreoptic endoscope for direct inspection of the upper gastrointestinal tract has revolutionized the investigation of dyspepsia. The oesophagus and the whole of the stomach and duodenum can be repeatedly examined under local anaesthesia with relatively little discomfort to the patient.

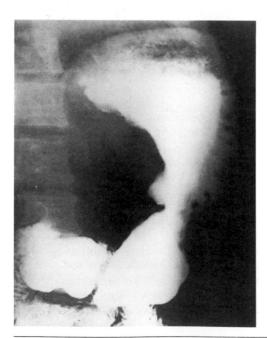

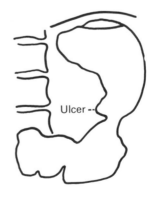

Ulcer --

**Fig. 4.29** Barium meal showing large penetrating ulcer on lesser curvature of the stomach.

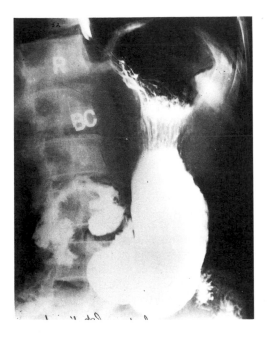

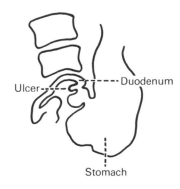

**Fig. 4.30** Barium meal showing large duodenal ulcer.

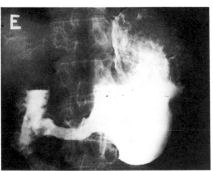

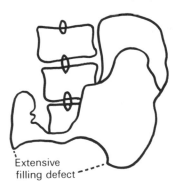

**Fig. 4.31** Extensive carcinoma of the lower third of the body of stomach.

A biopsy specimen may be taken from any visible abnormality for histological examination.

Cytological examination may also give valuable information, particularly in distinguishing between gastric carcinoma or ulcer.

Chemical investigation of the vomitus is only of value in cases of poisoning.

·The maximum hydrochloric acid output is obtained over a 1-h period after injection of the gastrin analogue pentagastrin. The aspiration should preferably be preceded by checking the position of the tube by X-ray screening and should be carried out by an experienced person so as to ensure that the gastric secretions are removed uninterruptedly and completely.

Gastric acid analysis is helpful in the following situations: (1) The absence of acid makes a diagnosis of peptic ulcer unlikely and suggests that a gastric ulcer, if present, is probably malignant. (2) The presence of acid excludes a diagnosis of pernicious anaemia. (3) Hyperchlorhydria is usual in ulcer. A very high acid production with a high ratio of basal- to maximal-output suggests a gastrin-producing tumour of the pancreas (Zollinger–Ellison syndrome.)

## THE SMALL INTESTINE

### Enteritis

Whether due to infected food usually with salmonella organisms, occasionally with staphylococci or dysentery, to mention only a few of many possible causes, all forms of enteritis (inflammation of the intestine) have colic and diarrhoea as their cardinal symptoms, with a few or no physical signs. The term *colic*, as applied to the intestine, means a pain of griping or twisting character lasting only some seconds at a time and corresponding with waves of peristalsis. Bacteriological examination of the stools is necessary for a complete diagnosis.

*Typhoid fever* deserves special mention as an example of an enteritis, affecting chiefly the ileum. In addition to local symptoms such as diarrhoea (pea-soup stools) or constipation, which may occur, there are well-developed constitutional symptoms and signs due to bloodstream infection. Notable points are the pyrexia, sometimes with bradycardia, the splenic enlargement and positive blood culture, the rash and positive agglutination reactions (Widal).

### The malabsorption syndrome

Defective absorption may be confined to one particular constituent of food, for example vitamin $B_{12}$ in pernicious anaemia. The term 'malabsorption syndrome' is usually reserved for those cases with multiple defects of absorption. It results either from diseases of the small intestine or from an inadequate supply of digestive enzymes (*see Table* 4.6). Coeliac disease is the commonest form of generalized malabsorption and is due to the flattening of the small intestinal villi brought about by contact with dietary gluten (gluten enteropathy). The clinical features include steatorrhoea (fatty stools) due to failure of fat absorption; anaemia resulting from inadequate absorption of iron, folic acid or vitamin $B_{12}$; osteomalacia and tetany due to calcium deficiency; wasting and oedema due to loss of protein; and various lesions of the skin, mucosae and nervous system resulting from a lack of vitamin B. Finger-clubbing may also occur (*see Table* 4.6).

### Crohn's disease

This is a chronic granulomatous process that most commonly affects the lower ileum ('regional ileitis') and colon (Crohn's colitis), but may appear in any part of the alimentary tract from the mouth (*see Fig.* 4.32) to the anus. There is diffuse infiltration and thickening of the bowel wall with narrowing of the lumen. Penetrating mucosal ulcers may lead to fistulae between loops of bowel, the pelvic viscera and the skin.

Symptoms and signs depend on the site of the lesion. Localized disease of the ileum may simulate appendicitis and present with colicky abdominal pain, fever and a tender mass in the right iliac fossa. More diffuse involvement of the small

| Table 4.6 | **The malabsorption syndrome** |
|---|---|

*Symptoms and signs*

| Symptoms and signs | Element not absorbed |
|---|---|
| Pale, bulky, greasy stools | Fat |
| Distended abdomen; frothy stools | Carbohydrate |
| Wasting, failure of growth, oedema | Protein |
| Anaemia | Iron; folic acid; vitamin $B_{12}$ |
| Pellagroid lesions of skin; ulceration of mouth; peripheral neuropathy | Vitamin-B group |
| Bone pains, fractures and deformities; tetany | Calcium |
| Haemorrhage | Vitamin K |
| Watery diarrhoea | Bile acids |
| Finger-clubbing | Cause unknown |

*Causes*

| Due to small intestine disease | Due to inadequate digestive enzymes |
|---|---|
| 1 Reduced mucosal surface area: extensive gastrectomy and similar operations are common causes in Western countries | 1 Lack of bile: obstructive jaundice |
| 2 Diffuse mucosal damage: gluten enteropathy (coeliac disease); intestinal ischaemia | 2 Lack of pancreatic enzymes: chronic pancreatitis; fibrocystic disease; carcinoma |
| 3 Diffuse mucosal infiltration: amyloid disease; reticulosis; Crohn's disease | 3 Poor mixing of enzymes: after gastrectomy |
| 4 Abnormal bacterial flora and infestations: 'blind loops'; tropical sprue; internal fistulae; after antibiotics | |
| 5 Impaired lymphatic drainage: intestinal lymphangiectasia | |

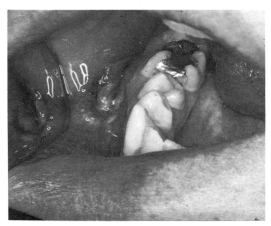

**Fig. 4.32** Ulceration of the buccal mucosa in a patient with Crohn's disease.

bowel or an entero-colic fistula can give rise to a malabsorption syndrome (*see* p. 112). Colonic disease may resemble ulcerative colitis with blood and mucus in the stools. Intestinal obstruction, fever and mucocutaneous ulceration or fistulae (especially perianal) are other typical features of the disease. The diagnosis may be established by demonstrating characteristic radiological changes in the small bowel and by the appearance in a biopsy specimen of non-caseating granulomas with giant cells.

## THE LARGE INTESTINE

### Ulcerative colitis

This is a non-specific inflammatory condition in which there is recurrent ulceration of the colonic and rectal mucosa. Unlike Crohn's disease, ulcerative colitis usually involves the rectum, spares the small bowel and does not produce fistulae. The complications include perforation, haemorrhage, stricture and, in some longstanding cases, carcinoma. There may also be systemic manifestations such as erythema nodosum or pyoderma gangrenosum, iritis, arthritis or finger-clubbing (*Fig.* 4.33).

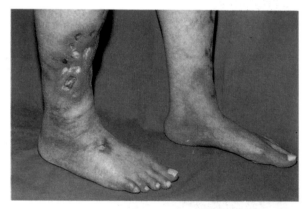

**Fig. 4.33** Pyoderma gangrenosum in a case of ulcerative colitis.

Ulcerative colitis may present insidiously with loose stools and abdominal discomfort or with an acute attack of fever, pain and bloody diarrhoea. The subsequent course is characterized by remissions and exacerbations which are sometimes related to emotional stress. In the established case, there are frequent loose stools with blood, mucus and pus, especially on waking, but often disturbing sleep. Rectal involvement results in tenesmus and the passage of blood and mucus alone, sometimes with constipation rather than diarrhoea. Physical signs may be lacking, but in patients with chronic extensive disease there is often anaemia and wasting and, rarely, the systemic features already listed. On proctoscopy, the rectal mucosa appears inflamed, bleeds easily and ulcers may be seen. The diagnosis is established and carcinoma exluded by endoscopy and a barium enema.

### Carcinoma

The colon and rectum are among the commonest sites for carcinoma. Symptoms and signs depend upon the position and malignancy of the tumour and whether it consists mainly of an ulcerative lesion or a stricture. Rectal carcinoma usually presents with blood, mucus and sometimes pus in the stool and can often be felt with the finger or seen through the proctoscope. Blood from an ulcerating carcinoma of the colon or caecum may not be visible in the stool, and in these cases the first symptoms are often anaemia and loss of weight. An abdominal tumour may be felt, but it must be remembered that the sigmoid colon, a common site for carcinoma, is not accessible to palpation. Alteration in bowel habit is an important symptom of the carcinoma especially when there is a stricture. Increasing constipation, sometimes alternating with diarrhoea, may be followed by colicky pains due to intestinal obstruction. Highly malignant or neglected lesions may first present with signs of peritoneal invasion or distant metastases. Radiography following a barium enema and endoscopy with biopsy are used to confirm the diagnosis.

### Diverticulitis

Diverticula are balloon-like protrusions of the colonic mucosa through parts of the wall where the muscle layers are weakened or absent. Diverticulosis is a common condition in elderly obese subjects, particularly in those who suffer from chronic constipation. Symptoms occur only if the diverticula are inflamed (diverticulitis) and include fever, colicky pain, diarrhoea sometimes alternating with constipation, haemorrhage and symptoms of cystitis if inflammation spreads to the bladder. A tender mass can sometimes be palpated, usually in the left iliac fossa.

### Irritable colon

This is the commonest gastrointestinal complaint in developed countries and is the result of a poorly understood disorder of motility that often affects not only the colon but also other parts of the gastrointestinal tract. Symptoms include constipation with fragmented pellet-like stools, diarrhoea (often alternating with constipation), abdominal pain, bloating, flatulence and the passage of mucus. The diagnosis is easy when symptoms are classical and of long-standing. However, it is important, particularly when symptoms are of recent onset, to exclude more serious causes such as carcinoma or inflammatory bowel disease. Furthermore, there are other less serious causes, such as the intolerance to certain foods. Apart from coeliac disease (p. 95), the most important of these is hypolactasia, an inability to split the disaccharide lactose in cow's milk which results in diarrhoea and flatulence.

### Intestinal obstruction

The small as well as the large intestine may be involved. When the cause is mechanical, as in strangulated hernia, mural growths or volvulus, constipation and colic are the initial symptoms. Soon, however, vomiting follows as a distinguishing feature in cases of acute obstruction. At first the vomitus consists of the stomach contents, later of bile regurgitated from the duodenum, and later still of the faeculent contents of the small intestine. In chronic cases of obstruction, especially of the large bowel, this characteristic vomiting is not present and the diagnosis must depend upon the history of constipation and colic and the special methods of examination. It must be emphasized again that the symptoms assume a special importance when they are persistent, for colic may arise from trivial disorders such as irritant food, temporary constipation or purgatives, but as a rule it passes away in such cases within a few days.

*Paralytic ileus* (adynamic ileus) is most common in cases of peritonitis but may occur in many painful thoracic and abdominal lesions. Constipation is associated with progressive abdominal distension, but colicky pain is uncommon. More rarely, vascular insufficiency (ischaemia) may give a similar clinical picture.

## SPECIAL INVESTIGATIONS

*A plain X-ray of the abdomen* may reveal distended loops of bowel with fluid levels in cases of intestinal obstruction. Abnormalities in the structure or activity of the intestines can be studied by radiographs taken over a 24-h period after a barium meal (*barium follow-through*). If small intestinal disease is suspected, a special barium preparation can be introduced in controlled amounts directly into the small bowel via a nasoduodenal tube (small bowel enema). The outline of the large intestine is better demonstrated by injection of barium via the anus (*barium enema*). The rectum and lower reaches of the sigmoid colon are poorly visualized in radiographs and such lesions as carcinoma, polyps, ulceration and haemorrhoids may be overlooked. Endoscopic methods are therefore employed for examination of the anal canal (*proctoscopy*) and for the lower sigmoid and rectum (*sigmoidoscopy*). The flexible fibreoptic endoscope (colonoscope) permits inspection of the mucosa throughout the whole length of the colon.

Examination of the faeces plays an important part in the diagnosis of intestinal diseases. *Inspection of the faeces* with the naked eye is described on p. 105. When foreign bodies such as gallstones and intestinal worms are anticipated, the stool should be washed repeatedly through muslin or a fine sieve. The most important chemical test applicable in the clinic room is that for occult blood. This is of great value in the detection of slight continual bleeding from ulceration or carcinoma of the stomach or intestines. Occult blood is recognized by smearing a little stool on a guiac-impregnated filter paper inside a plastic or cardboard wallet. A blue colour indicates a positive reaction produced by the pseudo-peroxidase activity of haemoglobin. *Microscopy of the faeces* may reveal pus cells, red cells, bacteria, ova and parasites such as *Entamoeba histolytica*. *Culture of the faeces* permits a more precise identification of pathogenic bacteria. These methods are used for the recognition of infections and infestations of the bowel and are thus essential to the investigation of diarrhoea. *Faecal fat excretion* is measured by chemical analysis of the total amount of faeces passed over a period of 3–5 days while the patient is taking a normal ward diet. An amount greater than 5 g daily indicates malabsorption of fat from the small intestine. Because of the unaesthetic nature of the laboratory analysis of faecal fats, there are continuing attempts to develop alternative tests for fat malabsorption, such as the $^{14}$-C triolein breath test. A useful qualitative side-room test is to add a lipophilic dye to a faecal smear and examine this microscopically for stained fat globules.

Failure to absorb other constituents of the diet can be detected by measuring their levels in the blood (e.g. *serum iron, vitamin B₁₂, folate, protein, calcium*) or the amount excreted in the urine after ingestion of the appropriate substance (e.g. *xylose excretion test, Schilling test*). In a patient with intestinal malabsorption, vitamin $B_{12}$ deficiency suggests a lesion in the lower ileum (where the vitamin is absorbed) or a blind loop syndrome. A normal xylose excretion test helps to distinguish pancreatic disease, in which only fat absorption is impaired, from intestinal causes of malabsorption.

A fragment of jejunal mucosa can also be obtained by means of a biopsy device which consists of a knife actuated within a small capsule at the end of a flexible tube (Crosbie capsule). Histological examination of the jejunal mucosa is of particular value in the diagnosis of adult coeliac disease (gluten enteropathy), in which there is marked atrophy of the villi.

## THE PERITONEUM

It is convenient to consider the peritoneum at this stage in view of its close association with the alimentary tract. In the description of abdominal pain it has already been pointed out that the peritoneum plays a great part in the production of pain in disease of individual viscera, and it is preferable to envisage such diseases as appendicitis and cholecystitis as diseases affecting the appendix and gallbladder with their enveloping visceral and neighbouring parietal peritoneum.

In some instances the involvement of the peritoneum is the most important aspect of the case. This is so in acute generalized peritonitis and in certain forms of chronic peritonitis.

### Acute generalized peritonitis

The examination of the 'acute abdomen' more frequently falls to the family doctor or surgeon than to the physician, but acute abdominal accidents are not infrequent in medical wards, and the condition therefore warrants some attention here. The symptoms are similar whatever the cause of the acute peritonitis (e.g. perforated ulcer, ruptured appendix abscess, acute pancreatitis). Intense, agonizing abdominal pain and circulatory collapse are the notable features. Other points of distinction are familiar to the surgeon, such as the less severe pain of a perforation into the lesser sac of the peritoneum, but only general features will be described here.

*Inspection* shows the abdomen to be fixed, exhibiting little if any movement with respiration. Breathing is of a thoracic type. The anxious distressed facies leaves no doubts as to the severity of the symptoms.

*Palpation* shows extreme abdominal tenderness and board-like rigidity of the abdominal muscles. The tenderness is often accompanied by hyperaesthesia of the skin. 'Rebound tenderness', a characteristic sign of acute peritonitis, can be elicited by gentle pressure on the abdominal wall followed by sudden withdrawal of the palpating hand.

*Percussion* – which, if employed, should be practised gently – may demonstrate tympanites due to the paresis of the intestinal musculature and the accumulation of gas in the intestines. Free gas may also be present in the peritoneal cavity, causing tympany in place of the usual liver dullness, and free fluid can sometimes be detected.

*Auscultation.* Bowel sounds may disappear completely in the later stages due to paresis of the intestinal musculature.

Several non-surgical conditions may simulate peritonitis quite closely, and when the signs are at all indefinite particular care should be taken to examine other systems. Severe abdominal pain may be caused by myocardial infarction, ketoacidosis in diabetes, aortic aneurysm, mesenteric arterial occlusion, diaphragmatic pleurisy, nerve root irritation, tabes dorsalis and acute porphyria, to mention only the more important lesions. If signs of disease are found in another system they must receive due consideration, but it is equally important that if they are trivial they should not be allowed to weigh against a correct diagnosis of peritonitis.

### Chronic peritonitis

Several types of chronic peritonitis are described but the most important is the *tuberculous form*, though even this has become rare in Western countries. Causes of chronic peritonitis include the carcinoid syndrome and certain drugs such as the beta-blocking agent practolol and methysergide used in the treatment of migraine. Chronic fibrosis of the peritoneum, especially of its posterior parts, can also occur without any evident precipitating cause. Chronic peritonitis is less common than peritoneal neoplasia, but the symptoms and signs are similar and the prognosis much more favourable in the former condition. This diagnosis should therefore always be considered in any patient presenting with the clinical features of chronic peritoneal disease.

The symptoms are indefinite and depend more upon mechanical interference with the stomach and intestines than upon the disease of the peritoneum itself. Thus colic, constipation and diarrhoea may occur. Constitutional symptoms of the causative disease are added, e.g. loss of weight, anaemia, and fever, in the case of tuberculosis. Peritoneal fibrosis can also lead to the symptoms and signs of chronic renal failure due to bilateral ureteric obstruction.

*Inspection* may show enlargement of the abdomen due to the presence of ascites (*see Fig.* 4.20) or of infiltrating masses in the peritoneum. The signs of ascites have been described. Peritoneal masses are most commonly seen in the upper abdomen lying in a transverse manner so that they may resemble an enlarged liver or a loaded transverse colon. Their contour, however, is more irregular and does not conform to the shape and size expected from these viscera.

*Palpation* helps to define a 'rolled omentum' of this kind from the liver and transverse colon.

### SPECIAL INVESTIGATIONS

The main investigations of value in the diagnosis of peritoneal diseases are paracentesis and peritoneoscopy. *Paracentesis* (needle aspiration of the peritoneal cavity) is sometimes used for the relief of ascites, and microscopic examination or culture of the ascitic fluid can be helpful in identifying the organism responsible for a chronic peritonitis (e.g. tuberculosis) and for demonstrating carcinoma cells in malignant cases. *Peritoneoscopy* (inspection of the peritoneal cavity through an illuminated tube) is sometimes used to determine the cause of ascites or liver enlargement when it is desirable to avoid laparotomy. *Peritoneal biopsy* may help to distinguish inflammatory from neoplastic disease.

## THE LIVER

Serious disease of the liver may be present without abnormal physical signs, as quite a small amount of liver tissue appears able to carry on the functions of the diseased portions.

A suspicion of liver disease may be aroused by enlargement of the organ especially if it is hard or irregular in outline (*see* p. 96); more rarely by diminution in size suspected by increased resonance over right lower ribs. Portal hypertension and hepatocellular failure also produce characteristic signs (*see Table* 4.7).

Many of the causes of liver enlargement and jaundice are not primarily those of liver disease and necessitate the examination of other systems for the discovery of their cause (*see* Chapter 8).

Three primary diseases of the liver need mention, namely infective hepatitis, cirrhosis and abscess.

### Infective hepatitis

This is due to a virus infection of the liver. The onset is characterized by marked anorexia, nausea, vomiting and depression, associated with evidence of general toxicity, e.g. fever and malaise. After a few days the nausea and toxicity lessen, but the patient then becomes jaundiced, the liver enlarges and some pain may occur in the right hypochondrium. Darkness of the urine and pallor of the faeces may be noticed before any change in the colour of the skin. The jaundice fades over the next week to ten days, and complete recovery in some weeks is the rule. In some rare fulminating cases there is an acute necrosis of the liver cells (acute hepatic necrosis) leading to *hepatic coma* in which the patient is usually deeply jaundiced, the liver decreases in size, and there is a characteristic foetor hepaticus. Hepatic cirrhosis may be a late complication of type B hepatitis whereas a type A infection produces no chronic sequelae.

### Cirrhosis of the liver

This condition is characterized by necrosis of hepatic cells followed later by fibrosis, nodular regeneration and abnormalities of the hepatic circulation. The commoner causes are as follows:

1. *Toxins*: These include alcohol and certain drugs (e.g. methyldopa). Alcohol probably accounts for most cases of cirrhosis in Western countries.
2. *Infections*: Hepatic cirrhosis occasionally follows severe or repeated attacks of viral hepatitis (*see above*).
3. *Auto-immune reaction* may take the form of primary biliary cirrhosis or chronic active hepatitis. *Primary biliary cirrhosis* is mainly a disease of middle-aged women and usually presents as an obstructive type of jaundice with troublesome pruritus. *Chronic active hepatitis* can occur at any age and in either sex and may simulate the clinical picture of a persistent or recurrent viral hepatitis (*see above*). In these forms of cirrhosis, auto-antibodies are usually present in the blood.
4. *Metabolic* causes of cirrhosis are rare but also important because effective treatment is available. *Haemochromatosis*, although it most often presents in middle-aged or elderly men, is probably a genetic abnormality of iron absorption. This results in iron deposition in the liver, pancreas, skin, gonads and

| Table 4.7 | Production of symptoms and signs in liver disease | |
|---|---|---|
| Pathological changes | Functional disturbance | Symptoms and signs |
| Mechanical factors (e.g. cirrhosis or congestive cardiac failure) | 1 Change in consistency and size | The liver may be enlarged or smaller, smooth or irregular, soft, firm or hard |
| | 2 Rapid stretching or involvement of capsule | Pain in right hypochondrium, intense nausea and vomiting |
| Portal hypertension | 1 Rise in portal vein pressure | Splenomegaly |
| | 2 Congestion of splanchnic vessels | Anorexia, nausea, flatulence and abdominal discomfort |
| | 3 Development of collateral circulation | Oesophageal varices and haematemesis, internal haemorrhoids and caput medusae (Fig. 4.34) |
| | 4 Intoxication of brain by crude nitrogen products from gut which have bypassed the liver filter in anastomotic channels | Hepatic encephalopathy manifested by personality changes progressing through stupor to coma. Also motor changes including a flapping tremor |
| Hepatocellular failure | 1 Reduction in serum albumin with resultant lowering of colloid osmotic pressure | Ascites and generalized oedema (Fig. 4.35) |
| | 2 Failure to excrete bilirubin glucuronide | Jaundice (Fig. 4.36) |
| | 3 Failure to store certain vitamins, e.g. vitamin K | Bleeding tendency |
| | 4 Impaired detoxication of various metabolites may lead to a raised blood level and toxic symptoms: | |
| | Oestrogens | Spider naevi (Fig. 4.37), palmar erythema, gynaecomastia, loss of body hair and testicular atrophy (see Figs. 4.38, 4.39) |
| | Aldosterone | Aggravation of oedema |
| | Crude nitrogenous products from the gut | Hepatic encephalopathy |
| | Morphine and barbiturates | Dangerous sensitivity to these drugs |

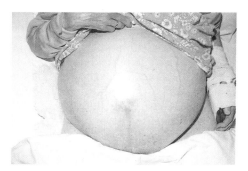

**Fig. 4.34**
Ascites and caput medusae.

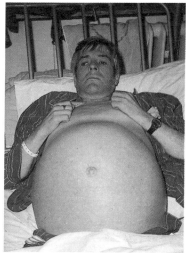

**Fig. 4.35**
Ascites and cirrhosis.

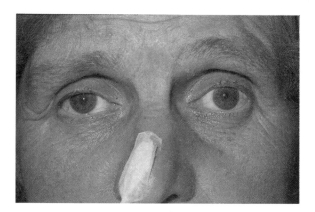

**Fig. 4.36** Jaundice.

joints to cause cirrhosis, diabetes, pigmentation, testicular atrophy and arthropathy. The condition can also result from excessive intake of iron from repeated blood transfusion and may respond to regular venesection. *Wilson's disease* (hepatolenticular degeneration) is also a congenital metabolic defect. Copper is deposited in the liver, brain and cornea. It usually shows itself in childhood with extrapyramidal or psychiatric features as well as cirrhosis, and may be recognized by the presence of Kayser–Fleischer rings in the cornea (*see* p. 40). Another rare metabolic cause for juvenile cirrhosis of the liver is congenital deficiency of $\alpha_1$-antitrypsin.

5. *Congestive changes* in the liver from chronic cholestasis ('biliary cirrhosis') or right-heart failure ('cardiac cirrhosis') are usually reversible if the cause is

removed and rarely lead to true cirrhosis as defined in the first paragraph of this section.

The chief symptoms and signs of cirrhosis can be attributed to three main causes: (1) enlargement of the liver, followed by shrinkage in the later stages — the surface is finely granular, but this can rarely be detected except through a very thin abdominal wall; (2) portal hypertension; and (3) hepatocellular failure. The symptoms and signs attributable to these last two causes are listed in *Table* 4.7 (*see also Figs.* 4.37–4.40). Nail changes of uncertain cause also occur in hepatic cirrhosis; these include clubbing and leukonychia (*Fig.* 4.40).

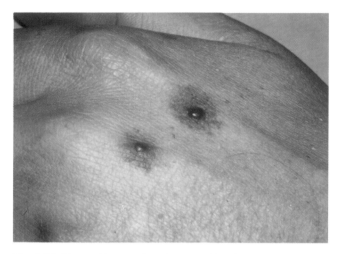

**Fig. 4.37** Giant spider naevi on dorsum of hand.

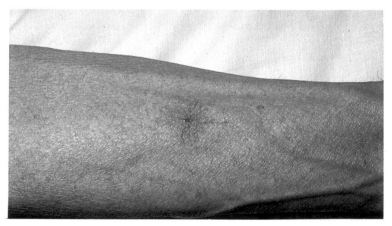

**Fig. 4.38** Spider naevus on the forearm of a patient with hepatic cirrhosis

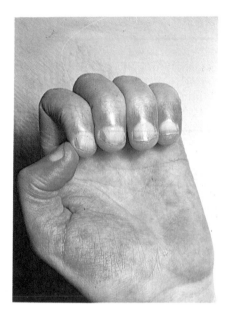

**Fig. 4.39**
Cirrhosis of the liver: palmar erythema and white nails (*see also Fig.* 4.40).

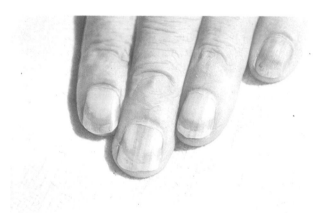

**Fig. 4.40** Cirrhosis of the liver. Increased whiteness of nails associated with hypoalbuminaemia.

### Liver abscess

*Multiple abscesses* of the liver may result from systemic infection, but, more commonly, from spread of suppurative processes through the portal system from some other part of the alimentary tract — e.g. the appendix. The latter condition is known as *portal pyaemia* and the liver symptoms are essentially secondary; it has become relatively rare since the introduction of broad-spectrum antibiotics. Diverticulitis and biliary tract sepsis are now the usual causes.

*Amoebic abscess* of the liver, although strictly speaking secondary to amoebic infection of the intestine, forms such a separate entity that it is considered here as a primary disease of the liver. Pain over the liver, toxaemia and fever are the characteristic symptoms. The liver is enlarged and tender, and irregularities in the surface of the organ are occasionally found. Examination of the stools may show the presence of *Entamoeba histolytica*, and a puncture of the liver itself through the abdominal wall or intercostal space enables the typical 'anchovy sauce' pus to be withdrawn (*see also* Chapter 12). The diagnosis may be made reliably by a serological fluorescent antibody test.

A rarer cause of liver abscess is actinomycosis, which is secondary to a focus elsewhere in the alimentary tract, usually in the ileocaecal region.

## SPECIAL INVESTIGATIONS
### Radiology

The liver cannot be displayed by conventional radiological techniques but is well shown by both ultrasound examination and computed tomography (CT scanning). Ultrasound is more widely available and is particularly useful for detecting filling defects in the liver substance (e.g. cysts, abscesses, tumours) and for diagnosing dilated hepatic ducts in extrahepatic obstruction. It is therefore valuable in establishing the cause of jaundice. As well as showing the presence of extrahepatic obstruction, ultrasound may show the level and nature of the block (e.g. carcinoma of the pancreas), but usually direct cholangiography will be needed to confirm this (*see below*).

In non-surgical jaundice a radionuclide scan of the liver is useful in showing filling defects greater than 2 cm in diameter, such as metastases, cysts and abscesses. Characteristic patterns of uptake may be seen in hepatocellular disease such as cirrhosis.

Portal hypertension may be diagnosed by the finding of oesophageal varices on barium swallow (*Fig*. 4.41) or at endoscopy which may show gastric varices (*Fig*. 4.42). The site of the obstruction can be identified by the injection of contrast medium into the spleen or, via the aorta, into the splenic artery, whence it fills the splenic and portal veins (*Fig*. 4.43).

Nuclear magnetic resonance of the liver appears more promising than either ultrasound or CT scanning for distinguishing diffuse abnormalities of the liver substance, e.g. different types of cirrhosis.

### Histology

Histological examination of the liver may be of value in the diagnosis of cirrhosis, tumours, infiltrations and infections of the liver, and for assessing the activity of a chronic hepatitis as in certain auto-immune disorders. A fragment of liver tissue can be obtained for this purpose by *percutaneous needle biopsy* and may be used for immunological tests, chemical estimations and enzymology.

## THE GALLBLADDER AND BILE DUCTS

### Cholecystitis

Inflammation of the gallbladder commonly results from gallstones, and its symptoms are often combined with those due to calculi. Occasionally acute

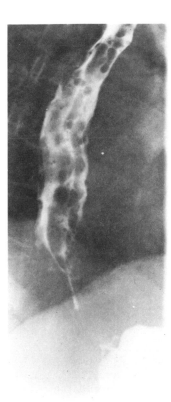

**Fig. 4.41**
Oesophageal varices. Note
the rounded filling defects
displacing the barium in the
oesophagus.

**Fig. 4.42** Gastric varices.

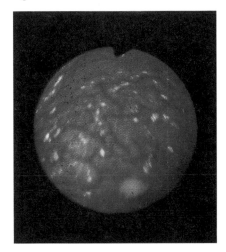

cholecystitis may occur without stones – acute acalculous cholecystitis. This is usually a surgical emergency terminating in gallbladder gangrene, and may be a complication of severe burns or follow major surgery.

Pain in the right hypochondrium and at the inferior angle of the right scapula is common. If the patient takes a slow, deep breath whilst the examiner's fingers are pressed firmly but gently over the right hypochondrium, there may be momentary interruption of breathing because of pain (Murphy's sign). Acute cholecystitis is accompanied by constitutional disturbances such as fever and leucocytosis, and on palpation there may be marked tenderness and guarding. The significance of the classical gallbladder symptoms of fat intolerance, flatulent dyspepsia and abdominal discomfort is now doubtful.

In acute cases greater constitutional disturbances such as pyrexia and leucocytosis are present together with more pronounced tenderness and guarding.

### Gallstones

These may produce the symptoms of cholecystitis just described. If a stone lodges in the neck of the gallbladder or passes into the cystic or common bile duct, a characteristic attack of *biliary colic* results (*see* p. 81). Obstruction of the common bile duct gives rise to jaundice (*see* p. 82). Although gallbladder

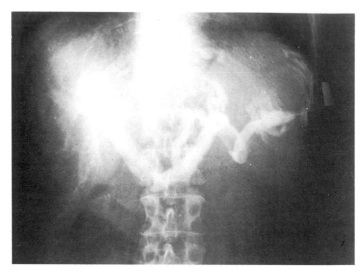

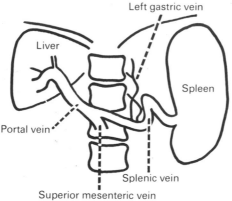

Left gastric vein

Liver

Spleen

Portal vein

Splenic vein

Superior mesenteric vein

**Fig. 4.43**
Porto-splenogram. A direct
injection into the spleen
demonstrating the dilated
gastric veins in portal
hypertension.

carcinoma is rare, when it is seen it is almost always in a gallbladder containing calculi.

## SPECIAL INVESTIGATIONS

The diagnosis of calculous gallbladder disease is made either by ultrasonography or cholecystography. About 20 per cent of calculi are calcified and will therefore show up on a plain abdominal X-ray (*Fig.* 4.44). If a stone is occluding the cystic duct, contrast material in bile cannot enter the gallbladder and it will be reported on oral cholecystography to be 'non-functioning'. Other causes of failing to opacify the gallbladder are poor hepatic function or jaundice and failure to swallow or absorb the cholecystogram tablets.

The bile ducts may be seen on ultrasound or CT scan (p. 450) but direct cholangiography is often necessary, and three methods are available. *Intravenous cholangiography* rarely gives a clear diagnosis, and is unsuccessful if there is more than

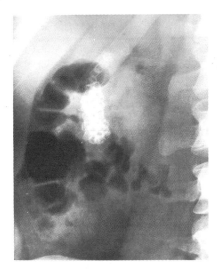

**Fig. 4.44**
Radio-opaque stones filling
the gallbladder and cystic
duct.

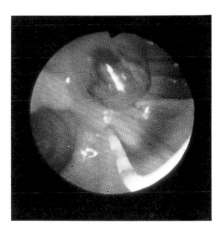

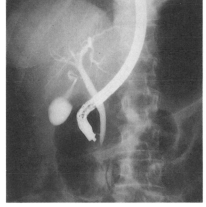

**Fig. 4.45**
Impacted stone in common
bile duct.

**Fig. 4.46**
ERCP via the
duodenoscope outlining
normal common bile duct,
gallbladder and cystic duct,
and hepatic duct.

minimal jaundice. Endoscopic retrograde cholangiography (ERCP) (*Figs.* 4.45, 4.46) and *percutaneous cholangiography* (PTC) give excellent visualization of the biliary system, although PTC may be difficult if the ducts are not dilated.

### THE PANCREAS

Three lesions may be mentioned as illustrative types of pancreatic disease.

### Pancreatitis

In acute pancreatitis there is intense agonizing upper abdominal pain with shock due to extravasation of blood and pancreatic secretions into the peritoneal cavity. An abdominal catastrophe is confirmed by the findings of severe tenderness and muscular rigidity and the diagnosis suggested by a raised serum amylase.

Chronic pancreatitis is nearly always alcohol-induced. The cardinal features are pain, exocrine insufficiency (protein malnutrition and steatorrhoea) and endocrine insufficiency (diabetes mellitus). The pain may be particularly severe and unrelenting, situated in the central abdomen, often radiating through to the back and eased by leaning forward.

### Cancer of the pancreas

The early symptoms are those common to many dyspepsias; pain, loss of appetite and flatulence. The pain is usually of a persistent boring type which radiates to the back and disturbs the patient's sleep. Just as in chronic pancreatitis it is sometimes partially relieved by bending forwards over a chair or bed, a posture not infrequently adopted by the patient. There are also symptoms of malignant disease, namely loss of weight, loss of strength and the development of cachexia. An important sign when present is *jaundice* of a persistent and increasing nature, due to the increasing constriction of the common bile duct by the growth. The tumour may be palpable in the epigastrium, especially if the patient is examined in the knee–elbow position. Painless jaundice and enlargement of the gallbladder may occur when the head of the pancreas is involved (*Fig.* 4.47). It is more difficult to diagnose lesions in other parts of the gland.

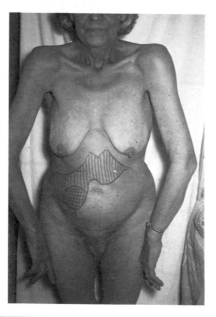

**Fig. 4.47**
Carcinoma of the pancreas. Note jaundice and emaciation. The shaded area indicates the outline of the enlarged liver and gallbladder.

Evidence of pancreatic insufficiency is often only slight until the late stages of the disease, and in many cases sufficient pancreatic tissue is left to carry on the functions of the organ. Because local functional and structural evidence of pancreatic carcinoma is often scanty, the tumour may first present with systemic manifestations of cancer such as unexplained weight loss, metastatic spread (e.g. lymphangitis carcinomatosa of the lung) or recurrent venous thromboses (thrombophlebitis migrans).

### Fibrocystic disease of the pancreas

This congenital abnormality of the pancreas is one manifestation of a diffuse disorder of exocrine glands and their secretions. The mucous glands of the bronchi, the sweat glands and the testes are also involved. The disease usually presents in infancy with recurrent bronchial infections associated with bronchiectasis and bulky fatty offensive stools due to steatorrhoea of pancreatic origin (*see* p. 504). Some victims die in childhood or adolescence, usually from respiratory infection, but with the advent of broad spectrum antibiotics an increasing proportion now survive to adult life. The males are usually infertile because of impaired testicular function. A diagnostic feature of the disease is the high salt content of the sweat.

### Endocrine disorders

Abnormalities of endocrine secretion relating to the pancreas are mentioned elsewhere and include diabetes mellitus, insulin-secreting tumour of the islet cells causing spontaneous hypoglycaemia (Chapter 11) and peptic ulcer with diarrhoea due to a gastrin-secreting adenoma (*see* pp. 82 and 107).

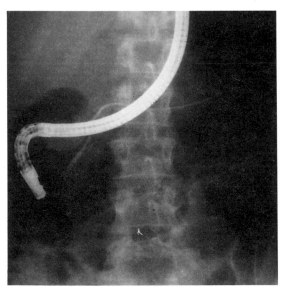

**Fig. 4.48** Retrograde pancreatography via the duodenoscope illustrating normal pancreatic duct systems.

## SPECIAL INVESTIGATIONS

Diseases of the pancreas, especially alcoholic chronic pancreatitis, are sometimes associated with calcification and this can be demonstrated in a plain radiograph of the abdomen. A barium meal X-ray may reveal widening of the duodenal loop in cases of carcinoma of the head of the pancreas. More recent techniques for delineating the physical contours of the pancreas include the use of ultrasound, computerized axial tomography and coeliac axis angiography. The anatomy of the pancreatic duct system can be demonstrated by cannulation of the ampulla of Vater and introduction of contrast medium at the time of fibreoptic duodenoscopy (retrograde pancreatography, *Fig.* 4.48). In diseases of the pancreas, there may be a deficiency of enzymes in the bowel as a result of obstruction to the pancreatic duct (e.g. in carcinoma) or an excess of enzymes, e.g. amylase or lipase, in the blood and urine due to leakage from pancreatic cells (e.g. in acute pancreatitis). A lack of lipase in the bowel leads to steatorrhoea due to excess of neutral fats in the stool, while lack of trypsin causes deficient protein digestion with the appearance in the stool of striated muscle fibres. Normally only small amounts of pancreatic digestive enzymes find their way into the bloodstream and appear in the urine. Pancreatic secretion can also be obtained for analysis by aspirating the duodenal contents after the injection of a pancreatic stimulant (e.g. secretin).

## Renal, urinary and genital systems

Symptoms suggesting diseases of the kidney and urinary tract include:
1. Disturbances in the act of micturition, including frequency, retention, incontinence and dysuria.
2. Alteration in the amount of urine.
3. Alteration in the appearance of the urine.
4. Pain: renal, ureteric, vesical or urethral.
5. General symptoms of abnormal renal function.

### Disturbances in the act of micturition

*Frequency* (without increase in the amount of urine) results from irritation of the bladder by infection, stone, tumour or blood; or from a reduction in the capacity of the bladder by fibrotic contraction or pressure from a pelvic tumour. In all these conditions, the patient's sleep is disturbed by the need to micturate (*nocturia*), whereas frequency due to emotional causes or cold is usually confined to the waking hours. Polyuria may also lead to frequency (*see below*).

*Retention* occurs in obstructive lesions of the urethra such as stricture and prostatic hypertrophy, in diseases of the spinal cord or sacral nerve roots and in coma due to various causes. Complete retention may be heralded by a phase of *hesitancy* (delay in starting micturition), by a poor or intermittent stream and by terminal dribbling.

*Incontinence* of urine is common when the mental faculties are impaired, especially in the elderly and in cerebrovascular lesions. In spinal cord diseases retention of urine is often followed by incontinence due either to overflow or to reflex evacuations of the bladder. Among the commoner neurological diseases resulting in incontinence are paraplegia, especially traumatic, and multiple sclerosis. Incontinence can also result from disease or deformity of the lower urinary tract such as a vesicovaginal fistula, a prolapsed uterus with cystocele, or muscular weakness in parous women. In these circumstances it is usually provoked by coughing or sneezing ('stress incontinence'). In men prostatic enlargement, benign or malignant, has the same result, which also occurs (fortunately rarely now) after prostatectomy. *Precipitancy*, the sudden onset of micturition without warning, is another cause of occasional incontinence, especially in neurological disorders.

*Dysuria* means difficulty in micturition and may thus include some of the symptoms already discussed. More commonly, however, the term is used to describe pain or discomfort during the act of micturition which usually results from disease of the bladder, prostate or urethra (*see below*).

### Alteration in the amount of urine

The urine volume may be increased (*polyuria*) or diminished (*oliguria*) or negligible (*anuria*).

**Polyuria** Large quantities of urine will be passed if the reabsorption of water from the tubular fluid is impaired in any way. Normally fluid is delivered to the tubules from the glomerular capillaries at a rate of 120 ml/min; 99 per cent of the water delivered to the tubules is reabsorbed secondarily to the reabsorption of sodium, chloride and other solutes. The formation of normal urine depends on the concentration gradient between the cortex, medulla and the papillae of the kidney; this gradient is determined by the functional anatomy of the loop of Henle, the secretion of antidiuretic hormone (vasopressin) by the posterior pituitary and the sensitivity of the tubular cells to vasopressin.

The urine volume is increased normally following the ingestion of large quantities of fluid, especially when this contains substances with a diuretic action (e.g. alcohol, tea, coffee). Polyuria may also result from nervousness (e.g. during medical examination). Diseases causing polyuria include the following:

a. Chronic renal failure: the solute load filtered and excreted by each of the few remaining nephrons is greatly increased, and there are not enough nephrons to maintain an effective medullary concentration gradient.
b. Diabetes mellitus: the osmotic effect of the unreabsorbed glucose prevents reabsorption of water from the tubular fluid.
c. Neurohypophysial diabetes insipidus: the secretion of vasopressin is impaired e.g. following trauma to the head.
d. Nephrogenic diabetes insipidus: where the tubules are insensitive to the action of vasopressin. This occurs primarily in a rare familial condition and secondarily in hyperparathyroidism and potassium depletion.
e. Oedematous states, such as cardiac failure, cirrhosis and the nephrotic syndrome treated with diuretics that primarily impair the tubular reabsorption of sodium choride and thence the reabsorption of water.

In chronic renal failure, diabetes mellitus, and diabetes insipidus, *thirst* and *polydipsia* result from the abnormal losses of water and are often the presenting symptoms of the underlying disorder.

**Oliguria and anuria** The urine volume is diminished physiologically under conditions of water deprivation. In a healthy subject the functions of the kidney can be maintained with the passage of as little as 500 ml of urine daily.

Oliguria may be defined as the passage of less than 500 ml of urine daily. This may occur in pre-renal conditions, such as shock, haemorrhage, dehydration and cardiac failure, when the kidney is not damaged but the renal blood flow and glomerular filtration rate are diminished. Oliguria is also found in established acute renal failure from primary renal disease such as acute glomerulonephritis.

Anuria can result from infarction of a single kidney or of both kidneys through massive embolization or dissecting aneurysm of the abdominal aorta with occlusion of the renal arteries. Other causes include bilateral cortical necrosis, which may follow severe postpartum haemorrhage, and complete obstruction of the ureters from bilateral stone or retroperitoneal fibrosis. Care must be taken to prove that failure to pass urine is due to anuria and not retention of urine. The lower abdomen must always be examined for a distended bladder and catheterization may be necessary to exclude obstruction of the urethra.

### Alteration in the appearance of the urine

This is considered more fully under the examination of the urine (p. 141). It is only necessary here to point out that the patient may first suspect urinary disease by noticing alteration in the colour and general appearance of the urine, e.g. red or smoky brown in haematuria, cloudy with an offensive smell when infected, frothy with proteinuria and dark orange or brown in obstructive jaundice. Various drugs may colour the urine, causing alarm or sometimes delight if the patient thinks it reflects the efficacy of treatment.

### Pain

In acute glomerulonephritis there may be a dull ache in the lumbar regions, but pain is usually absent in this and other glomerulonephropathies. By contrast, pain is common in acute pyelonephritis and is usually localized to the renal angle on the side of the affected kidney. Pain is particularly associated with any obstruction of the ureter, either at its origin in the pelvis of the kidney, during its course in the abdomen or at its entrance into the bladder. Obstruction may be caused by stones or by solid material such as blood or pus in urinary infections. An obstruction of uncertain nature is sometimes present in hydronephrosis; hence pain is also common in this condition. Only rarely is the obstruction caused by stricture or kinking of the ureter (e.g. by an aberrant renal artery). In some of these instances the characteristic pain of *renal colic* may be present (*Fig.* 5.1). This consists of intense sharp pain generally referred in the first place to the lumbar region, i.e. at the renal angle (outer edge of erector spinae and the lower border of the 12th rib). It radiates forwards into the abdomen and downwards into the groin, the testis or the thigh. This spread is due to *ureteric colic*. Vomiting,

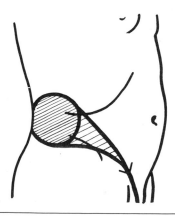

**Fig. 5.1**
Renal colic. Pain starts in the loin and radiates to the groin, and sometimes into the genitalia and thigh.

sweating and great prostration generally accompany these attacks, which may last for several hours, especially when calculus is the cause of the obstruction. Although certain movements may aggravate the pain, the patient is often restless and rolls from side to side in an effort to gain relief. In this regard, the pain of renal colic differs from that of peritonitis in which the patient prefers to lie still. Between attacks or renal colic a dull ache may be present in the loin.

*Pain arising from the bladder or urethra* may be due to the passage of solid material such as pus, blood or stone and will then be similar in character to renal colic. Such pain is usually referred to the lower abdomen, the perineum and in the male to the glans penis. The term *strangury* is sometimes used if the urine is passed painfully, drop by drop. A burning or scalding discomfort is felt when there is inflammation of the lower urinary passages (e.g. cystitis or urethritis), especially if the urine is excessively acid. These pains generally occur during or at the end of micturition (*see also* 'Dysuria').

## General symptoms

**Renal oedema** In acute glomerulonephritis the oedema may be slight and short-lived, chiefly occurring in the face, though sometimes in dependent parts. In the nephrotic syndrome the oedema may be generalized, extreme and longstanding. In severe chronic renal failure the development of oedema indicates that the failing kidney can no longer maintain homeostasis with respect to sodium and water and that the terminal stage of the illness is not far away. In all cases, renal oedema results from the inappropriate retention by the kidney of sodium chloride and water. In acute glomerulonephritis, the reduction in glomerular filtration rate with continued reabsorption of sodium and water by the tubules is probably to blame. In the nephrotic syndrome the massive loss of proteins in the urine results in a fall in their plasma concentration. This leads to a reduction in the colloid osmotic pressure of the plasma and so to increased transudation of fluid into the tissues. The plasma volume is thus reduced, and in compensation the renal tubules reabsorb sodium chloride and water to expand the extracellular fluid volume until the plasma volume is restored. In chronic renal failure the tubular reabsorption of sodium is proportionately increased, but the glomerular filtration rate and the filtered load of sodium are reduced. Oedema often develops when more than 95 per cent of nephron function is lost and the glomerular filtration rate expressed as creatinine clearance falls below 5 ml/min. Renal oedema is not confined to the dependent parts as in heart disease and may be generalized (*see Fig.* 5.12, p. 151). In most patients the effect of gravity is apparent, ankle oedema developing at the end of the day in the ambulant patient and sacral oedema in the patient who rests in bed.

**Symptoms due to high blood pressure** (*see* p. 210) Many of the symptoms occurring in renal disease are due to associated hypertension, which may lead to disturbance of the cerebral circulation. In most patients the rise in blood pressure is caused by the retention of sodium chloride and water with an increase in plasma volume and not by an increased secretion of renin.

In acute nephritis there is often a sharp rise in blood pressure during the early stages so that convulsions and signs of cardiac failure may appear, but these are often indistinguishable from the effects of salt and water retention. Hypertension in chronic renal disease may be associated with headaches, vomiting and left ventricular failure.

**Renal failure** The clinical features of renal failure are as varied as the functions carried out by the normal kidney. The kidney has a considerable functional reserve, and the body has a surprising tolerance of the nitrogenous waste metabolites normally excreted in the urine. In most patients the failing kidney can maintain homeostasis with respect to body water and ionic concentrations of electrolytes as the glomerular filtration rate declines over a tenfold range from 100 ml/min to only 10 ml/min. When more than 90–95 per cent of nephron function has been lost, or when the system is stressed by trauma or by intercurrent illness, the manifold features of the *uraemic syndrome* appear. These have defied explanation in terms of a single identifiable uraemic toxin. Many can be attributed to the imbalance in fluid and electrolyte metabolism. Generally, the patient feels tired, listless and breathless on exertion. These features can often but not always be explained by *anaemia* which is frequently present and which reflects a decrease in erythropoietin secretion by the kidney. There may be *purpura* and bleeding from the gastrointestinal tract due to defective platelet function.

*Urogenital* symptoms include thirst, polydipsia, polyuria and nocturia. In both sexes there is loss of libido and infertility, with impotence in men and secondary amenorrhoea in women.

*Cardiovascular* symptoms include precordial pain from pericarditis, ankle swelling, breathlessness on exertion and paroxysmal nocturnal dypsnoea from hypertension, with salt and water retention.

The *alimentary* system is disturbed by anorexia, nausea, vomiting and sometimes diarrhoea. The breath has an ammoniacal odour from the breakdown in the mouth of urea to ammonium carbonate under the influence of bacterial urease. The patient loses weight.

The *respiratory* system is implicated in the hyperventilation that results from metabolic acidosis, and which the patient often does not notice (Kussmaul's breathing).

*Central, peripheral and autonomic nervous system* involvement leads to an inability to concentrate, muscle twitching, restlessness of the legs, paraesthesiae and pareses due to peripheral neuropathy and autonomic neuropathy with hypohidrosis, impotence and postural syncope due to hypotension.

The *skeleton* is affected in patients with long-standing renal disease even when renal function is only moderately impaired. Bone pain and pathological fractures indicate defective mineralization and secondary hyperparathyroidism. These may result from a failure of the kidneys to synthesize the active metabolite of vitamin D and from their failure to excrete phosphate. Both may depress the plasma concentration of ionized calcium and thus stimulate increased secretion of parathyroid hormone and hypertrophy of the parathyroid glands.

Ultimately there is extreme prostration, drowsiness, mental confusion, convulsions and coma, gastrointestinal haemorrhage and haemorrhagic pericarditis with cardiac tamponade. Death may also result from hyperkalaemia or severe acidosis.

# ■ PHYSICAL SIGNS: EXAMINATION OF THE RENAL, URINARY AND GENITAL SYSTEMS

Examination comprises the following routine procedure.

1. *General examination* of the patient, with particular attention to the cardiovascular system, nervous system and retinae.

2. *Examination of the abdomen* to detect any enlargement of the kidneys or any tenderness over these or over the ureters or bladder. Occasionally it may be possible to palpate a thickened ureter or tumours arising from the bladder.

3. *The external genitalia* should also be examined especially for evidence of enlargement, neoplastic or inflammatory signs in the testis or epididymis and abnormalities in the urethra.

4. *Examination of the pelvic organs* through the rectum or vagina.

5. *Examination of the urine* by chemical and microscopical methods.

## GENERAL EXAMINATION

The presence or absence of *oedema* should be noted in every case. The colour of the patient is important, as *anaemia* is a common secondary effect of nephritis. Undue dryness of the skin and haemorrhages should also be noted, as they are common in uraemia. In these cases the skin often has a dirty brownish appearance like fading sunburn. This may be due to the retention of urinary pigments or to the failure of the kidney to degrade melanocyte-stimulating hormone from the pituitary.

*Systematic examination* should include measurement of blood pressure and a search for signs attributable to hypertension such as a thrusting left ventricular impulse, crackles at the lung bases, evidence of cerebrovascular disease and retinal vascular changes (*Fig.* 5.2) (*see also* Chapter 10, p. 349). Signs of uraemia

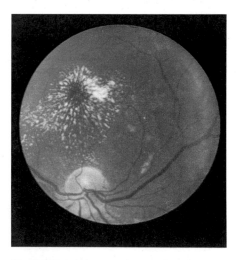

**Fig. 5.2** Ophthalmoscopic appearance in renal disease showing hard retinal exudates and the 'macular fan'.

may be found in the respiratory system (Kussmaul's breathing), heart (pericardial friction rub), nervous system (twitching, drowsiness, peripheral neuropathy) and alimentary tract (dry coated tongue, bloody diarrhoea).

## EXAMINATION OF THE ABDOMEN

### The kidneys

Palpation of the kidneys is best carried out with the patient in the recumbent position and the head slightly raised on a pillow. One hand is placed under the loin with the tips of the fingers resting against the erector spinae, while the other is placed flat on the abdomen with fingers pointing upwards towards the costal margin (*Fig.* 5.3). The patient is then instructed to take a deep breath, and firm pressure is exerted by both hands at the height of inspiration, so that if the kidney is palpable it moves down into the space between the examining hands and is 'trapped'. When the organ can be felt in this way it is recognized as a swelling with a rounded lower pole, and if sufficient of it can be grasped between the hands, the characteristic reniform shape with a medially placed notch (the hilum) can be recognized, though this is difficult. The consistency of the swelling should be firm without hardness. It is not uncommon to feel the right kidney in women, and in some cases both kidneys may be freely movable and can be manipulated into different parts of the abdomen (floating kidney).

'*Tumours*' of the kidney when of moderate size retain the characteristic kidney

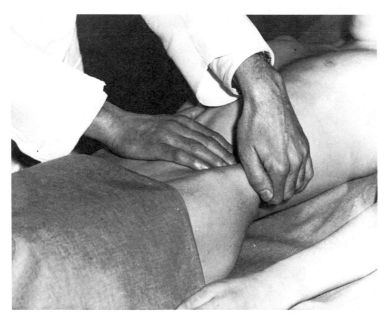

**Fig. 5.3** Palpation of the kidney. One hand is placed on the abdomen with the fingers pointing towards the costal margin, the other is pressed firmly against the loin. If the kidney is enlarged or mobile it moves downwards on inspiration and is sandwiched between the two hands.

shape, but with experience can be recognized as larger than normal. Those commonly recognized on abdominal examination are hypernephromas and polycystic kidneys; the former may be unduly hard and somewhat irregular, while in the latter cystic swellings may be palpable as characteristic bosses.

Inspection and percussion are of lesser importance, but tumours may show as a bulge in the loin which is dull on percussion and is best seen with the patient sitting up. Colonic resonance occurs in front of a renal tumour on the left side, thus distinguishing it from a splenic tumour. The character of the skin in the loin should also be noticed, as redness and oedema may be present in perinephric infection.

### The bladder

If distended with urine the bladder can be seen as a rounded or pyriform swelling arising from the pelvis (*Fig.* 5.4) and extending upwards, sometimes as far as the umbilicus. Its outline is confirmed by palpation and percussion and its lower margin cannot be felt. A distended bladder must be distinguished from a pregnant uterus or an ovarian cyst which may be of similar consistency. Proof that it is the bladder is obtained by catheterization, but voluntary evacuation should always be attempted first.

### THE EXTERNAL GENITALIA

The external genitalia may provide some important clues to the diagnosis (*see also* Chapter 3, p. 56).

### Male

Meatal ulcer is a common cause of painful micturition, haematuria and retention in babies and infants. It is a sequel to circumcision and may lead to

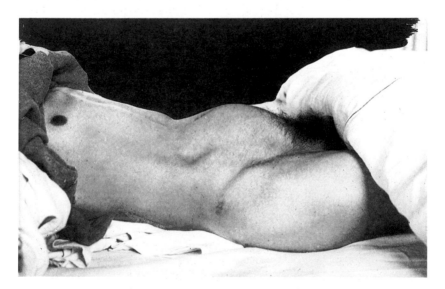

**Fig. 5.4** Distended bladder.

meatal stenosis. A purulent discharge in the adult is diagnostic of urethritis and in company with swelling and tenderness of the epididymis suggests gonorrhoea, but infection with *Escherichia coli* is now at least as common. Strictures can be palpated in the penile urethra. The epididymis which is moderately enlarged, craggy and only slightly tender suggests genito-urinary tuberculosis, while tethering of the scrotal skin posteriorly and sinus formation are diagnostic. The ductus deferens (vas) is frequently thickened, but beading is uncommon. Swellings of the testis itself are more likely to be neoplastic, though orchitis occurs in mumps, and gummas are still occasionally seen. Hydrocele may be a sign of some other disease, inflammatory or neoplastic, involving the tunica vaginalis.

### Female

Vulvovaginitis due to monilial, trichomonal or gonococcal infection will explain scalding in the adult and urethral caruncle scalding and tenderness in the elderly. A cystocele large enough to protrude from the vulva can cause retention; smaller cystoceles are often associated with stress incontinence. Vulval itching (pruritus vulvae) is an important early symptom of diabetes mellitus.

## EXAMINATION OF THE PELVIC ORGANS

### Male

Rectal examination is necessary in all cases of suspected urinary disease. The left lateral or dorsal positions are used, the latter permitting bimanual examination, though the former is more commonly employed. When it is used, and the finger has been inserted with its dorsum towards the bladder, it should be gently rotated, so that the more sensitive pulp of the finger palpates tissues and organs anterior to it (*Fig.* 5.5).

The prostate (*Fig.* 5.6) can normally be felt as an elastic swelling with a median groove terminating in a notch at the top. Gross adenomatous enlargement of the gland makes it more difficult to feel the upper surface or the notch, but the consistency is rubbery or even spongy. The apparent size of the gland is often exaggerated by a distended bladder. The malignant prostate has lateral infiltration so that it is difficult to identify the lateral margins. There is no 'give' when the finger pushes the prostate forwards. Irregularity and hardness in the prostate suggest malignant disease or occasionally prostatic calculi. Prostatic massage may give smears which are useful in the diagnosis of prostatitis and occasionally in malignant prostate.

The seminal vesicles lie above the prostate, running upwards from its outer margins, but can only be felt if they are full. Thickening due to tuberculous infiltration is sometimes an important diagnostic point in suspected urinary tuberculosis.

### Female

Inspection of the vulva (*Figs.* 5.7, 5.8) should first be made. Such common conditions as vaginal discharge, prolapse or urethral caruncle may at once be apparent. The vagina and cervix can then be inspected with a bivalve speculum in the dorsal position or a duck-bill speculum in the left lateral position. Differentiation between the types of vulvovaginitis will be facilitated, and

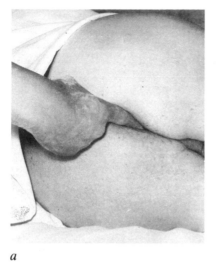

*a*

*b*

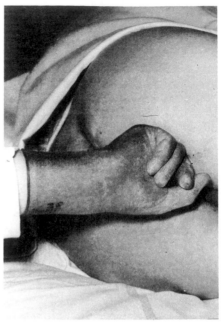

**Fig. 5.5**
Rectal examination. The finger is inserted
as shown in *a*, and then gently rotated to
define the prostate.

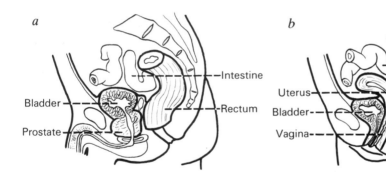

**Fig. 5.6** Shows the anatomical situation of structures which
can be palpated per rectum or per vaginam.

urethral, vaginal and cervical swabs taken for bacteriological confirmation. Cystocele may be disclosed as a cause of frequency (*Fig.* 5.8). An advanced cervical
carcinoma might explain uraemia, due to ureteric obstruction, or incontinence if
a vesical fistula is demonstrated. Obstruction to the passage of the speculum by
a complete vaginal septum (frequently miscalled an 'imperforate hymen') will
explain acute retention in the adolescent due to haematocolpos. Diverticulum of the
urethra or paraurethral abscess may explain dysuria and dribbling incontinence.

Vaginal examination in the dorsal position permits bimanual assessment of the
uterus and its appendages. Softening of the cervix and body of the uterus and

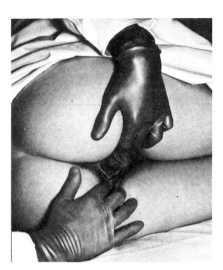 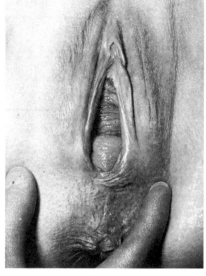

**Fig. 5.7**
Inspection of vulva and
vaginal entrance.

**Fig. 5.8**
Inspection of vulva showing
cystocele and rectocele.

enlargement of the latter, due to pregnancy, may explain urinary frequency without scalding. Tenderness in the renal angles during the second half of pregnancy, especially when accompanied by fever and vomiting, suggests pyelitis. Acute retention is uncommon in women, but with the exception of hysteria is due to intrapelvic masses, such as an impacted retroverted gravid uterus, uterine fibroids, ovarian cyst or haematocele due to ectopic gestation. In contrast to the male, genital tuberculosis is not usually accompaned by urinary tuberculosis. Calculi in the terminal portion of the ureter are palpable per vaginam.

## EXAMINATION OF THE URINE

Examination of the urine is pre-eminently the method by which the diagnosis of urinary diseases is established.

### Inspection

Inspection shows the *colour* of the urine and any *deposit Fig.* 5.9.
**Colour** Highly concentrated urine usually has a dark amber colour inclining to orange. It frequently results from loss of fluid through other channels, as by sweating or diarrhoea. It also occurs in heart failure. These conditions lead to increased concentration of the urine, but a deeper colour may also result from changes in diet as increased proteins and purines favour the excretion of uric acid derivatives. Pale urine, on the contrary, is found when the concentration of solids diminishes and the urine is of large amount and usually of low specific gravity. It therefore occurs after excessive intake of fluids, alcohol and other diuretics, and in certain types of chronic renal disease; also in diabetes insipidus, in which the

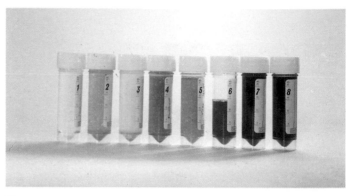

**Fig. 5.9** Coloured urines. 1, yellow, normal; 2, pink, phenolpthalein or rhubarb; 3, orange, rifampicin; 4, red, haematuria; 5, orange, obstructive jaundice; 6, claret red, porphyria; 7, black, alkaptonuria; 8, black, melanuria.

volume of urine is increased and its concentration diminished. A pale urine of high specific gravity (owing to the presence of sugar) occurs in diabetes mellitus.

Abnormal constituents may produce a complete change in the colour of the urine. Bile gives it a dark greenish-orange appearance, blood a red, reddish-brown or smoky colour, haemoglobin a deep red, and melanin and alkapton a very dark appearance, sometimes black. Red urine or one which darkens on standing may suggest the rare but important condition of porphyria. The possibility of excreted drugs modifying the colour of urine has been mentioned, among them riboflavin, rifampicin and phenindione (Dindevan), an orange to orange-pink colour, while brighter pink may result from santonin or phenolphthalein. Even food and drink may cause a similar colour, e.g. beetroot and rhubarb.

**Deposit** Fresh urine rarely has much deposit if it is normal, but on standing deposits of phosphates or urates may produce a cloudiness or even a thick heavy layer. Phosphates are usually a white or light buff colour and disappear if the urine is acidified, whilst urates vary from a buff colour to a pink or brick-red disappearing on heating. These constituents have no pathological significance. A fainter cloudiness may be produced by bacteria, giving the urine an opalescent or shimmering appearance. Pathological constituents such as pus and blood also produce turbidity, increasing in some cases to a thick deposit.

### Specific gravity (relative density)

The normal specific gravity or urine is generally about 1·015 to 1·025 (conveniently styled 1015 or 1025), but wide variations are found in health, according to the quantity of fluid ingested and the amount lost through the skin and bowels. A persistently low specific gravity (1010 or rather less) suggests chronic renal disease if rarer causes such as diabetes insipidus can be excluded. Very high specific gravities (1030–1060) are rarely found except in the presence of large amounts of sugar in the urine in diabetes mellitus. When a specific gravity of over 1050 is found, the possibility of artefact must be excluded.

### Reaction

The urine may be acid or slightly alkaline in health. It is frequently alkaline for a short period during the digestion of food, the so-called 'alkaline tide'. Decomposition on standing and the liberation of free ammonia also render it alkaline, especially when the urine is heavily charged with bacteria. The type of diet may also alter the reaction, vegetables and fruit tending to make it alkaline, meat acid.

### Smell

A strong ammoniacal smell is frequently found in infants and after decomposition when the urine has been left standing. Infection with *Escherichia coli* imparts a fishy odour, while certain foods, notably asparagus, also give rise to a characteristic smell.

### Quantity

The amount of urine passed in 24 hours should be recorded. In health it averages 1500 ml.

### Chemical examination

Rapid and simple tests for the presence in the urine of protein, glucose, ketones, bilirubin, urobilinogen and blood are now available. These tests can be carried out at the bedside and should be regarded as a part of the physical examination of the patients rather than as a special investigation. Each test is based upon a colour change in a strip of stiff absorbent cellulose which has been impregnated with the appropriate reagent. A fresh specimen of urine is collected in a clean test-tube free of contaminants (especially detergents and acids). The change in colour of the strip after contact with urine is compared with a colour chart in a bright white light. Single strips for the simultaneous detection of a number of abnormal urine constituents are available for routine urine testing (*Fig.* 5.10).

The chemical principles underlying the colour reactions illustrated in *Fig.* 5.10 are as follows:

*pH test*: This test is based on a double indicator principle which gives a broad range of colours covering the entire urinary pH range. Colours range from orange through yellow and green to blue.

*Protein test*: This test is based on the protein error of indicators principle which means that at a constant buffered pH, the development of any green colour is due to the presence of protein. Colours range from green–yellow for 'negative' through yellow–green and green to green–blue for 'positive' reactions.

*Glucose test*: This is a double sequential enzyme reaction. The reaction utilizes the enzyme glucose oxidase to catalyse the formation of glucuronic acid and hydrogen peroxide from the oxidation of glucose. In turn, a second enzyme, peroxidase, catalyses the reaction of hydrogen peroxide with a potassium iodide chromogen to oxidize the chromogen to a green–brown colour.

*Ketone test*: This reaction is based on the purple colour developed with acetoacetic acid or acetone and nitroprusside. The components are stabilized in a dry reagent containing glycine as the nitrogen source and a strongly alkaline buffer.

1. Completely immerse reagent area of the strip in FRESH, well-mixed uncentrifuged urine and remove immediately.

2. Tap edge of strip against the side of the urine container to remove excess urine. Hold the strip in a horizontal position to prevent possible soiling of hands with urine, making sure that the test area faces upwards.

3. Compare test area closely with corresponding Colour Charts on the bottle label at the times specified. HOLD STRIP CLOSE TO COLOUR BLOCKS AND MATCH CAREFULLY.

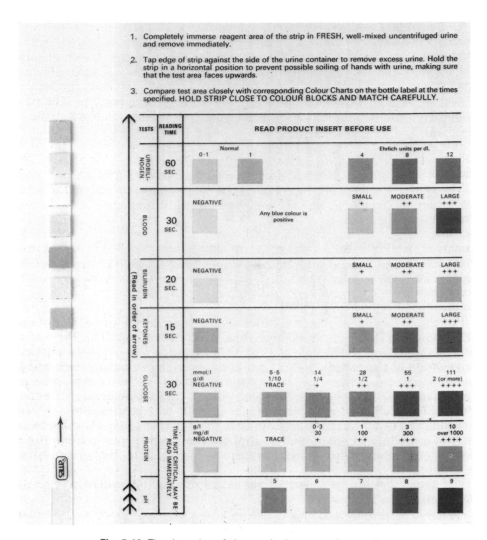

**Fig. 5.10** The detection of abnormal urinary constituents, by colour reaction. The strip carrying seven different reagents (left of picture) is immersed in the urine and any colour changes are compared with those in the control chart after the appropriate time interval. (*Reproduced by courtesy of Ames Company, Division of Miles Laboratories Ltd, Slough, England.*)

*Bilirubin test*: This reaction is based on the coupling of bilirubin with diazotized dichloraniline in a strong acid medium. The colour developed is a tan-to-purple shade.

*Blood test*: The detection of occult blood is based on the peroxidase-like activity of haemoglobin which catalyses the reaction of peroxide and the chromogen orthotolidine to form blue oxidized orthotolidine.

*Urobilinogen test*: This test area is based on the Ehrlich reaction in which paradimethylaminobenzaldehyde reacts with urobilinogen in a strongly acid medium to form a red colour.

False-positive results for protein may occur with alkaline highly buffered urine, for ketones if the urine contains L-dopa metabolites and for bilirubin in patients taking chlorpromazine. A false-negative result for blood may occur with infected samples of urine and those of high specific gravity and also in the presence of ascorbic acid.

It is important that the instructions which accompany the reagents should be followed exactly. The information given here is intended only as a general guide; the details are not necessarily applicable to all the available reagents.

The common abnormal constituents indicating the presence of urinary tract disease are protein, blood and pus.

**Proteinuria** The presence of protein in the urine may vary from a trace to 10 g per litre or more. Very small amounts may be derived accidentally from the urinary passages, particularly from the vagina and prepuce. Protein derived from these sources is inconstant and has no pathological significance. Diseases of the kidney, the bladder and the urethra, in which pus or blood is produced, are also accompanied by proteinuria, and the possibility of these should be considered before attributing proteinuria to nephritis.

Protein excreted into the urine by the kidneys otherwise falls into two classes: (1) Physiological proteinuria; (2) Pathological proteinuria. The distinction between these two is not always easy.

*Physiological proteinuria* This generally occurs in children or young adults, and the amount of protein is usually small, though occasionally considerable. It appears in the urine in significant circumstances. Usually it is absent in the early morning specimen, but appears after the patient has been up for an hour or two; sometimes it appears only after exercise. Various names have been applied to the different types of physiological proteinuria, such as *orthostatic* or *postural* when it seems to be dependent upon change in posture of the individual.

It is thought that this harmless form of proteinuria is due to venous congestion of the kidneys chiefly from altered posture, especially with lordosis. Repeated examination is often necessary before proteinuria can be called 'physiological'. Its inconstancy is an important point, and also the fact that it usually disappears after 24 hours' rest in bed. It is not accompanied by other evidence of nephritis, as is shown by good response to the renal efficiency tests and the absence of casts (occasionally a few hyaline casts may occur) in the urine.

*Pathological proteinuria* Although heavy proteinuria suggests organic renal disease, the amount of protein may be quite small even when the kidneys are badly damaged and functioning poorly. The persistent presence of more than 1 g/l of protein in the urine generally indicates the presence of nephritis, unless pus or blood is responsible. In chronic pyelonephritis proteinuria is generally mild, whereas in the nephrotic syndrome the loss of protein in the urine usually exceeds 5 g per 24 h and can reach 20–30 g in severe cases. Proteinuria may occur as a manifestation of systemic disease affecting the kidneys. Thus in cardiac failure and febrile states, small amounts of protein (up to 1 g per 24 h) may be lost in the urine without any real kidney disease, but this disappears if treatment is successful. Proteinuria occurs in eclampsia, amyloidosis and diabetes mellitus and also following the ingestion of certain chemical poisons. Bence Jones protein, consisting of fragments of light chains of the immunoglobulin molecule, is found in the urine in certain cases of multiple myelomatosis. It can be demonstrated by heating a specimen of urine, acidified with acetic acid, in a tube to which a thermometer is attached. The protein is precipitated between temperatures of 40 and 60 °C, almost disappears as boiling point is approached, and reappears on cooling.

**Haematuria** Blood in the urine may vary in amount from large quantities visible to the naked eye to a few red corpuscles detectable only by microscopial examination. The blood may be derived from any part of the urinary tract—the kidneys, rarely the ureters, the bladder or the urethra. When derived from the kidney it has an opportunity to become intimately mixed with the urine, which is correspondingly reddish-brown in colour ('smoky') or evenly pink, but when derived from the bladder or urethra it may remain separate from the urine, and have the bright-red appearance of pure blood. Clots may appear, sometimes stringy if casts of the ureter are caused by excessive bleeding from the kidney. Blood from the urethra may be dislodged by the urinary stream and thus precedes the urine. The reverse is the case when the bleeding is taking place in the bladder.

Haematuria may be due to haemorrhagic conditions, to disease of the kidney itself or to lesions in the lower urinary tract. Haemorrhagic conditions can cause bleeding from the kidney as one part of a generalized disorder of the blood (e.g. thrombocytopenia, prothrombin deficiency) or the blood vessels (e.g. scurvy, allergic purpura, certain acute fevers). The renal diseases producing haematuria include the acute forms of nephritis, trauma, infarction, malignant hypertension, congenial cystic kidney, nephrotoxic drugs (e.g. sulphonamides), calculus, neoplasm, tuberculosis and acute bacterial infection. These last four conditions are also the main causes of bleeding from the bladder and, less commonly, from the ureters or urethra.

**Pyuria** A few pus cells in the urine have little significance, especially in women, as they may derive from the vagina. Larger quantities of pus usually indicate an inflammatory lesion of the urinary tract, and in most cases organisms are to be found on microscopical examination and on culture. Quantitative estimations of the number of pus cells passed per hour can vary from a few hundred in normal persons to 1 000 000 or more in heavy urinary infections. In all cases in which pus is found, therefore, a specimen of urine collected aseptically is a necessity both to establish the presence and nature of the organisms and the fact that the pus has a urinary origin. The urethral meatus is swabbed with a weak antiseptic and a midstream specimen of urine is then collected in a sterile receptacle. A catheter should be used only if, for any reason, this procedure is impracticable (e.g. in the unconscious patient).

Cystitis, pyelitis and suppuration in the kidney substance are important causes of pyuria, but smaller amounts of pus may occur from prostatitis and urethritis in men. While protein and blood are the usual abnormal constituents in cases of nephritis, pus cells are not uncommonly found, especially in acute nephritis. Pus may also be derived from extrinsic causes such as diverticulitis of the colon or the rupture of an appendix abscess into the bladder.

**Pneumaturia** Gas is rarely expelled with the urine, but pneumaturia may occasionally prove of considerable diagnostic value, suggesting a communication between the urinary tract (usually the bladder) and the alimentary tract (the colon). It is occasionally found, for example, in cases of diverticulitis in which the diverticulum has become adherent to the bladder. Carcinoma of the colon is the next most common cause. Rarely, faeces may be passed with the urine.

### Microscopical examination

The urine should always be examined microscopically. Apart from the presence of small numbers of red corpuscles and pus cells which may not be recognizable by chemical tests, microscopical examination may show the presence of casts, crystals, foreign bodies, micro-organisms and parasites.

*Casts* (cylinduria) in appreciable numbers are most commonly found in cases of nephritis. They are formed by protein being precipitated in the tubules and moulded into cylindrical shape with the incorporation of any cellular elements or debris that may also be present. Red cells in the tubular lumen can only have come from the glomerular capillaries. Their presence in casts is thus pathognomonic of glomerulonephritis, and the recognition of red cell casts in the urine provides an important contribution to the differential diagnosis of patients with haematuria. Their reddish-brown colour may be lost, but they can still be recognized by comparison with free red cells elsewhere in the urinary sediment. A fresh specimen must be examined since red cell casts degenerate rapidly if the urine is left to stand. Leucocyte casts are found in chronic pyelonephritis, and epithelial cell casts are produced by desquamation of the renal tubular epithelium from any cause. Granular casts may result from the degeneration of cellular casts or from the incorporation of debris. Hyaline casts reflect the severity of proteinuria and are found most commonly when the urine contains few cells.

*Crystals* are often found in the urine but are rarely of diagnostic importance. It is important to recognize the hexagonal crystals of cystine which are found in patients with a rare congenital metabolic defect (cystinuria) associated with recurrent stone formation.

Many other bodies may be seen in urine, and some of these need experience for their recognition. They are rarely indicative of urinary or any other form of disease. They include vaginal epithelium, spermatozoa, urates, phosphates and all manner of foreign bodies.

**Bacteriuria** As catheterization is now avoided, when possible, to prevent trauma and consequent risk of urinary infection, the midstream technique is used to provide a suitable specimen of urine for all purposes.

This may be handled in any hospital laboratory to ascertain the bacterial count, but in domiciliary practice a simple 'dip-inoculum' enables the doctor to send the specimen through the post to a laboratory. High bacterial counts (100000 per ml or more) may be found as the only urinary-tract abnormality.

Parasites in the urine are rare in Great Britain, but *Trichomonas vaginalis* is sometimes found even in catheter or midstream specimens. Of the more exotic parasites, *Bilharzia haematobia* is the most important; the large ova are easily recognized under low magnification (*see* Chapter 12).

### Special investigations

Special investigations of value in the elucidation of urinary-tract disease include radiography, cystoscopy, chemical examination of blood and urine, tests of renal function and renal biopsy.

**Radiography** A direct radiograph of the abdomen will usually reveal the size and contour of the kidneys. The urinary conduit including the renal pelvis, ureters and the bladder, are best outlined by the intravenous injection of a radio-opaque dye which is excreted in the urine—intravenous pyelography (IVP) or intravenous urography (IVU) (*Fig.* 5.11). If the dye cannot be excreted because of poor renal function, it may be injected through a ureteric catheter inserted at cystoscopy (retrograde pyelography). Alternatively, when the ureteric orifice is blocked, a needle may be inserted percutaneously into a dilated renal pelvis under ultrasound guidance (antegrade pyelography). Ultrasound examination is a safe, non-invasive technique to estimate the shape, size and consistency of the kidneys and is particularly useful in distinguishing a benign cyst from a solid and probably malignant swelling. CT scanning may demonstrate the spread of a renal tumour into the renal veins and para-aortic lymph nodes as well as perinephric swellings. Renal angiography outlines abnormalities of the renal arteries and arterial, capillary and venous changes in the kidney itself.

**Cystoscopy** This is mainly of value in the diagnosis of bladder disease (e.g. tumours) by direct vision and by biopsy. Cystoscopy also permits catheterization of the two ureters for pyelography or for studies of differential renal function.

**Blood and urine chemistry** Disordered renal function is most simply assessed by measurement of urea, creatinine and electrolyte (sodium, potassium and bicarbonate) concentrations in plasma and urine. The commonest abnormality is an increase in plasma urea and creatinine concentrations, but as renal function deteriorates metabolic acidosis results in a fall in plasma bicarbonate, and ulti-

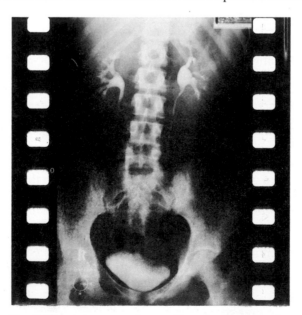

**Fig. 5.11** Intravenous pyelogram. Normal appearance of renal pelves, ureters and bladder.

mately there is a rise in plasma potassium which can be fatal. The plasma sodium concentration reflects a change in body water as often as a change in sodium balance, being increased in dehydration and decreased in water intoxication. The additional measurement of plasma calcium, phosphorus and alkaline phosphatase concentrations in patients with moderately severe renal failure provides useful information on the response of the skeleton to disordered vitamin D metabolism and to changes in parathyroid hormone concentrations.

Three main aspects of renal function and disease can be studied: glomerular filtration, the control of renal tubular reabsorption and the differential function of the two kidneys.

Glomerular filtration rate can be assessed most conveniently in terms of the creatinine clearance, using a timed collection of urine which is usually made over a 24-h period. The creatinine clearance is derived by dividing the excretion rate of creatinine by the plasma creatinine concentration. The quantity of protein excreted per day can be measured on the same 24-h sample of urine. In patients with glomerulonephritis the differential clearance of two proteins of high and low molecular weight is measured to obtain an index of selectivity of the proteinuria. In some cases, only proteins of low molecular weight such as albumin and transferrin escape the glomerular filter. In others, larger quantities of proteins of high molecular weight, such as the immunoglobulins and fibrinogen, pass through the glomerular basement membrane and the proteinuria is termed 'unselective'.

Tubular reabsorption of water is assessed in terms of the ability of the kidney to alter the specific gravity or osmolality of the urine in response to water deprivation and loading. Defective tubular reabsorption of sodium, potassium or magnesium can be revealed by limiting the oral intake of these substances and measuring the ability of the kidney to compensate in terms of reducing their urinary excretion rates.

The differential function of the two kidneys was assessed at one time by comparing the composition of urine samples obtained from the two sides by ureteric catheterization. Such information can now be obtained non-invasively from intravenous pyelography or by scanning the two kidneys with an external counter following the intravenous injection of a radio-isotope which is excreted in the urine (isotope renography).

**Renal biopsy** The histological diagnosis of diffuse renal disease can often be established by needle biopsy. This method is of particular value in determining the cause of a nephrotic syndrome.

■     ## THE DIAGNOSIS OF RENAL AND URINARY TRACT DISEASES

Sometimes the symptoms already enumerated—frequency, dysuria, pain, oedema and so forth—attract attention to the urinary system, but not infrequently, especially in cases of nephritis, the onset is insidious and silent, and routine examination of the urine may first throw light on the cause of a patient's poor health. This is one of a number of reasons for making the examination of the urine a necessary part of every medical examination, a measure often throwing unexpected light on an obscure case and saving the examiner from making serious mistakes in diagnosis.

The more common diseases of the urinary system follow. Some of them fall more frequently within the province of the surgeon but are discussed briefly as they may overlap into that of the physician.

# ■ DISEASES OF THE KIDNEYS

Many renal disorders ultimately result in total renal failure with the clinical features of uraemia already described. Common causes of chronic renal failure are listed in *Table* 5.1. The development of techniques to replace renal function by mechanical means or by kidney transplantation, and the limited availability of these dramatic measures, means that accurate diagnosis is essential. This has been facilitated by a greater understanding of pathophysiological mechanisms and by classifications based on analysis of renal biopsy material.

| Table 5.1 | **Causes of chronic renal failure** |
|---|---|
| | Glomerulonephritis (primary and secondary) |
| | Chronic pyelonephritis |
| | Renal vascular disease |
| | Polycystic kidneys |
| | Chronic obstructive uropathy (e.g. prostatic) |
| | Congenital nephropathies |
| | Analgesic nephropathy |
| | Diabetes mellitus |

*Diseases affecting the glomeruli*, whether primary or secondary to systemic disorders, account for well over half of all patients developing chronic renal failure, as well as for many patients with self-limiting conditions. Renal biopsy, used in conjunction with laboratory indices of disordered immunological function, has helped to identify distinct patterns of disease in a field which was previously greatly confused. Five distinct clinical syndromes can be recognized.

## Acute glomerulonephritis

Acute glomerulonephritis (or acute nephritic syndrome) was common in children but, like rheumatic fever, is now seen infrequently. Both are apparently immunological responses to streptococcal infections, generally of the throat in Western countries but sometimes of the skin in the tropics or where living standards are poor.

An acute nephritic syndrome may also complicate systemic lupus erythematosus, Henoch–Schönlein purpura and subacute bacterial endocarditis. The glomeruli are congested with cellular proliferation and deposition of immune complexes of antigen, antibody and complement in the capillary walls. The clinical picture consists of haematuria, albuminuria, casts, oedema (especially facial, *Fig.* 5.12), with associated hypertension and sometimes uraemic symptoms. The course of the illness is usually benign leading to full recovery within a few months. A few cases are fulminating, leading to death within months.

## Recurrent haematuria

Recurrent haematuria with insignificant proteinuria, normal blood pressure and normal renal function, often within 1–3 days of an upper respiratory

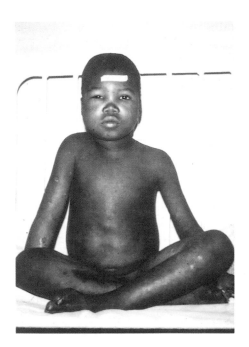

**Fig. 5.12**
Acute glomerulonephritis.
Note facial oedema causing
narrowed palpebral fissures,
oedema of legs and septic
skin lesions.

tract infection, can develop in some patients. The condition is commoner in children, resolves spontaneously within a week, and in most cases carries a good prognosis. Renal biopsy reveals focal proliferation of mesangial cells in some of the glomeruli, with mesangial deposition of immunoglobulins, especially IgA. This association was recognized by Berger in 1968, and the condition now bears his name.

### Rapidly progressive glomerulonephritis

A small but significant number of patients develop proteinuria, oedema, mild hypertension and progress to end-stage renal failure within weeks or months of their presentation. Some cases follow a viral or bacterial infection. Occasionally the lungs are involved with haemoptysis from alveolar haemorrhage, an association recognized by Goodpasture in 1919. In the kidney the glomerular capillaries are compressed and eventually obliterated by a crescent of proliferating epithelial cells which line Bowman's capsule. In Goodpasture's syndrome the glomerular damage is caused by a circulating antibody formed against a protein in the capillary wall, possibly shared by the alveolar capillaries. In other patients, circulating immune complexes are to blame.

### Asymptomatic proteinuria

Many patients have no symptoms but are found to have proteinuria or an increased blood pressure on routine medical examination. Renal function may be normal or variably impaired, and the glomeruli may show proliferation of cells or fibrosis. In some patients the proteinuria continues with no deterioration in renal function, whereas others slowly progress to fatal renal failure.

## Nephrotic syndrome

The triad of oedema, hypoalbuminaemia and heavy proteinuria can arise from a variety of diseases affecting the glomeruli. The common pathogenetic factor is the magnitude of the protein loss. This is usually greater than 5 g daily in adults or 0·1 g/kg in children, and this amount exceeds the capacity of the liver to compensate by increased synthesis. An increased plasma cholesterol is also found. Patients present with the insidious onset of oedema and some notice frothy urine. Some primary and secondary causes of the nephrotic syndrome are listed in *Table* 5.2. In minimal lesion glomerulonephritis the glomeruli appear normal on light microscopy, although with the electron miscroscope loss of pedicle structure can be seen. The condition occurs more commonly in children, the proteinuria is highly selective, and most case respond to treatment with corticosteroids. In membranous, proliferative and mesangiocapillary glomerulonephritis there is deposition of immunoglobulins and complement in the glomeruli, with thickening of the basement membrane or proliferation of cells, or a combination of the two. Hypertension is more common and remissions less frequent than in the minimal lesion type and many patients progress slowly to chronic renal failure. Among conditions in which glomerular damage occurs secondarily, quartan malaria deserves mention as possibly the commonest cause of nephrotic syndrome in the world.

| Table 5.2 | **Causes of nephrotic syndrome** |
|---|---|
| A | *Primary or idiopathic glomerulonephritis* (minimal lesion, membranous, proliferative, mesangiocapillary) |
| B | *Secondary* (a) Infections or disordered immunity: quartan malaria, infective endocarditis, systemic lupus erythematosus (*Fig.* 5.13), Henoch–Schönlein purpura (*Fig.* 5.14) |
|  | (b) Drugs and other chemicals: mercury, gold, penicillamine, probenecid |
|  | (c) Glomerular infiltrations: amyloidosis, diabetes mellitus, myelomatosis |
|  | (d) Tumours: myelomatosis, lymphomas, bronchogenic and other solid tumours |

## Renal vascular diseases

The most important of these is *malignant* or *accelerated hypertension*. This may complicate either essential or renal forms of hypertension (*see also* Chapter 7) and generally develops rapidly over a matter of months presenting with albuminuria, casts, high blood pressure readings and papilloedema.

The renal changes in the malignant phase are due to a necrotizing arteriolitis, and the end result (apart from vascular complications) is renal failure. At this stage it is difficult to be sure of the origin of the condition, whether in fact the hypertension is primary or secondary. This may be shown diagrammatically (*Fig.* 5.15).

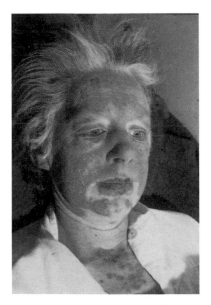

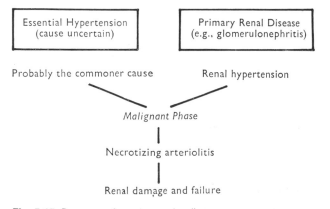

**Fig. 5.13**
Systemic lupus
erythematosus. This patient
developed nephrotic
syndrome.

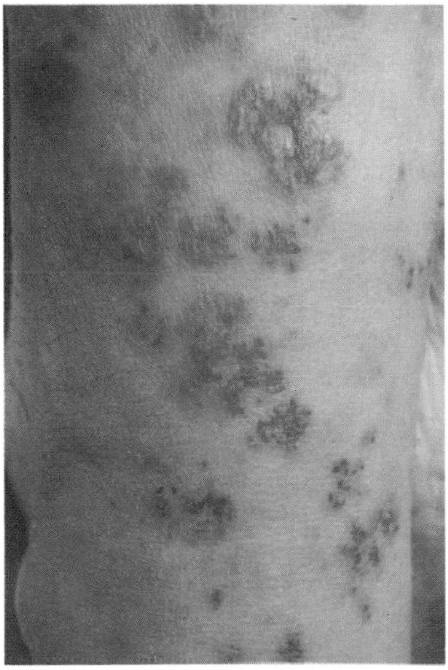

**Fig. 5.14**
Henoch-Schönlein purpura on
the leg of a patient passing
10 g protein a day.

Essential Hypertension
(cause uncertain)

Primary Renal Disease
(e.g., glomerulonephritis)

Probably the commoner cause

Renal hypertension

*Malignant Phase*

Necrotizing arteriolitis

Renal damage and failure

**Fig. 5.15** Progress of renal vascular disease.

## Acute tubular necrosis

This condition may be regarded as vascular in origin resulting from shock, especially in association with crush injuries or postpartum haemorrhage. Acute failure of renal function occurs with oliguria, anuria and uraemic symptoms. Spontaneous recovery may occur in a few weeks: if the patient is maintained by dialysis, function may be restored in about 10 days.

### Renal artery stenosis

Renal artery stenosis (*Fig.* 5.16) is occasionally responsible for hypertension and, if proved by arteriography, may offer chances for surgical relief.

### Renal vein occlusion

Thrombosis of the leg veins may extend through the inferior vena cava to involve the renal veins. The ensuing clinical picture is usually that of the nephrotic syndrome (p. 152) or acute renal failure.

### Pyelonephritis

This is the most serious manifestation of urinary-tract infection. The organism commonly responsible is *Escherichia coli*, as in the case of cystitis (*see* p. 158).

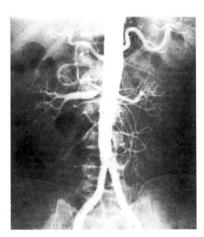

**Fig. 5.16**
An aortogram carried out by catheterization of the femoral artery showing stenosis of the mouth and proximal end of the right renal artery.

In the acute form the classic syndrome includes pain in the loin, on one or both sides, marked loin tenderness, with high fever, rigors and frequency of micturition. There may be recurrent attacks of this kind and the disease may become chronic. In such cases radiological changes due to cortical scars and clubbing of the calices may be found. The urine generally shows a high content of the infecting organism (100 000 per ml or more), pus cells and granular or leucocyte cases. An increase in antibody titres against the O antigen of *Escherichia coli* may also be found.

Pyelonephritis is particularly common during pregnancy and may have been preceded by a high bacteriuria, possibly dating back to childhood. It is now considered that chronic pyelonephritis may exist without clinical symptoms; this may result in a pathological kidney which is difficult to distinguish from other forms of renal disease and indeed may terminate in renal failure.

### Analgesic nephropathy

The regular consumption over many years of mild analgesics containing phenacetin and aspirin can result in necrosis of the renal papillae (papillary necrosis) and interstitial nephritis with ultimately the development of chronic renal failure. The condition is common in Australia where the endemic consumption of analgesics is high while the hot climate encourages the formation of small volumes of highly concentrated urine.

### Renal tuberculosis

The primary lesion is cortical and remains subclinical until the calices and pelvis are affected, when symptoms begin to appear. It is often associated with tuberculous lesions in other parts of the urinary system, e.g. the bladder or epididymis. A tuberculous focus may be found elsewhere, as in the chest or spine.

Constitutional symptoms are rare and the patient remains in good condition. Of the local symptoms, frequency of micturition is most important and progressive; it may be accompanied by pain on micturition. Haematuria may also be a presenting sign. Pyuria is generally recognized if microscopic examination of the urine is made, but special methods of investigation, particularly examination and culture for tubercle bacilli in the urine, cystoscopy and pyelography, may be necessary to establish the diagnosis.

### Renal calculus

Stones may be present in the kidneys without symptoms. Sometimes a dull ache may occur, and if the stone becomes dislodged and passes down the ureter, an attack of colic results (*see* Pain, p. 133).

The traumatic effects of the stone, especially when in movement, often result in haematuria, and the urine should be examined microscopically for red corpuscles.

Calculi may lead to infection of the kidney, affecting the pelvis (pyelitis) or kidney substance (pyelonephritis). A stone impacted at the junction of the pelvis and ureter may cause hydronephrosis or pyonephrosis (*Fig.* 5.17). The impaction of a stone may also cause temporary anuria.

A tendency to form renal calculi may reflect a disturbance in calcium, uric acid or, more rarely, cystine metabolism. Symptoms and signs of hyperparathyroidism (p. 478) should especially be sought.

### 'Tumours' of the kidney

Kidney 'tumours', i.e. swellings or enlargement, generally have the shape of the normal organ (*see* p. 137), but if very large may fill the whole loin or spread into other parts of the abdomen. They vary in consistency from that of normal renal tissue to the extreme hardness of some malignant growths. The more important tumours are hydronephrosis, polycystic disease and hypernephroma. It should be remembered that a normal right kidney is quite commonly palpable, especially in women.

*Hydronephrosis* is a ballooning of the kidney calices and pelvis by retained urine, due to intermittent or partial obstruction of the ureter, in some cases idiopathic and due to neuromuscular disturbance, in some due to calculus. The kidney retains its normal shape but is occasionally large enough to be palpable. Bilateral hydronephrosis results from obstruction to the urethra by a stricture or prostatic enlargement.

*Polycystic disease* is characterized by the development of numerous cysts in the kidney which destroy its substance. The affection is generally bilateral, and the

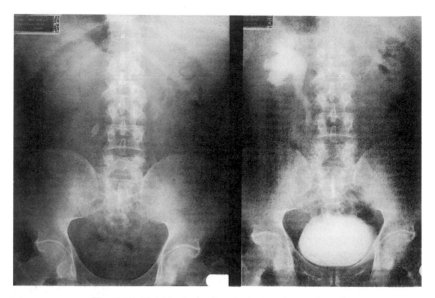

**Fig. 5.17** Right hydronephrosis due to obstruction of ureter by stone illustrated on plain radiograph and intravenous pyelogram.

kidneys are palpable as large 'bossed' reniform tumours. Other symptoms suggest the presence of chronic renal disease (polyuria, proteinuria, high blood pressure, etc.). Haematuria is sometimes a symptom. The condition is often familial, and if it is not recognized in infancy, symptoms may be delayed until middle life.

*Hypernephroma*, the commonest malignant tumour of the kidney, is generally recognized by the presence of a renal tumour with haematuria which is often painless, thus distinguishing it from calculus. It may also show itself by metastases in bone or lungs, and corresponding symptoms such as pain or cough, or by malignant ascites.

## DIALYSIS AND TRANSPLANTATION

Chronic renal failure is fatal, but many patients can now be treated successfully by dialysis and by transplantation. These therapeutic activities have created a new range of extraordinary physical signs to replace the traditional features of severe uraemia.

The patient with a functioning transplant will not usually be anaemic but may show features of mild Cushing's syndrome from taking corticosteroid drugs to prevent graft rejection. There will be an easily palpable, firm, non-tender kidney in either the right or left iliac fossa under the scar of a healed surgical wound (*Fig.* 5.18). During rejection there will be fever and hypertension; the graft will enlarge and become tender, the urine volume falls and renal function deteriorates.

Patients on haemodialysis are more commonly anaemic and pass little or no urine. They usually have an arteriovenous fistula (*Fig.* 5.19) in one arm or forearm with distension of the proximal veins, scars from frequent venepuncture and a palpable thrill with audible bruit over the anastomosis. In some patients the veins may become greatly distended over the years (*Fig.* 5.20). A few patients still have

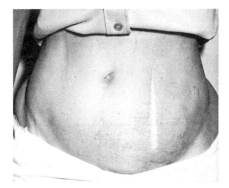

**Fig. 5.18**
Renal implant beneath a scar
in the left iliac fossa.

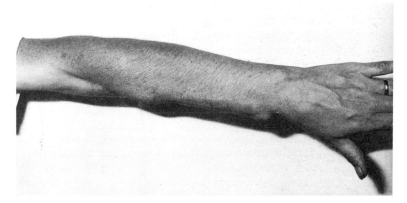

**Fig. 5.19** The swelling just above the wrist is the site of an
arteriovenous fistula created for haemodialysis.

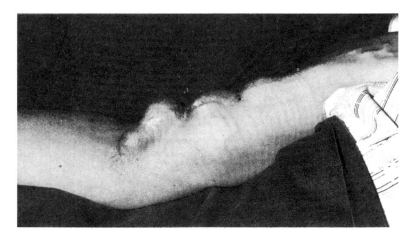

**Fig. 5.20** Gross venous distension in the upper arm resulting
from a long-standing arteriovenous fistula.

indwelling arterial and venous cannulae, joined externally with siliconized latex rubber (silastic) tubing to form a shunt. These are used less commonly now owing to the high incidence of infection and clotting. Some patients are maintained on long-term peritoneal dialysis. In these cases an indwelling soft silastic cannula will be found emerging from the anterior abdominal wall below the umbilicus, usually slightly to one side of the midline.

# ■ DISEASES OF THE BLADDER

## Cystitis

Frequency of micturition and dysuria are the characteristic symptoms of cystitis. Fever is rarely marked. The diagnosis is completed by the finding of pyuria, by the discovery of some causal factor such as prostatic enlargement or vesical calculus and sometimes by cystoscopic examination, which may be necessary to determine the essential nature of the cystitis. Special forms of cystitis causing severe symptoms, especially in women, include Hunner's ulcer (interstitial cystitis) and urethro-trigonitis. Symptoms of recurrent apparent cystitis are common in women and may be due to a chronic urethritis, the so-called 'urethral syndrome'. The aetiology is obscure but is probably multifactorial and includes trauma and prolapse, bacterial infection and hormonal factors.

## Calculus

Calculus in the bladder may cause dysuria and haematuria. Its presence generally requires instrumental (cystoscopy) or radiological methods for its recognition. As it is nearly always secondary, a decision must be made as to whether it has come down from the kidney, or whether it complicates prostatic enlargement or a diverticulum of the bladder.

## Tumours

Tumours (papillomas and carcinomas) usually cause haematuria, and require cystoscopy for their diagnosis. Adenomatous or carcinomatous enlargements of the prostate may project as tumours into the bladder and cause uninary obstruction. This may be recognized by rectal examination. Enlargement of the prostate should always be considered as a cause of urinary symptoms in elderly men, especially when the symptoms resemble those of chronic renal disease (nocturia and slight proteinuria).

# The respiratory system

## ■ SYMPTOMS OF RESPIRATORY DISEASE

### Cough

Cough may be either a voluntary act or a reflex response to irritation of the respiratory mucosa mediated through a centre in the medulla. It consists of a forceful expiratory effort with the glottis closed, followed by the sudden explosive release of the pent-up air along with sputum or other irritant matter.

The student must note whether a cough is dry or productive of sputum, whether it is short or paroxysmal, the times at which it tends to occur and finally the character of the sound. A dry cough occurs when the mucous membrane of the larynx, trachea or bronchi is congested with little or no exudate, as in the early stages of respiratory infections and following the inhalation of irritant dusts or fumes, e.g. tobacco smoke. A 'loose' or productive cough indicates free exudate in the respiratory passages, as in chronic bronchitis and bronchiectasis.

A short cough is usual in upper respiratory infections such as the common cold and when respiratory movements are suppressed by pleuritic pain.

Prolonged or paroxysmal coughing is characteristic of chronic bronchitis and also of whooping-cough, in which a rapid series of coughs is followed by a deep inspiration through a partially closed glottis. A foreign body may be responsible for the abrupt onset of paroxysmal cough, and this possibility must always be considered, especially in children, from whom no history may be forthcoming. A severe paroxysm may be followed by vomiting or by syncope, the latter being due to the raised intrathoracic pressure interfering with venous return to the heart and thus diminishing cardiac output.

Any tendency for cough to occur at particular times should be noted. Cough and expectoration of sputum are often most troublesome on rising in the morning and going to bed at night, especially in chronic bronchitis and bronchiectasis. This may be due to the change in posture moving secretions from damaged insensitive areas of mucosa to more sensitive parts. A change of temperature, as in moving from a warm room to the cold outside air, also provokes cough in patients with chronic bronchitis. For this reason, and also because of the greater frequency of respiratory infections, the cough is worse in winter than in summer. Cough waking the patient at night, although quite common in chronic bronchitis, should always suggest the possibility of pulmonary congestion due to left heart failure or mitral stenosis (*see* p. 268). Other causes of nocturnal cough include asthma (especially in children), secretions running down the larynx from the posterior nares in patients with chronic infections of the nose or sinuses and the inhalation of oesophageal or gastric contents due to oesophageal obstruction or hiatus hernia.

Finally, the character of the actual sound produced by the cough should be observed. Intrathoracic tumours, especially aneurysm, can press on the trachea and cause cough with a metallic, hard quality described as 'brassy'. If a tumour involves the recurrent laryngeal branch of the vagus and interferes with the normal movements of the vocal cords, the cough loses its explosive character and becomes prolonged and wheezing, like that of a cow; it is then known as a 'bovine' cough. Diseases of the larynx responsible for cough (e.g. neoplasm) are sometimes identified by the hoarseness of the cough and the accompanying stridor.

### Sputum

Quite apart from the laboratory examination of sputum, much important information can be gained by naked-eye inspection. The patient should be instructed to expectorate into a sputum cup, and the amount measured after 24 h. The student should note the amount, consistency and colour of the sputum. Large amounts may be found in bronchiectasis and pulmonary abscess or when an empyema ruptures into a bronchus. The expectoration of large quantities of sputum on change of posture is particularly characteristic of bronchiectasis and pulmonary abscess, and in these conditions the sputum may sometimes have an offensive smell due to infection by anaerobic organisms. A large amount of thin, colourless sputum is seen in the relatively rare alveolar cell carcinoma of the lung.

The consistency and colour of the sputum may be of diagnostic value. Thick, viscid sputum, which sometimes takes the shape of bronchial casts, occurs in asthma, especially the kind associated with bronchopulmonary aspergillosis (*Fig.* 6.1). Thin, watery sputum suggests pulmonary oedema. Green coloration indicates pus while a yellow colour may be due to pus or to a high eosinophil content. Blood in the sputum may give a rusty appearance in pneumonia, a diffuse pink staining in pulmonary oedema or it may appear as streaks or clots (*see below*).

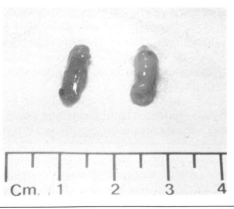

**Fig. 6.1**
Bronchial casts consisting of viscid sputum and fungal mycelia from a patient with asthma associated with bronchopulmonary aspergillosis.

## Haemoptysis

Expectoration of blood is known as haemoptysis. The amount may vary from streaks to several pints and may consist of pure blood or be mixed with sputum or salivary secretions. From the patient's history it is not always easy to determine whether the blood has been coughed up or vomited. The important differences between haemoptysis and haematemesis are summarized in *Table* 6.1.

The staining of the sputum for some days after the haemorrhage is perhaps the most convincing point of distinction between haemoptysis and haematemesis.

If it is definitely established that the blood has been spat up, the mouth and throat should be examined for any local cause, such as epistaxis, bleeding gums or a congested pharynx, which may cause small amounts of blood to appear in the mouth. However, haemoptysis must never be attributed to these causes until a chest radiograph has been proved normal.

The most serious common causes of haemoptysis are bronchial carcinoma, bronchiectasis, mitral valve disease, tuberculosis and pulmonary infarction.

| Table 6.1. | **Diagnosis of haemoptysis and haematemesis** |
|---|---|
| *Haemoptysis* | *Haematemesis* |
| Cough precedes haemorrhage | Nausea and vomiting precede haemorrhage |
| Blood frothy from admixture with air | Generally airless |
| Sputum bright red in colour and may be stained for days | Blood often altered in colour by admixture with gastric contents, usually dark red or brown |
| History suggests respiratory disease | Previous history of indigestion |
| Confirmed by bronchoscopy | Confirmed by gastroscopy |

## Dyspnoea

**Physiological aspects** Dyspnoea, or breathlessness, may be defined as an undue awareness of respiratory effort or of the need to increase this effort.

The awareness of respiratory effort has been related to the force used to ventilate the lungs. This force is increased when the thoracic cage or pleura is abnormally rigid, the pleural cavity filled with fluid or air, airways resistance increased, or the lungs less distensible than normal; this also occurs when there is an increased demand for breathing as a result of hypoxia, anaemia, acidosis or thyrotoxicosis. Dyspnoea may also take the form of an awareness of the need to increase respiratory effort, as in breath-holding and paralysis of the respiratory muscles (e.g. poliomyelitis).

The sensation of dyspnoea is probably derived from two main sources: receptors sensitive to stretch and deflation in the thoracic cage and lungs, and chemoreceptors in the aorta and carotid arteries and in the reticular substance of the medulla which are sensitive to oxygen lack, carbon dioxide excess or changes in pH. The relative importance of these thoracic and central sources of dyspnoea is not known, but experimental work suggests that stimuli arising from receptors in the respiratory muscles themselves are the main immediate cause of dyspnoea even when there is no increase in respiratory movements.

**Clinical aspects** An attempt should be made to assess the severity of the dyspnoea by noting whether it is present at rest, with gentle activity such as undressing or walking on level ground, during moderate exertion, such as climbing stairs, or only on more strenuous exercise. The ability of the patient to carry out routine tasks at work or in the home should also be recorded.

Dyspnoea may be due to disease of the bronchi, lungs, pleura or thoracic cage, to cardiac failure, to an increased central demand for respiration or to psychogenic causes.

1. Dyspnoea due to *disease* of the bronchi, lungs, pleura or thoracic cage is usually brought on by exertion. Dyspnoea which develops suddenly at rest suggests pulmonary embolism or pneumothorax.

2. The dyspnoea of *cardiac failure* is due to an increased stiffness of the lungs resulting from engorgement with blood when the mitral valve is diseased or the left ventricle fails. The dyspnoea is provoked by exertion and relieved by rest, but it is also influenced by posture. When the patient lies flat, gravitational effects increase the congestion of the lungs. This causes dyspnoea when the patient lies down ('orthopnoea', or 'upright breathing'), and sometimes a violent attack of breathlessness may waken him from his sleep ('paroxysmal nocturnal dyspnoea'). These attacks may be accompanied by cyanosis and the expectoration of large amounts of thin, frothy sputum stained pink with blood due to pulmonary oedema. Attacks of cardiac dyspnoea unassociated with effort or changes in posture can also result from myocardial infarction or a rapid dysrhythmia (*see also* Cardiovascular System, Chapter 7).

3. Dyspnoea can result from an *increased demand* for respiration even when the heart, lungs and thoracic cage are healthy. This increased demand arises from stimulation of central receptors by hypoxia (e.g. high altitudes, anaemia), acidosis (e.g. diabetes, uraemia), or when metabolism is increased (e.g. fever, thyrotoxicosis). Other signs of the disease causing the dyspnoea will usually be apparent; the pallor of anaemia should especially be looked for in all patients complaining of breathlessness.

4. *Psychogenic dyspnoea* should never be diagnosed until all possible organic causes have been excluded. This form of dyspnoea is quite common because any discomfort in the chest may be interpreted as breathlessness by the nervous patient. Such discomfort may be due to anxiety about the heart or lungs, ectopic beats, muscular symptoms such as a 'stitch' or gastric flatulence. These relatively innocent conditions in an apprehensive patient may result in sighing respirations and a desire to take frequent deep breaths; the dyspnoea occurs as often at rest as on exertion and especially while talking. These patients may ventilate in excess of metabolic requirements, thus lowering the arterial tension of carbon dioxide to produce such symptoms as dizziness, paraesthesiae and tetanic cramps in the hands due to respiratory alkalosis (*see also* p. 465).

### Pain (*see also* Pain, p. 7)

Lung tissue is insensitive and pain in the chest is always the result of conditions which affect the surrounding structures. When the pleura is involved, pain is a prominent feature. The pain is usually described as 'cutting', 'stabbing' or 'tearing' on deep breathing or coughing. Most commonly it is felt in the axillae and beneath the breasts, but it may occur in regions remote from the chest and cause difficulty in diagnosis. The parietal pleura, including that covering the outer portion of the diaphragm, is innervated through the thoracic roots (intercostal nerves), the lower six of which are responsible for the supply of skin areas on the abdominal wall and back. Pleural pain is therefore frequently referred to the abdomen and lumbar regions, and has given rise to a mistaken diagnosis of acute abdominal lesions.

The innervation of the central portion of the diaphragm by the phrenic nerve (3rd and 4th cervical) occasionally leads to referred pain in the neck and shoulder-tip in diaphragmatic pleurisy.

In lesions of the apex of the lung such as Pancoast's syndrome (bronchial carcinoma causing Horner's syndrome with involvement of the 8th cervical and 1st dorsal nerve roots), all the pain may be referred to the arm.

Finally, it must be mentioned that many pains that occur in the chest are not associated with respiratory disease. These include pains due to disease of the heart (*see* Chapter 7), oesophagus and upper abdominal viscera (e.g. hiatus hernia), osteoarthritis of the spine, lesions of the ribs, sternum and intercostal muscles, herpes zoster and diseases of the breast.

### Upper respiratory tract symptoms

These include sneezing, nasal obstruction and discharges, facial pain due to disease of the nose or paranasal sinuses, and hoarseness or aphonia resulting from laryngeal disease.

### Extrathoracic symptoms of respiratory diseases

Diseases of the respiratory system can produce symptoms in other parts of the body:

1. 'Constitutional' symptoms such as loss of appetite and weight, lassitude, sweats and dyspepsia, as in tuberculosis and carcinoma.

2. Symptoms of hypoxia and carbon dioxide retention ('hypercapnia'), including mental disturbances, headaches, sweats, tremors, convulsions and coma (*see also* Bronchitis, p. 186).

3. Evidence of pulmonary heart disease ('cor pulmonale'): oedema, jugular venous engorgement, liver distension and ascites (*see also* p. 244).

4. Finger clubbing and painful swellings in the limbs due to pulmonary osteo-arthropathy, as in bronchial carcinoma and bronchiectasis (*see* p. 165).

5. Distal manifestations of bronchial carcinoma also include the symptoms of metastases in other organs and, more rarely, various forms of myoneuropathy and endocrine disorder (*see also* Bronchial Carcinoma, p. 187).

---

■      **PHYSICAL SIGNS: EXAMINATION OF THE RESPIRATORY SYSTEM**

---

Certain signs may be noted before the systematic examination of the chest is made, namely, the character of any sputum (p. 160), the presence of cyanosis or clubbing of the fingers and the condition of the neck.

---

## Cyanosis

**Physiological aspects** Cyanosis, a blue coloration of the skin or mucosae, occurs when there is an excess of desaturated haemoglobin or of certain abnormal haemoglobins in the capillaries. Desaturated haemoglobin rarely causes cyanosis until it amounts to more than about 5 g/dl (30 per cent of the total amount of haemoglobin in the capillaries), and even then there is great variation in the ability of different observers to recognize cyanosis. Moreover, desaturation does not happen until there is already considerable hypoxia because haemoglobin only gives up its oxygen when the tension in the blood has fallen below about 10·6 kPa (80 mmHg) (normal 13·3 kPa, 100 mmHg). It is apparent, therefore, that cyanosis is usually a sign of severe oxygen deficiency.

Cyanosis may be classified according to its cause:

1. *Peripheral cyanosis*. This is due to a diminished capillary blood flow allowing more time for the removal of oxygen by the tissues. There are two types of peripheral cyanosis:

   *a.* Cyanosis due to a reduced cardiac output (e.g. mitral stenosis, shock, etc.).

   *b.* Cyanosis due to local vasoconstriction (e.g. cold).

2. *Central cyanosis*. In this form of cyanosis there is an excess of desaturated haemoglobin in the blood leaving the aorta. There are three types of central cyanosis:

   *a.* Cyanosis due to deficient oxygenation of the blood in the lungs resulting from inadequate ventilation of perfused areas of lung (e.g. pneumonia; chronic bronchitis), from a reduction in the total amount of air ventilating the lungs as a whole (e.g. poliomyelitis); or from impaired oxygen transfer across the alveolar capillary membrane (e.g. fibrosing alveolitis).

   *b.* Cyanosis due to a right-to-left shunt of blood bypassing the lungs through a septal defect in the heart (e.g. Fallot's tetralogy) or between a pulmonary artery and vein (arteriovenous aneurysm) (p. 292). A shunt effect may also occur through a lobe or segment of lung of which the bronchus is occluded (e.g. bronchial carcinoma).

   *c.* Cyanosis due to an absolute excess of desaturated haemoglobin, the percentage saturation being normal. This occurs in primary polycythaemia.

3. *Cyanosis due to abnormal pigments (Enterogenous cyanosis)*. This form of cyanosis, which results from the presence in the red cells of an excess of either sulph-haemoglobin or methaemoglobin, sometimes imparts a mauve or brownish tinge to the skin. It is unaccompanied by dyspnoea or other respiratory symptoms, but headache, lassitude and constipation are common. Enterogenous cyanosis is usually due to the ingestion of substances that favour the combination of haemoglobin and sulphur absorbed from the bowel or the reduction of haemoglobin to methaemoglobin (e.g. sulphonamides, phenacetin and other analgesic drugs). These abnormal haemoglobins can be identified by spectroscopic examination of the blood.

**Clinical aspects** The patient or a relative may report that cyanosis is present all the time or only during exertion or exposure to cold. Cyanosis must be looked for in the extremities (the fingers and toes, nose, lips and ears) and also in the oral mucosa. If there is doubt, cyanosis can be brought to light by exercise, which increases the removal of oxygen by the tissues. Peripheral and central cyanosis can be distinguished by warming the hands in a bowl of hot water or by inspection of a naturally warm part such as the oral mucosa: heat increases capillary blood flow and thus abolishes peripheral cyanosis. If cyanosis persists in a warm part, then it must be either central or enterogenous. The effect of breathing pure oxygen for 10 minutes should then be observed: cyanosis due to lung disease or polycythaemia will disappear while cyanosis due either to a right-to-left shunt bypassing the lungs or to abnormal pigments will remain (*see Table* 6.2).

| Table 6.2 | **The effects of local heat and breathing oxygen on the different types of cyanosis** | |
|---|---|---|
| *Cause of cyanosis* | *Local Heat* | *Breathing oxygen* (for 10 min) |
| *Peripheral* | Abolished | Remains |
| *Central*: Pulmonary | Remains | Abolished |
| Polycythaemic | Remains | Abolished |
| Right-to-left shunt | Remains | Remains |
| *Enterogenous* | Remains | Remains |

## Clubbing of the fingers (*Fig.* 6.2)

This is an important sign of certain diseases of the lungs and also of the heart and alimentary system; rarely it may be congenital in origin. It can be recognized by a bulbousness of the soft terminal portion of the fingers and by an excessive curvature of the nail in both the longitudinal and lateral planes. An early sign of clubbing is loss of the normal angle at the base of the nail, seen best in the lateral view. Later the nail may become loose in its bed so that movement can be elicited when light pressure is exerted over the nail base ('fluctuation'). Sometimes, the finger ends are also cyanotic and the nails abnormally shiny.

Finger clubbing may be associated with similar changes in the toes and, in bronchial carcinoma especially, with a painful swelling over the ends of the long bones. This last condition is known as 'hypertrophic pulmonary osteoarthropathy'

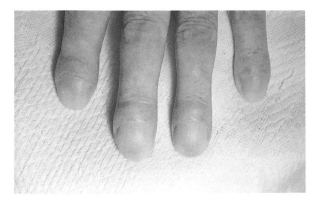

**Fig. 6.2** Finger clubbing due to bronchial carcinoma.

and must always be considered when a patient with finger clubbing complains of symptoms that suggest arthritis in the wrists and ankles. The exact cause of clubbing and osteoarthropathy remains uncertain, but the local changes are probably due to an overgrowth of the soft tissues and subjacent periosteum associated with an increased peripheral blood flow (*Fig.* 6.3). These changes will sometimes regress if the primary cause is removed.

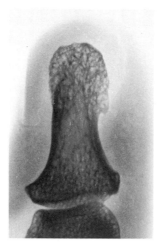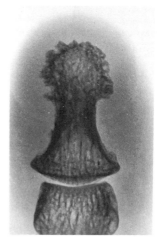

**Fig. 6.3** Radiograph of a clubbed finger (*right*) compared with the normal (*left*). Note soft tissue swelling and overgrowth of subperiosteal bone.

## The neck

Examination of the neck may reveal important signs of respiratory system disease. The student should inspect the neck for engorged jugular veins and accessory respiratory movements and then palpate the trachea and lymph nodes.

**The jugular veins** These may be overfilled, not only in congestive cardiac failure (p. 268) but in superior mediastinal obstruction due, for example, to bronchial carcinoma (*Fig.* 6.4). These two causes can be distinguished by the presence of pulsation in cardiac failure and its absence in mediastinal obstruction (p. 193). Filling of the jugular veins during expiration and emptying during inspiration may result from raised intrathoracic pressure in patients with expiratory airways obstruction (e.g. asthma).

**Accessory respiratory movements** Inspiratory contraction of the sternomastoid muscles may occur with respiratory distress of any kind, but is particularly associated with overinflation of the lungs due to chronic airways obstruction. The sternomastoids are best examined by drawing them backwards between thumb and forefinger to see if they become taut with inspiration. Abnormal recession of the suprasternal and supraclavicular fossae may also be observed during inspiration in these patients.

**The trachea** This is palpated in the suprasternal notch for lateral displacement

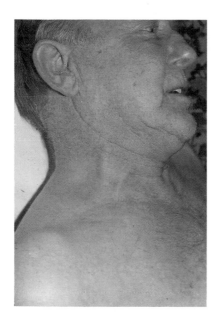

**Fig. 6.4** Mediastinal tumour. Engorged veins in the neck.

(p. 175). The length of trachea which can be felt between the cricoid cartilage and sternal notch (normal: 3–4 fingerbreadths) may be reduced by elevation of the sternum in patients with chronic overinflation of the lungs. Also in these patients, the downwards pull of the diaphragm can cause descent of the trachea and larynx during inspiration; this can be detected by resting the tip of the index finger on the thyroid cartilage. A downwards pull on the larynx may also occur during systole in patients with aortic aneurysm ('tracheal tug').

**Lymph nodes** These may be enlarged from secondary bronchial carcinoma, lymphoma, tuberculosis or sarcoidosis. Careful palpation of the supraclavicular fossae is especially important in cases of lung disease since the scalene nodes are the most commonly affected and also because carcinoma of the lung apex (Pancoast tumour) may be felt at this site.

### The larynx

Examination of this structure should be made in all cases of chronic respiratory disease. Changes in the voice and special types of cough should be noted. The laryngoscope may show tuberculous ulceration in association with the pulmonary disease or vocal cord paralysis, especially in cases of mediastinal tumour and malignant disease of the lung.

### INSPECTION OF THE CHEST

The skin over the chest wall should be noted as in the inspection of any part of the body. Particular attention should be directed to the presence of engorged veins (*Fig.* 6.5) or subcutaneous nodules (*see also* p. 330).

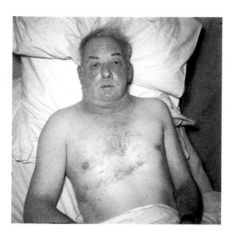

**Fig. 6.5**
Superior mediastinal
obstruction. Note swelling of
neck, dilated veins on the
chest and dusky tint of face.

## Position of the apex beat and trachea

Except in very thin patients, the trachea can rarely be seen, and obesity may also mask the impulse of the heart apex; palpation is therefore necessary to confirm their position. The heart and trachea may be displaced to the opposite side by pleural effusion or pneumothorax, or drawn to the same side by pulmonary fibrosis. Displacement of the heart towards the left axilla may give a false suggestion of cardiac enlargement. Displacement to the right causes the cardiac impulse to appear well within the nipple line, and the maximal pulsation may even be to the right of the sternum.

## Character of respiratory movements

**Expansion of the chest** The degree of the expansion of the chest may be measured by placing a tape measure just below the nipples, with its zero mark at the middle of the sternum, and instructing the patient to breathe in and out as deeply as possible. In women mammary tissue should be avoided by making the measurements above or below the breasts. It is important that several readings should be taken, as the initial respiratory efforts are often shallower than subsequent ones.

Particular note should also be made of the equality of expansion of the two sides. In the absence of skeletal changes, such as scoliosis or the effects of poliomyelitis, a definite inequality signifies disease of the bronchi, lungs or pleurae. The affected side, whatever the pathology, usually moves less than the sound side. Generalized restriction of expansion is more commonly seen in emphysema, though it occurs in extensive bilateral disease and in ankylosing spondylitis.

**Manner of breathing** The manner of breathing should next be noted. In men the diaphragm is more freely used than the intercostal muscles, and its downward excursion with inspiration leads to free movements of the abdominal wall—abdominal respiration. Similar breathing is characteristic of children.

In women, on the other hand, the movements of the chest are greater than those of the abdomen, because respiration is chiefly accomplished by use of the intercostal muscles—thoracic respiration. Various mixtures of these two types of breathing—diaphragmatic and costal—are found in health, but a sudden change in the type of breathing may be significant of disease. Thus, acute peritonitis by limiting the abdominal movements produces a costal type of breathing, while pain from pleurisy or other cause may lead to restriction of the chest movements. When the diaphragm is paralysed, the upper part of the abdomen may be drawn in during inspiration.

**The rate and depth of respiration** The rate and depth of respiration should be observed without the patient's knowledge, as consciousness of the act of breathing tends to make it irregular. The rate varies in normal individuals between 16 and 20/min at rest, but is faster in children and slower in old age. It bears a definite ratio to the pulse rate of about 1:4, which is usually constant in the same individual. The depth of breathing, or tidal ventilation, is about 500 ml at rest, but some form of spirometer is needed to make this measurement (*see* Pulmonary Function Tests, p. 198).

The rate and depth of breathing are regulated by the respiratory centre through reflexes deriving from receptors in the thorax and great vessels (*see also* Dyspnoea, p. 161). They usually increase or decrease together, but rate may increase at the expense of depth when deep breathing is inhibited by a pleuritic pain or by gross reduction of the vital capacity (e.g. extensive pulmonary fibrosis, poliomyelitis). Conversely, slow deep breathing is sometimes seen in airflow obstruction and cerebral conditions associated with coma. An increased rate ('tachypnoea') and depth ('hyperpnoea') occur when there is an increased demand for ventilation, as in exercise, fever, thyrotoxicosis, acidosis and diseases of the heart or lungs associated with hypoxia or hypercapnia (*see also* Dyspnoea, p. 161). A decrease takes place during sleep and when the respiratory centre is depressed by cerebral disease or narcotic drugs.

**Abnormal types of breathing** When there is great dyspnoea the accessory muscles of respiration may be called into play. During inspiration, the sterno-mastoid and other neck muscles contract, the nares are dilated by the alae nasi (especially in children) and there are often gasping movements of the mouth. During expiration the abdominal muscles contract and patients with airways obstruction may purse their lips; this probably serves to prevent collapse of the airways during expiration by raising the intrabronchial pressure (*Fig.* 6.6) (*see also* Emphysema, p. 194). In-drawing of the intercostal spaces during inspiration may be seen in patients, children especially, with severe airways osbstruction. Multiple fractures of the ribs or sternum can result in a flail chest with paradoxical breathing, the unsupported chest wall being drawn in by the negative intrathoracic pressure during inspiration.

A special variety of breathing known as Cheyne–Stokes respiration consists of a temporary cessation of breathing (apnoea) followed by respirations which gradually increase in magnitude to a maximum and then diminish until apnoea occurs once more. This phenomenon is usually found in illnesses which interfere with the function of the respiratory centre, such as hypoxia, raised intracranial pressure, uraemia and advanced heart disease (*see also* Chapter 7). In nervous subjects, breathing may be irregular in rate and depth and interspersed with deep sighing breaths.

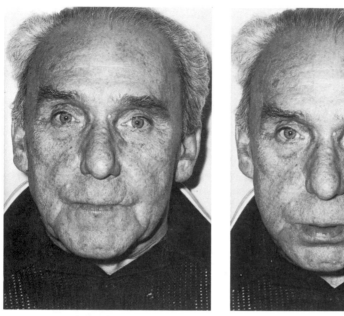
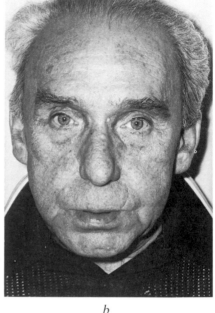

*a*                                                          *b*

**Fig. 6.6** Lip pursing in a patient with emphysema. *a,* Lips tightly apposed at height of inspiration. *b,* Lips held narrowly apart during expiration.

### Chest deformities

Abnormalities of the chest wall are not infrequently present without disease of the thoracic contents. The softness of the bones in childhood renders the chest liable to deformities if the normal relationship between intrathoracic pressure and that of the atmosphere is disturbed. For example, nasal obstruction due to adenoids and broncial narrowing due to asthma or bronchitis may produce gross alteration in the configuration of the chest. Many types of chest deformity exist, amongst which may be mentioned:

1. *Harrison's sulcus,* a groove running horizontally from the sternum outwards in the lower part of the chest.

2. *Pigeon-chest,* in which there is marked bulging of the sternum; this is a common sequel to asthma in childhood (*see Fig.* 6.31, p. 186).

3. *Funnel breast,* an exaggeration of the normal depression seen at the lower end of the sternum. This is often congenital in origin (*Fig.* 6.7). Combinations of these three are sometimes present. Rickets favours their production by making the bones abnormally soft, and sometimes leaves further traces as a 'rickety rosary', a series of knob-like projections on the chest wall at the junction of the ribs with the costal cartilages. Deformities of the thoracic cage can also result from osteomalacia due to malabsorption from the bowel (*see* Malabsorption Syndrome, p. 112).

4. The *barrel-shaped chest,* in which the chest is fixed in the inspiratory position

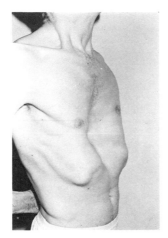

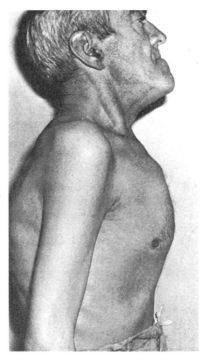

**Fig. 6.7**
Funnel sternum.

**Fig. 6.8**
Barrel-shaped chest of
emphysema. Note especially
the great increase in
anteroposterior diameter, the
gentle kyphosis and the
prominent sternal angle. Note
that the sternomastoid is
acting as an accessory
muscle of inspiration.

(*Fig.* 6.8). This deformity may occur in emphysema but is not a constant or diagnostic sign of this disease.

5. *Spinal deformities*: ankylosing spondylitis restricts the expansion of the chest by immobilizing the costovertebral joints, while kyphoscoliosis (*Fig.* 6.9) may so diminish the volume of the lungs as to cause cardiac and respiratory failure in middle life.

6. Localized bulging or recession of the chest wall may result from aneurysm, empyema, cardiac hypertrophy, local disease of the ribs or sternum and fibrotic changes in the lungs and pleura.

### Anatomical landmarks (*Figs.* 6.10, 6.11)

It will be convenient before leaving the examination of the chest by inspection to recall a few important facts in thoracic anatomy.

The *sternal angle* is formed by the junction of the manubrium with the body of the sternum, and corresponds with the attachment of the second costal cartilage to the sternum. It is a convenient bony point from which to count the ribs and intercostal spaces. It serves as a guide to the position of the thoracic viscera by marking the level of the bifurcation of the trachea, the meeting of the lung borders and the upper limit of the atria.

Posteriorly, the *scapulae* cover a large area of the chest which is relatively

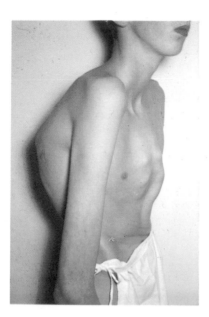

**Fig. 6.9**
Congenital kyphoscoliosis and sternal deformity (Marfan's syndrome).

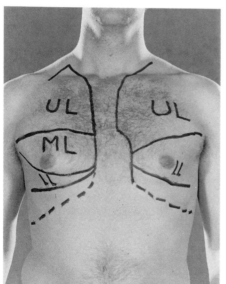

**Fig. 6.10** Anatomical landmarks of the lungs and pleurae as seen from the front. The lobes of the lungs are marked out by plain black lines. The lower limit of the pleura is marked by the dotted line. UL, upper lobe; ML, middle lobe; LL, lower lobe.

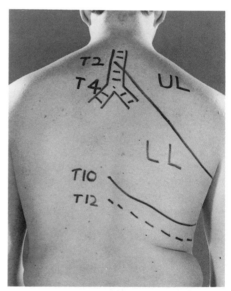

**Fig. 6.11** Anatomical landmarks of the lungs and pleurae as seen from the back. The right side only is marked. The plain lines indicate the upper and lower boundaries of the lower lobe of the lung. The dotted line indicates the lower limit of the pleura. The trachea and its bifurcation and the positions of the spines of the 4th, 10th and 12th dorsal vertebrae are shown. UL, upper lobe; LL, lower lobe.

inacessible to examination. The spine of the scapula is usually at the level of the 2nd thoracic vertebra, its angle reaching to the 7th vertebra. The roots of the lungs lie in the interscapular region at the level of the spines of the 4th, 5th and 6th thoracic vertebrae.

The *lobes of the lung* are separated by the oblique fissure, above which lies the upper lobe (and the middle lobe on the right side), and below it the lower lobes.

The fissure runs roughly in the line of the fifth rib, being slightly above at the back and a little below in the front. The upper margin of the right middle lobe is defined by a line from the 4th costal cartilage to the fifth rib in the mid-axilla: the lingula of the left upper lobe is a little higher in front but extends to a similar point in the axilla.

It will be recognized that the upper lobes are principally accessible from the front, and the lower lobes from the back: in the axillae important segments of all lobes are open to examination. Further, it will be appreciated that there are five bronchopulmonary segments above the fifth rib, and on the right side at least, five below. The radiological identification of these segments is important in defining more accurately the extent of a pulmonary lesion with a lobe (*Figs.* 6.12, 6.13).

The apices of the upper lobes rise about 2–3 cm above the clavicles. From this point the inner margins of the lungs and their covering pleurae slant towards the

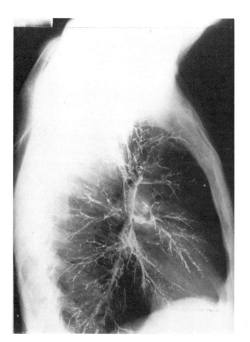
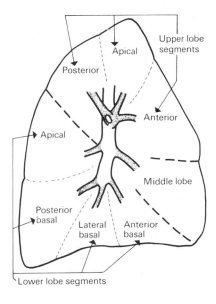

**Fig. 6.12** Bronchogram and diagram of bronchopulmonary segments of right lung. The middle lobe embraces a medial and a lateral segment. The lower lobe also has a medial basal segment which lies on the mediastinal aspect of the lobe and is therefore not shown in this lateral view.

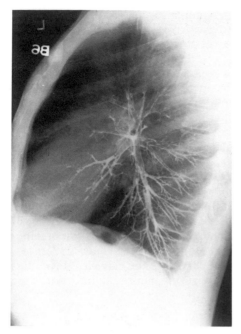
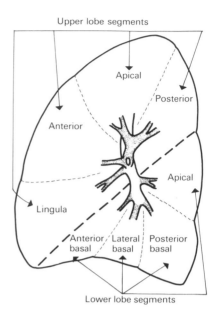

**Fig. 6.13** Bronchogram and diagram of bronchopulmonary segments of left lung. Note that the apical and posterior segments of the left upper lobe arise from a common bronchus so that they are usually described together as the 'apicoposterior segment'.

sternum, meeting each other in the midline at the sternal angle. On the right side this margin of the lung continues down the sternum as far as the sixth costal cartilage, where it turns outwards and downwards to meet the midaxillary line about the eighth rib, the scapular line at the tenth rib, and the paravertebral line at the spine of the 10th thoracic vertebra. On the left side the landmarks are the same, with the exception that the lung border turns away from the sternum at the fourth instead of the sixth costal cartilage, owing to the position of the heart, which lies closely in contact with the chest wall over this region. At the apices, and along the inner margins of the lungs, the pleura lies so close to the lungs as to follow the same surface markings, but at the lower borders of the lungs the pleura extends farther, lying 4–5 cm below the lung borders anteriorly and posteriorly, and as much as 9–10 cm below in the axillae. These costodiaphragmatic recesses of the pleural cavity may be filled up with lung substance during deep inspiration.

## PALPATION

For successful palpation the hands must be warm and used as gently as possible. They should be placed over the two apices, and by looking over the patient's shoulders, with his chin dropped on the chest, the movement of the upper lobes can be compared. The lower lobes may similarly be examined by

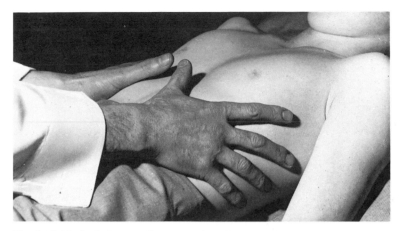

**Fig. 6.14** Method of comparing expansion of the two sides of the chest.

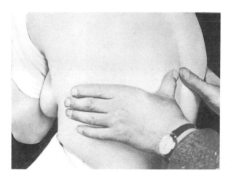

**Fig. 6.15**
Palpation of the bases behind. The thumbs meet at the vertebral spines during expiration and the fingers extend towards the axillae.

placing the hands around the costal margins, in the lower parts of the axillae or over the bases of the lungs at the back (*Figs.* 6.14, 6.15).

Examination of the vocal fremitus may then be made at the same areas.

The position of the apex beat and of the trachea should be confirmed by palpation (*Fig.* 6.16). To determine the position of the trachea the finger should be inserted above the suprasternal notch. The finger will slip to one side if the trachea is deviated.

The axillae and supraclavicular fossae should be examined for hard lymph nodes which may be the only evidence of malignancy. Palpation also detects subcutaneous emphysema, which has a characteristic spongy feeling and usually results from injury to the lung due to fracture of the ribs, drainage of a pneumothorax or rupture of the oesophagus. If it is overlooked and the area auscultated, crepitations may be wrongly diagnosed. The sternum, ribs and intercostal spaces should be palpated for abnormal swellings or tenderness.

### Vocal fremitus

This special sign consists in detecting vibrations transmitted to the hand from the larynx through the bronchi, lungs and chest wall. The patient is

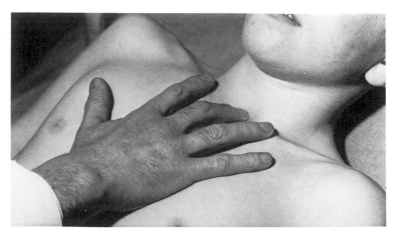

**Fig. 6.16** Tracheal position: method of palpation.

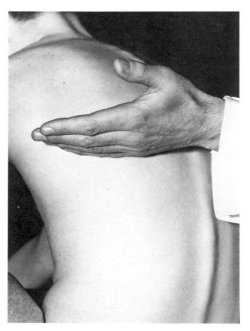

**Fig. 6.17**
Vocal fremitus. For accurate comparison of the vocal fremitus in different parts of the chest the ulnar border of the hand should be used. Compare ribs with ribs, and intercostal spaces with intercostal spaces.

asked to say 'ninety-nine', or 'one, one, one', and the same hand is placed on the chest in identical places on the two sides in turn. The flat of the hand may be used, or for more accurate localization the ulnar border of the hand, which is more sensitive (*Fig.* 6.17).

An increase or decrease in vocal fremitus has the same significance as the corresponding change in vocal resonance (*see below*).

## PERCUSSION

Percussion consists in setting up artificial vibrations in a tissue by means of a sharp tap, usually with the fingers. The middle finger of the left hand is placed in close contact with the tissues, in this case the chest wall. A blow is then made on the second phalanx of this finger with the middle finger of the right hand. The striking finger must be kept at right-angles to the other finger as it falls, and the blow must be made by movements of the wrist only; no movement of the shoulder is necessary (*Figs.* 6.18–6.21). The striking finger must be lifted clear immediately after the blow to avoid damping the resulting vibrations. If the organ or tissue to be percussed lies superficially, percussion should be light, but if it lies

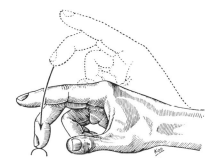

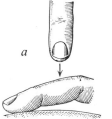

**Fig. 6.18**
Correct method of percussion. Note the movement of the wrist and the vertical position of the terminal phalanx of the percussion finger as it strikes the other.

**Fig. 6.19**
Errors in percussion. a, Incorrect—the striking finger is not making close contact with the tissue to be percussed. b, Correct position.

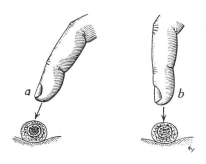

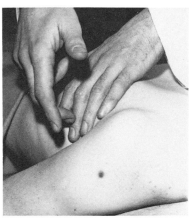

**Fig. 6.20**
Errors in percussion. a, Incorrect—the finger is not vertical as it strikes the other. b, Correct method.

**Fig. 6.21**
Percussion of the axilla.

deep or should it be desired to set into vibration a large mass of tissue such as the base of one lung, heavy percussion must be employed. Light percussion on the clavicles (*Fig.* 6.22) is a useful method of determining changes in the character of the lung substance at the apices. Heavy percussion may be accomplished by using two fingers instead of one, or by using several fingers without any intermediate finger (*Fig.* 6.23).

The percussion note is altered by change in the structure of the underlying tissues. Thus hyper-resonance is found when air fills the pleural cavity (pneumothorax), or is contained unloculated in a large lung cyst. Dullness may be found when the normal air-containing lung tissue becomes solidified, as in

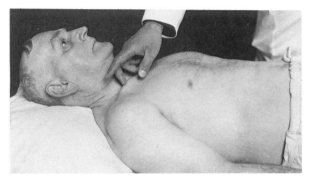

**Fig. 6.22** Percussion on the clavicle. Sometimes changes in the character of the lung tissue at one apex, e.g. consolidation, produce a change of note on percussion over the corresponding clavicle.

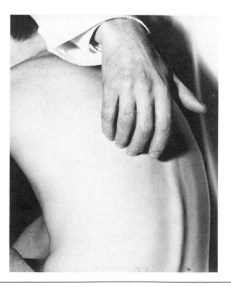

**Fig. 6.23**
Heavy percussion. The fingers are used direct.

pneumonia, new growth and fibrosis, while absolute or stony dullness is present over pleural effusions or occasionally over solid lung if the bronchus is blocked. Overinflation of the lungs, as in emphysema, may abolish the normal liver and cardiac dullness. The student should familiarize himself with these various notes by percussing the appropriate parts of his body (lung for normal resonance, lower abdomen for hyper-resonance or tympany, liver for dullness and thigh for stony dullness).

## AUSCULTATION

Before using the stethoscope the student should listen carefully to the patient's breathing. The breathing of a healthy resting subject cannot be heard at a distance of more than a few inches from the face. Audible breathing at rest can be an important early sign of airways disease. It may be caused by vibrations of airways tissues or secretions, or by turbulent airflow due either to increased velocity of flow or to airways narrowing.

A variety of breathing sounds of diagnostic relevance can be detected by the unaided ear.

1. *Stertorous breathing*. This is due to vibrations of the soft tissues of the naso-pharynx, larynx and cheeks resulting from loss of muscle tone. It may occur in coma from any cause and in some subjects during sleep (snoring).

2. *Rattling breathing* due to vibration of mucus retained in the main airways. This indicates ineffectual cough due to suppression of the cough reflex or to general weakness.

3. *Gasping, grunting and sighing*. These sounds are mainly due to increased velocity of airflow and can be normal responses to a variety of physical and emotional stimuli: exercise, pain, cold, fear and grief. When persistent, however, they may reflect some form of chronic anxiety state.

4. *Hissing* (Kussmaul's) breathing is produced by the patient taking deep breaths through a nearly closed mouth. This probably signifies hyperventilation without dyspnoea and therefore without reflex opening of the mouth during inspiration. It is a sign of severe acidosis, as in diabetic ketosis, uraemia and salicylate poisoning.

5. *Wheezing* is usually louder on expiration than on inspiration and denotes narrowing of the bronchi as in asthma. As already mentioned, airways narrowing of lesser degree can lead to audible breathing without wheeze.

6. *Stridor* is of lower pitch than wheeze and more closely resembles a voice sound. It can be simulated by partial closure of the vocal cords while breathing deeply. Unlike wheeze, stridor is at least as loud in inspiration as in expiration for two reasons: first, because it usually results from narrowing of the extrathoracic airways (trachea or larynx), which are not subject to intrathoracic pressure changes; secondly, because the narrowing is often due to a rigid lesion such as tumour, which prevents fluctuation in airways diameter during the respiratory cycle.

### Use of the stethoscope

Quietness is essential for good auscultation, and some experience is necessary in learning to disregard noises which come through the stethoscope but which are not the direct result of respiration or cardiac contraction. Hair on the chest produces crackling noises which may be mistaken for lung sounds. Unless all clothes are removed from the chest, sounds will inevitably be heard from their friction against the chest wall or on stethoscope tubing, and care should be taken to see that blankets put around the shoulders are not allowed to move. If the patient is nervous or cold, shivering will produce sounds similar to those heard over a contracting muscle. In general, low pitched sounds are best heard with the bell resting lightly on the skin and high pitched sounds with firm pressure from the diaphragm.

As in other methods by which the chest is examined, identical points on the two sides must be compared, particularly beneath the clavicles and in the supraspinous fossa to examine the upper lobes, and over the lower ribs (seventh to tenth) at the back for auscultation of the lower lobes, and in the axillae where there is access to parts of all the lobes.

Auscultation must be carried out with definite objectives in mind:

1. To determine whether the breath sounds are equal on the two sides.
2. To ascertain the character of the breath sounds.
3. To detect any added sounds and decide their nature, and whether they are intra- or extrapulmonary.
4. To compare the voice sounds over different parts of the lungs.

### Breath sounds (*Figs.* 6.24, 6.25)

Breath sounds are due to fluctuations in intraluminal pressure and oscillation of solid tissues which result from turbulent gas flow in the trachea and

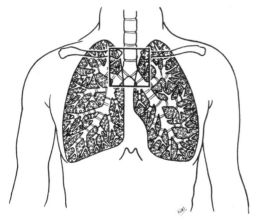

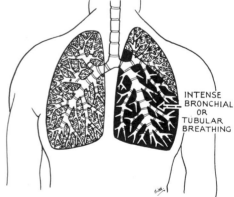

INTENSE BRONCHIAL OR TUBULAR BREATHING

**Fig. 6.24**
Breath sounds in normal lung, anterior aspect. The square marks the area of broncho-vesicular breathing, which is found also over the corresponding part of the back. Over other areas normal vesicular breath sounds are heard.

**Fig. 6.25**
Breath sounds in solid lung, such as occurs in pneumonia. Lung alveoli airless, bronchi patent, breath sounds bronchial or tubular. Lower lobe only shown as affected.

proximal bronchi. In the small peripheral airways and alveoli, gas flow is of lower velocity and laminar in type and is therefore silent.

The type and intensity of breath sounds are modified by the filtering effect of tissues between source and stethoscope. Breath sounds from which high frequencies have been filtered by normally inflated alveoli are described as *vesicular* (the vesicles, or alveoli, acting as the filter, not the source, of the sound). This is a rustling noise, louder and more prolonged in inspiration than in expiration (*Fig.* 6.26). The less the filtering, the more closely will the sound approximate to its source in the trachea and bronchi, i.e. to *bronchial* breathing. This is a higher pitched clearer sound than vesicular breathing, inspiration and expiration are of equal length and there is a distinct gap between them. When this type of breathing is found over the lungs themselves it is invariably abnormal, although a modified form (*bronchovesicular*) may be heard when the stethoscope is placed near to the trachea in the midline of the chest.

 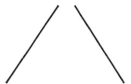 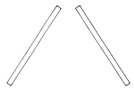

*Vesicular*
Rustling quality Expiration shorter and softer than inspiration and continuous with it

*Bronchial*
Loud and clear. Expiration and inspiraton of same duration and intensity, and separated by a pause

*Cavernous*
As for bronchial, but more 'hollow' in quality

**Fig. 6.26** Breath sounds.

**Abnormal breath sounds** Thoracic diseases may either diminish the intensity of breath sounds or alter their quality to give bronchial breathing.

A generalized reduction in the intensity of the sound may result from obesity or overinflation of the lung and also from hypoventilation. A localized reduction in breath sounds occurs when there is diminution of air entry (e.g. bronchial occlusion) or when the bronchial source of the sound is deflected at interfaces between media with different acoustic properties, as in the case of pleural effusion and pneumothorax.

Bronchial breathing is heard when the medium interposed between the bronchi and stethoscope is a good conductor of sound and, unlike normal alveoli, permits the passage of high frequencies. This occurs when the alveoli contain fluid instead of air (consolidation), when there is collapse or fibrosis of the lung with patent bronchi and sometimes over a thin layer of pleural fluid (e.g. at the top of a pleural effusion). Bronchial breathing may also occur when for any reason the trachea or main bronchi are so displaced as to be physically nearer to the stethoscope.

Rarely, a bronchus may communicate directly with a large abnormal air space either in the lung (cavity) or pleural space (pneumothorax). This can give rise to a hollow resonating breath sound known as *cavernous* or *amphoric* breathing (*Figs.* 6.27, 6.28).

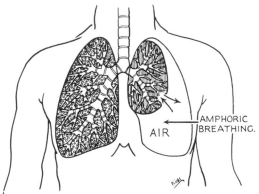

**Fig. 6.27**
Breath sounds in open pneumothorax. Amphoric breath sounds. Lung collapsed. Bronchi partially obliterated. Communication at arrows between lung and pleural sac. (For other effects of pneumothorax, such as mediastinal displacement, *see Fig.* 6.38).

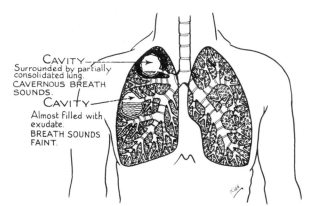

**Fig. 6.28**
Breath sounds in cavitation. Cavernous breath sounds. If the cavity is well filled no abnormal breath sounds will be heard, though breathing may be faint.

## Voice sounds

Normal lung filters out high frequency vowel sounds so that speech (e.g. 'ninety-nine') is heard through the stethoscope as a low-pitched mumble. When the lung is airless as in consolidation, fibrosis or collapse with a patent airway, the vowel sounds come through to produce intelligible, syllabic speech. This sound is termed *bronchophony* and its acoustic basis is the same as for bronchial breathing.

Whispering is a high frequency sound produced by turbulent airflow in upper airways. This sound is therefore filtered out by normal lung and, like bronchophony, can be heard through the stethoscope only when the lung is airless and the airways patent – *whispering pectoriloquy*.

At the upper limit of a pleural effusion, where the fluid layer is thin, the voice sounds are reflected with loss of the low frequency elements. This gives rise to a high-pitched sound with a nasal bleating quality – *aegophony*.

## Added sounds (*Fig.* 6.29)

Chest diseases can give rise to three kinds of added sound: *wheezes*, *crackles* and *pleural friction*. *Wheezes* are due to the oscillation of airways and other tissues set into motion by an impediment to airflow.

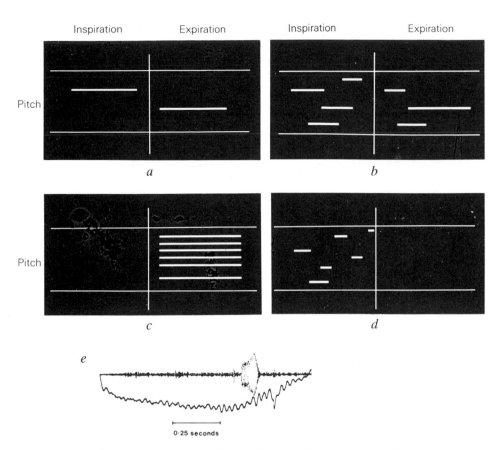

Inspiration     Expiration     Inspiration     Expiration

Pitch

*a*       *b*

Pitch

*c*       *d*

*e*

0·25 seconds

**Fig. 6.29** *a*, Fixed monophonic wheeze. *b*, Randon monophonic wheezes. *c*, Expiratory polyphonic wheeze. *d*, Sequential inspiratory wheezes (squawks). *e*, Pneumograph of a squawk (immediately preceded by a crackle). The lower curved line indicates the rate of inspiratory airflow. (*a – d*, reproduced from *Lung Sounds*, by kind permission of Dr Paul Forgacs and Ballière Tindall; *e*, by kind permission of Dr John Earis.)

**Fixed monophonic wheeze** This is a single note of constant pitch, timing and site. It results from air passing at high velocity through a localized narrowing of one airway. Bronchial carcinoma is the commonest cause. *Stridor (see* p. 179) is a special example of this sound.

**Random monophonic wheezes** These are random single notes which may be scattered and overlapping throughout inspiration and expiration and are of varying duration, timing and pitch. They signify widespread airflow obstruction, as in asthma or bronchitis.

**Expiratory polyphonic wheeze** This is a complex musical sound with all its component parts starting together and continuing to the end of expiration. It is probably due to expiratory dynamic compression of large central airways and is therefore audible at the mouth. When unaccompanied by inspiratory wheezes, it usually indicates emphysema in which the central airways are narrowed by the positive pressure which has to be exerted to empty the inelastic lungs.

**Sequential inspiratory wheezes ('squawks')** A series of sequential (not overlapping) inspiratory sounds or sometimes a single sound (*Fig.* 6.29*e*), due to the opening of airways which had become abnormally apposed during the previous expiration. These tend to occur in deflated areas of lung and are therefore heard in various forms of pulmonary fibrosis, especially fibrosing alveolitis. The mechanism is similar to that of crackles and these often precede the squawk.

**Crackles (*Fig.* 6.30)** These result from the explosive equalization of gas pressure between two airway compartments when a closed section between them suddenly opens. Expiratory closure of airways is gravity-dependent, so that crackles are mainly basal in site.

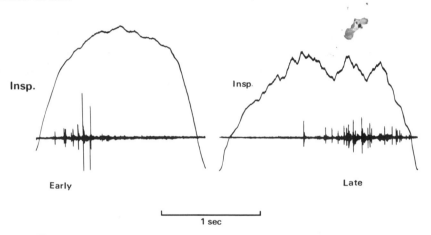

**Fig. 6.30** Phonopneumograph of early (*left*) and late (*right*) inspiratory crackles. (The upper curved lines indicate the rate of air flow.) (By kind permission of Dr Leslie Capel and *Thorax*.)

*Early inspiratory and expiratory crackles* signify abnormal expiratory closure of proximal intrapulmonary airways with re-opening later in expiration or early in inspiration. They tend to be scanty, low-pitched, audible at the mouth and unaffected by posture. Those that disappear after a few deep breaths are common in the elderly and of little pathological significance. Otherwise, they are usually indicative of bronchitis.

*Late inspiratory crackles* are generally due to restrictive conditions of the lung itself, resulting in expiratory closure of the small peripheral airways with re-opening at the end of inspiration. In contrast to early inspiratory crackles, they are usually fine, profuse, high-pitched, inaudible at the mouth and may vary with posture. They are heard especially in patients with fibrosing alveolitis, pneumonia and pulmonary oedema.

**Pleural friction** Oscillations arising from frictional resistance between two layers of inflamed or roughened pleura produce a creaking sound: the pleural friction rub. This tends to recur in the same part or parts of each respiratory cycle. The intensity of the sound may be increased by firm pressure of the stethoscope.

## EXAMINATION AFTER EXERCISE

Examination of the patient after exercise is essential to the assessment of the respiratory system. Exercise may take the form of running, in the case of younger patients, climbing flights of stairs or, if the equipment is available, riding a static bicycle or walking on a treadmill. The following observations should be made after exercise:

1. The amount of exercise needed to induce dyspnoea, or the distance walked in a given time.

2. The respiratory and heart rate and the time needed for these to return to the pre-exercise level.

3. Whether cyanosis appears during exercise.

4. Whether wheeze develops after exercise (*see* p. 186).

---

## ■ THE DIAGNOSIS OF RESPIRATORY DISEASES

For convenience in describing their symptoms and signs, the common diseases of the respiratory organs may be grouped under the following headings—those affecting (1) the bronchi, (2) the lungs, (3) the pleura and (4) the mediastinum.

### THE BRONCHI

The symptoms and signs of bronchial disease can be attributed to:

1. Irritation of the bronchial mucosa with increased secretions causing cough and expectoration.

2. Narrowing of the bronchial lumen, which results in dyspnoea, stridor, wheeze, early inspiratory and expiratory crackles and the signs of overinflation of the lungs (*see also* Emphysema, p. 194).

3. Complete occlusion of the lumen causing the symptoms and signs of collapse of the lung (*see* p. 190). The bronchi may be narrowed or occluded by exudate or foreign bodies in the lumen, by mucosal oedema, tumour or spasm arising in the bronchial wall, or by pressure from without by enlarged lymph nodes.

It is convenient to consider diseases of the bronchi according to whether they affect the whole of the bronchial tree or are localized to one part of it. Generalized bronchial disease includes asthma and bronchitis and usually reveals itself by auscultatory signs with few changes in the radiograph. In localized disease, such as bronchiectasis and bronchial carcinoma, physical signs are often lacking and a radiograph is then needed to make a diagnosis.

### Bronchial asthma

Bronchial asthma usually starts in childhood, but may not appear until middle age ('late-onset asthma'). It is characterized by attacks of wheezing dyspnoea due to narrowing of the bronchi by spasm, mucosal oedema or mucous secretions. These attacks are brought on by a variety of factors, including allergy to certain inhaled dusts (e.g. house dust, pollens), respiratory infections, emotional upsets or physical exertion ('exercise-induced asthma'). A history of other 'allergic' manifestations, such as hay fever and infantile eczema, or a family history of these conditions, is common in those with an early onset of the disease.

The patient may be quite free of symptoms and abnormal signs between the attacks, but the illness can become continuous. Cough usually occurs only during the attacks, when it may be associated with the expectoration of viscid mucoid sputum; nocturnal cough is a characteristic presenting symptom of asthma in childhood.

Physical examination reveals laboured breathing associated with a prolonged expiratory wheeze, activity of the accessory muscles of respiration, signs of overinflation of the lung due to trapping of air during expiration (*see also* Emphysema, p. 194) and, in a severe attack, cyanosis may also be seen. In children, there may be permanent deformity of the chest wall (pigeon chest, *Fig.* 6.31). Bronchial asthma must be differentiated from the paroxysmal dyspnoea of left heart failure (*see* Chapter 7) and from localized wheezing due to partial bronchial obstruction by neoplasm.

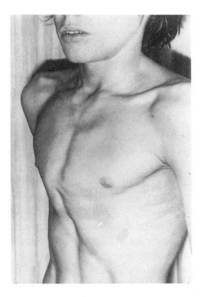

**Fig. 6.31**
Pigeon chest in a 15-year-old boy with asthma since infancy.

## Bronchitis

Acute bronchitis usually complicates an acute infection of the upper respiratory tract. Chronic bronchitis may be associated with chronic respiratory infections, but more often it can be related to cigarette smoking or to environmental causes such as air pollution. The principal symptom is cough, with mucoid sputum, which is worse in the morning and during the winter months. Acute exacerbations are provoked by adverse climatic conditions such as fog, and also by respiratory infection, when fever, purulent sputum and wheezing dyspnoea are additional symptoms. The main physical signs are expiratory wheeze and early inspiratory crackles. The signs in acute cases are similar to those of asthma. Chronic bronchitis in men is often complicated by emphysema in middle life (*see* p. 194). Other important complications in severe chronic cases are respiratory and cardiac failure, the combination of cyanosis and oedema producing the 'blue-bloater' syndrome (*see also* the 'pink-puffer' syndrome of emphysema, p. 194).

### Bronchiectasis

This most commonly results from tenacious plugs of mucus formed during an attack of pneumonia or acute bronchitis (often associated with measles, whooping-cough or cystic fibrosis) in early childhood; bronchiectasis will occur if the lung collapses and irreversible damage is done to the bronchi before the plug has been dissolved or expelled. Bronchiectasis may also complicate bronchopulmonary aspergillosis and auto-immune disorders in adult life. The dilatation of the bronchi, and the loss of ciliary action and cough reflex due to damage to their mucosa, causes retention and infection of secretions. These secretions are responsible for the chief symptom of bronchiectasis which is the expectoration of large amounts of purulent sputum, sometimes stained with blood. The main physical sign is coarse crackles, usually over the lower lobes of the lungs. In the absence of active infection (as in the treated case), however, there may be no abnormal signs, and then the diagnosis must depend upon radiological examination, including bronchography. Finger clubbing and, rarely, amyloidosis occur in the more advanced cases and the disease may also be complicated by recurrent pleurisy, pneumonic consolidation and by fibrosis in the surrounding lung (*see below* and p. 189).

### Bronchial carcinoma

Carcinoma of the bronchus is the commonest form of malignant tumour in men. Heavy cigarette smoking is an important causative factor.

The most frequent early symptoms are cough and haemoptysis, although it may present with a feverish pneumonic illness which tends to persist or relapse, pleuritic pain, dyspnoea on exertion or with various manifestations outside the chest (*see below*). As in other forms of malignant disease, there is progressive wasting leading to cachexia and death within a few months to a year in the untreated case.

The commonest signs are those of collapse, consolidation and effusion, or a combination of all three. The finding of pleural effusion without mediastinal displacement suggests either that there is also an underlying collapse of the lung or that the mediastinum has been invaded and fixed by tumour. This disease is often associated, and may even present, with signs outside the chest. These include anaemia and loss of weight, the signs of metastases to other organs (e.g. bone or brain), finger clubbing and painful swellings of the hands and feet due to osteoarthropathy, engorgement of the face due to mediastinal obstruction, and, more rarely, various forms of myoneuropathy and endocrine disorder, presumably due to chemical substances secreted by the tumour (*see also* p. 459).

## THE LUNGS

The more important pathological changes which may take place in the lungs include congestion, oedema, consolidation, cavitation, collapse, fibrosis and emphysema (*see Table* 6.3). These changes are found in various combinations in different lung disease.

| Table 6.3 | Physical signs in chest diseases* | | | | | |
|---|---|---|---|---|---|---|
| | Consolidation | Collapse | Fibrosis | Emphysema | Effusion | Pneumothorax |
| Mediastinal shift | None | Towards | Towards (with chest wall retraction) | None | Away | Away |
| Vocal fremitus | Increased | Usually diminished | Diminished | Diminished | Diminished | Diminished |
| Percussion note | Dull | Dull | Dull | Hyperresonance. Loss of liver and heart dullness | Flat or stony | Tympany |
| Breath sounds | Bronchial | Absent or bronchial | Diminished or bronchial | Diminished. Prolonged expiration | Diminished (bronchial above) | Diminished or amphoric |
| Voice sounds | Bronchophony. Whispering pectoriloquy | Diminished or bronchophony | Diminished or bronchophony | Diminished | Diminished (aegophony above) | Diminished |
| Added sounds | Fine inspiratory crackles (in the early stages and during resolution) | None | Coarse crackles (if bronchiectatic) | Expiratory wheeze | Friction rub (in early stages) | 'Metallic' crackles. Succussion (if fluid present) |

* It must be noted that two or more of these conditions often occur together, e.g. consolidation and collapse. The signs of both conditions may then be found.

### Congestion and oedema

The term 'congestion of the lung' has been used rather loosely in the past. It should be reserved to describe the state resulting from engorgement of the pulmonary veins and capillaries. Oedema is a later stage of the same process and consists of actual transudation of fluid into the walls and lumina of the smaller air spaces in the lungs. The commonest causes of congestion and oedema are left ventricular failure and mitral stenosis (*see* Chapter 7, pp. 255–257), but more rarely it can be due to acute inflammation of the lung (e.g. influenza) or to the inhalation of an irritant gas (e.g. phosgene, nitric oxide).

The main symptoms of congestion and oedema are dyspnoea, which in the cardiac case is worse when the patient lies flat ('orthopnoea'), cough and haemoptysis. The chief difference between the two stages is that, in congestion, the lungs are dry and the signs are usually those of asthmatic wheezing, while in oedema the transudate results in a copious pink, frothy sputum, and crackles, both fine and coarse, can be heard.

### Consolidation (*Fig.* 6.32)

This is a condition in which the alveoli are filled with an exudate from the blood, either inflammatory (e.g. pneumonia) or haemorrhagic (e.g. infarction due to occlusion of a pulmonary artery).

The symptoms are those of the cause. Pneumonia is characterized by dry cough, sometimes with rusty sputum, pleuritic pain, fever with rigors and, if consolidation is extensive, dyspnoea and cyanosis. The symptoms of infarction are similar, but the onset is usually more sudden, fever of lesser degree and frank haemoptysis is common.

The physical signs of consolidation are diminished expansion (especially when there is pleuritic pain), moderate impairment of percussion note (less than in

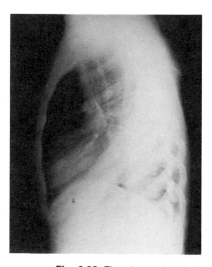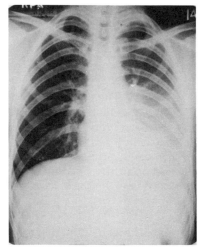

**Fig. 6.32** The chest, showing lobar pneumonia of the left lower lobe.

effusion), increased vocal fremitus, bronchial breathing, bronchophony, whispering pectoriloquy and late inspiratory crackles. An overlying pleural friction rub is common. The mediastinum remains central.

### Collapse

Pulmonary collapse or atelectasis may occur as a congenital abnormality but will be discussed here only in its acquired form.

Collapse results from bronchial obstruction preventing air from entering the lung, so that the air which remains is absorbed into the bloodstream. The symptoms vary in intensity according to the rapidity with which the collapse occurs. Breathlessness is the principal sympton and, in cases of sudden collapse, e.g. bronchial occlusion by a foreign body, it is extreme. In the more gradual collapse from bronchial carcinoma, dyspnoea may be noticed only on effort.

Inspection may reveal some flattening and reduced expansion over the affected part, but gross retraction of chest wall structures suggests fibrosis. In upper lobe collapse the trachea is displaced to the affected side (*Fig.* 6.33) and in lower lobe

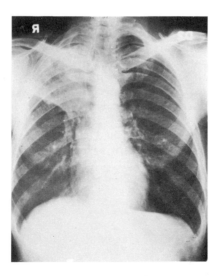

**Fig. 6.33**
Pulmonary collapse. Note that the right upper lobe is airless. The trachea is deviated to the right and the fissure between the upper and middle lobe is elevated.

collapse, the heart. The percussion note is dull because the lung is airless. Breath sounds and voice sounds are diminished or absent because the bronchus is occluded. However, the lung may remain collapsed and perhaps consolidated after the obstruction has been relieved (e.g. after the expectoration of a mucus plug). In such cases, bronchial breathing and bronchophony will be heard. These signs may also occur if, as a result of the collapse, the trachea or a main bronchus has been drawn over to one side and thus lies nearer to the stethoscope.

### Fibrosis

Pulmonary fibrosis may be the result of many inflammatory diseases of the lung. Localized fibrosis is most often due to tuberculosis (*Fig.* 6.34), bronchiectasis or to a destructive form of pneumonia (e.g. staphylococcal).

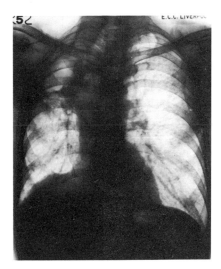

**Fig. 6.34**
Note tuberculous cavity at
right apex with deviation of
trachea and elevation of
diaphragm due to fibrosis.

The eventual results of localized fibrosis of the lung are in some ways comparable to those of pulmonary collapse, for the lung becomes shrunken in volume, contains little air and draws in the chest wall on the affected side and the mediastinum from the opposite side. The results are, however, produced in a much more gradual manner, and, although the chief symptom is again breathlessness, it is rarely so urgent as in acute forms of pulmonary collapse. Cough and expectoration occur if the fibrosis is associated with bronchiectasis.

The signs of fibrosis (*Fig.* 6.35) depend on the shrinkage of the lung and its consequent drag on surrounding tissues, and on the diminished amount of air entering and contained in the lung. The chest is retracted and smaller in volume, and the heart and trachea are pulled towards the affected side. The ribs are often

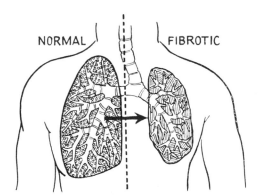

**Fig. 6.35** Pulmonary fibrosis. The shoulder is lower and the
chest wall retracted on the affected side. The lung is shrunken
and the bronchi compressed. The signs are therefore: limited
movement; diminished vocal fremitus and vocal resonance
(variable); percussion note impaired; breath sounds faint
(sometimes bronchial); mediastinal contents (trachea, heart
etc.) displaced in direction of arrows.

closer together, and expansion is limited or absent. The percussion note is dull because of the relatively airless state of the lung. The breath sounds are faint and may be bronchial, as in the case of pulmonary collapse when the bronchus is patent or drawn nearer to the stethoscope. Added sounds when present are generally due to associated changes, e.g. bronchitis, tuberculosis or bronchiectasis.

A more generalized form of fibrosis can result from sarcoidosis and from the inhalation of irritant dusts such as silica or asbestos. A special form of generalized fibrosis known as *fibrosing alveolitis* may be due to the inhalation of an allergen, as in the case of farmer's lung ('extrinsic allergic alveolitis'), or to some intrinsic process of unknown cause ('cryptogenic fibrosing alveolitis'). The clinical features are dyspnoea, cyanosis, finger clubbing, rapid shallow breathing and fine late inspiratory crackles.

## THE PLEURA

### Pleurisy

*Inflammation* of the pleura can result from various diseases of the underlying lung, especially pneumonia, infarction or neoplasm, and more rarely from diseases in other sites (e.g. oesophagus; subphrenic abscess). In the early stages, friction between the two layers of the pleura gives rise to pleuritic pain and an audible friction rub. Later, if fluid forms between the two layers of the pleura, the pain and rub may be replaced by the features of pleural effusion (*Fig.* 6.36).

*Pleural effusion* may take the form of an *exudate* from the causes already mentioned. The fluid has a high protein content, may contain inflammatory cells or blood and sometimes consists of pus (empyema). In cases of cardiac failure, or hypoproteinaemia due to renal disease, the fluid is a clear, watery *transudate* with a low protein and cell content and usually forms without preceding pleural friction. A rare form of pleural effusion is that which results from impaired lymphatic drainage. Obstruction to the thoracic duct causes a fatty or 'chylous' effusion. In congenital hypoplasia of the lymphatics, pleural effusion is accompanied by a yellow discoloration of the finger nails (*Fig.* 6.37). Patients with pleural effusion

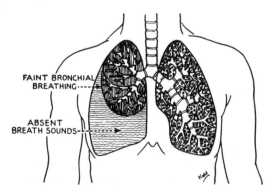

**Fig. 6.36** Breath sounds in pleural effusion. Lung compressed, therefore relatively solid. Bronchi narrowed by compression. (*See also Fig.* 6.33 for other signs of pulmonary collapse.)

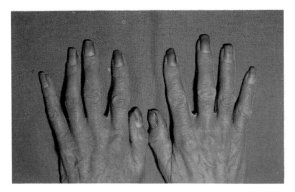

**Fig. 6.37** Yellow nails.

complain of gradually increasing dyspnoea and the signs consist of mediastinal shift towards the opposite side and stony dull percussion note with diminished vocal fremitus, breath sounds and voice sounds at the affected lung base. Broncho-phony and aegophony may be heard over the upper part of the effusion.

### Pneumothorax (*Fig.* 6.38)

Air in the pleural cavity is known as pneumothorax. The air gener-ally enters through a communication between the lung and the pleural cavity.

Spontaneous pneumothorax is usually due to the rupture of a subpleural bulla of congenital or inflammatory origin and is commonest in young men. It also occurs as a serious complication of generalized emphysema in older patients. The condition usually occurs suddenly with the production of dyspnoea and pain which may resemble that of myocardial infarction (*see* pp. 252, 254) when the pneumothorax is large, or it may be pleuritic in type. If the air leaks gradually, the symptoms may be unnoticed and the condition discovered only by radiography.

The mediastinum is displaced towards the opposite side when the pneumotho-rax is large. The most characteristic sign is impairment of breath and voice sounds in the presence of a well-preserved or even hyper-resonant percussion note. Rarely, the breath sounds have a hollow 'amphoric' quality due to the resonating properties of the pneumothorax. In cases of left-sided pneumothorax, the dis-placement of air trapped in the mediastinal pleural space can cause a clicking sound, synchronous with each heart beat.

### THE MEDIASTINUM

### Mediastinal obstruction

This may be caused by inflammatory and neoplastic processes of which the commonest is bronchial carcinoma invading the mediastinum directly or by metastatic involvement of lymph nodes. There may be pressure effects upon the superior vena cava, the sympathetic, recurrent laryngeal and phrenic nerves, and sometimes on the trachea, main bronchi and oesophagus (*Fig.* 6.39, *Fig.* 6.5, p. 168).

The resulting symptoms and signs thus include engorgement of veins in the

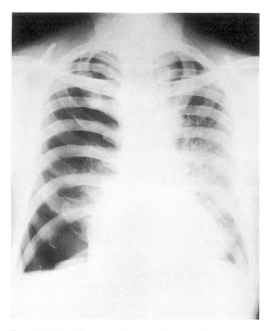

**Fig. 6.38** Air fills the right pleural cavity. Note the lack of lung markings compared with the normal side. The edge of the partly deflated lung can be seen as a thin white line.

neck, arms and chest with suffusion and oedema of the face and 'bursting' headaches on lying or bending, Horner's syndrome (*see* p. 358), hoarseness, dyspnoea, stridor and dysphagia.

### Emphysema

This is a condition characterized by permanent overinflation of the distal air spaces of the lung with disruption of their walls. These changes are associated with expiratory airways obstruction and loss of elasticity of the lungs. Emphysema is seen most often in middle-aged men who have suffered for many years from chronic bronchitis, but it may develop without any preceding respiratory illness. Rarely, emphysema is associated with an inherited deficiency of $\alpha_1$ antitrypsin. It presents with increasing breathlessness on exertion, with more severe disability provoked by respiratory infection in the winter months.

Inspection reveals a distended chest fixed in the inspiratory position ('barrel chest') (*Fig.* 6.8, p. 171): the sternum is displaced outwards and the ribs and clavicles are more horizontal than normal. Expansion is limited and inspiration can only be achieved with the aid of the accessory muscles of the neck elevating the clavicles. Expiration is greatly prolonged and is often accompanied by pursing of the lips (*Fig.* 6.6, p. 170).

On percussion, the note is hyper-resonant and the normal areas of dullness over the heart and liver are obliterated by the distended lung. On auscultation,

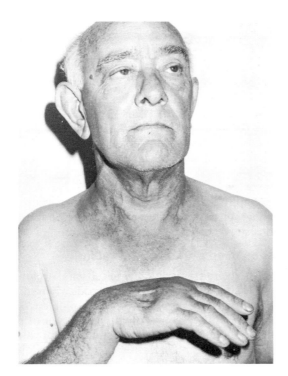

**Fig. 6.39** Mediastinal obstruction from bronchial carcinoma. Note pitting oedema of hand, engorged neck veins and right-sided ptosis.

the breath sounds are diminished, and expiration is prolonged and wheezing, but the wheeze may only be apparent during a forced expiration.

The disease may be complicated by the formation of bullae on the surface of the lung, which sometimes rupture to form a pneumothorax (*see* p. 193).

The resulting disturbance in respiratory function is responsible for the chief symptom, dyspnoea, and also for various extrathoracic manifestations in the later stages of the disease. These include the symptoms and signs of hypoxia, of carbon dioxide retention (*see* p. 163) and of right heart failure (*see* p. 224), the last being due in part to hypoxic constriction of the pulmonary arterioles and in part to obliteration of the capillaries surrounding the overinflated alveoli. In the non-bronchitic forms of emphysema, these signs of respiratory and cardiac failure are relatively uncommon, the patients remaining well oxygenated at the cost of considerable hyperventilation and dyspnoea. This is known as the 'pink-puffer' syndrome (see also the 'blue-bloater' syndrome of chronic bronchitis, p. 187).

## ■ SPECIAL INVESTIGATIONS

### Radiography

A radiograph of the chest must be regarded as routine in all patients complaining of persistent respiratory symptoms. Special radiological investigations include fluoroscopy (or screening) of the lung and diaphragmatic movements; lateral, oblique and apical views; X-rays focused at different depths in the lung (tomography) to detect local lesions, such as a cavity or tumour; and the introduction of a radio-opaque medium into the bronchial tree (bronchography) to demonstrate bronchiectasis or bronchial narrowing (*Fig.* 6.40), or into the pulmonary artery (angiography) to demonstrate arterial occlusions by embolism. Computerized axial tomography (the "CAT Scan") may be used to define the precise size, site and consistency of an intrathoracic lesion.

### Examination of sputum and pleural fluid

Microscopy of the sputum may reveal cells and organisms of various kinds. These include tubercle bacilli, appearing as red rods when stained by Ziehl–Neelsen's method, malignant cells or an excess of eosinophil leucocytes, suggesting an allergic state. More rarely, evidence of the inhalation of a noxious dust may be found, e.g. asbestos bodies. Culture of the sputum is of value in detecting the dominant infecting organism and its sensitivity to the available antibiotics, but special techniques are needed to grow tubercle bacilli. These observations on the sputum apply also to the pleural fluid, but in this case additional help can be obtained by a cell count and by measuring the specific gravity and protein content of the fluid. A high value for any of these three suggests an exudate (e.g. tuberculosis) rather than a transudate (e.g. congestive cardiac failure). The type of cell in a pleural exudate should also be noted: a predominance of red cells is commonest in carcinoma, pus cells indicate empyema, while a lymphocytic effusion favours a chronic infection such as tuberculosis. Fat globules may be seen in the chylous effusion of thoracic duct obstruction.

### Pulmonary function tests

The commonly used tests of respiratory function can be considered under two headings: ventilation of the lungs and gas exchange in the lungs. Tests in the first category include measurements of lung size (e.g. vital capacity, VC), the patency of the airways (e.g. forced expiratory volume, FEV), and the amount of air used to ventilate the lungs during normal breathing at rest and on exercise (minute and alveolar ventilation). These tests can all be made by simple spirometric methods. Gas exchange is examined by measuring the tensions of oxygen and carbon dioxide in arterial blood and by calculating the gas transfer factor or diffusing capacity using a carbon monoxide uptake technique (*see Table* 6.4).

### Endoscopy and biopsy procedures

*a*. Direct inspection of the larynx (laryngoscopy) and the bronchial tree (bronchoscopy) by a rigid or flexible fibreoptic instrument to detect carcinoma or other abnormality in the wall or lumen of the airways (*Fig.* 6.41).

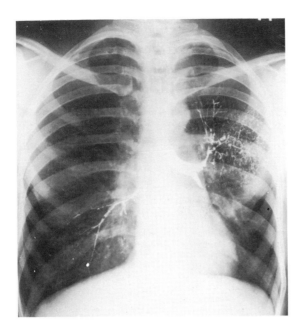

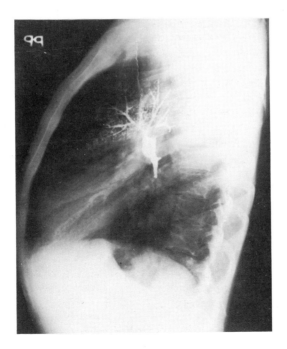

**Fig. 6.40** The chest, showing carcinoma of the left lower bronchus—narrowing demonstrated by radio-opaque fluid.

| Table 6.4 | **Commonly used tests of lung function** | |
|---|---|---|
| Test | Definition | Conditions in which it is most commonly used |
| **1  Spirometric Tests of Ventilation** | | |
| Vital capacity (VC) | The volume of air which can be expelled after a maximal inspiration Normal: 3–5 l | Decreased in conditions restricting the expansion of the lungs (e.g. deformities of thoracic cage, pleural thickening or effusion, lung fibrosis) |
| Maximum voluntary ventilation (MVV) | The amount of air which can be shifted in 1 min by maximal respiration. Normal: 120–160 l per min | Decreased in diffuse airways obstruction (e.g. asthma, bronchitis, emphysema) |
| Forced expiratory volume (in 1 s) (FEV₁) | The amount of air which can be expelled in 1 s after a maximal inspiration. Normal: 75 per cent of vital capacity | Decreased in diffuse airways obstruction (e.g. asthma, bronchitis, emphysema) |
| Minute and alveolar ventilation | Minute ventilation The amount of air breathed in 1 min during normal respiration, i.e. tidal volume × respiratory rate. Normal at rest: 6–8 l per min  Alveolar ventilation The amount of air ventilating the alveoli in 1 min during normal respiration, i.e. (tidal volume minus anatomical dead space*) × respiratory rate. Normal at rest: 4–6 l per min | Increased in many lung diseases (e.g. pneumonia) and metabolic disorders (e.g. acidosis, thyrotoxicosis). Decreased in cerebral and neuromuscular diseases (e.g. narcotic drugs, poliomyelitis) |
| **2  Tests of Gas Exchange** | | |
| Arterial oxygen saturation (See also Cyanosis, p. 164) | The oxygen content of arterial haemoglobin as a percentage of the content when blood is exposed to air. Normal: 97 per cent | Decreased in hypoventilation (e.g. cerebral and neuromuscular disorders) Continued perfusion of under ventilated parts of lung (e.g. in emphysema) Impaired diffusion (e.g. fibrosis due to dust diseases) Shunts of blood bypassing the lungs (e.g. Fallot's tetralogy) |
| Arterial oxygen tension ($Pa_{O_2}$) | The partial pressure of oxygen in arterial blood. Normal: 100 mmHg | |
| Arterial $CO_2$ tension ($Pa_{CO_2}$) | The partial pressure of $CO_2$ in arterial blood. Normal: 40 mmHg | Increased in hypoventilation. Reduced in hyperventilation. (Less affected by diffusion impairment or shunts because of the relatively high diffusibility of $CO_2$) |

\* Normal (approximately): 100 ml in women, 150 ml in men.

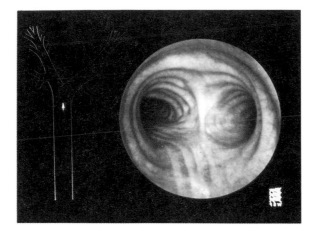

*a*

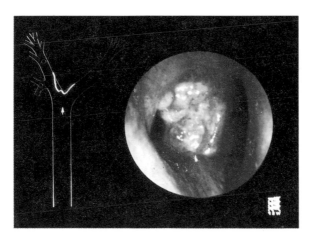

*b*

**Fig. 6.41** Bronchoscopic view of the bifurcation of the trachea into the two main bronchi. *a*, Showing normal appearances and *b*, carinal infiltration due to carcinoma. (By kind permission of Dr Peter Stradling.)

*b*. Various secretions or tissues can be procured for laboratory examination. Pleural fluid is collected by aspiration of the pleural cavity with a needle, while bronchoalveolar secretions and samples of the bronchial mucosa or lung can be obtained during bronchoscopy. Percutaneous biopsy of the pleura or of the lung can be carried out with a special needle or by means of an open surgical procedure.

### Immunological tests

Sensitivity to certain respiratory allergens may be inferred in atopic subjects by skin prick tests producing a weal and flare reaction or occasionally proved by the inhalation of the appropriate antigen. Measurement of serum IgE and RAST (radio allergo absorbent test) will confirm the atopic status of many asthmatics and measurement of IgA, IgG and IgM levels may sometimes reveal low or absent values in bronchiectasis. Autoantibodies such as rheumatoid factor and antinuclear antibody are present in some cases of fibrosing alveolitis not associated with rheumatoid arthritis and specific precipitating antibodies can be detected in the sera of patients with extrinsic allergic alveolitis, such as farmer's lung and bird fancier's lung, as well as bronchopulmonary aspergillosis and aspergilloma.

The tuberculin test for tuberculosis consists of the intradermal injection of killed tubercle bacilli. A positive reaction appears within 72 h as a raised weal in the skin indicating the body's past experience of tubercle bacilli, but it does not necessarily indicate active infection (*Fig.* 6.42). The Kveim test for sarcoidosis must be biopsied 6 weeks after the intradermal injection of Kveim antigen and examined microscopically for characteristic granulomata.

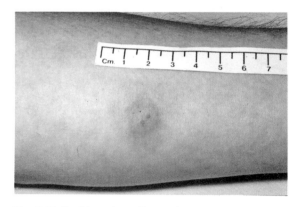

**Fig. 6.42** Positive tuberculin reaction.

## The cardiovascular system

■      **SYMPTOMS OF HEART DISEASE**

The patient with heart disease may complain of many different symptoms, some of which may apparently be unconnected with the cardiovascular system. Often there are no symptoms and a cardiac lesion is found by routine examination.

Certain symptoms are, however, constantly found in cardiovascular disease, and though they may have other causes, careful attention should be paid to them in order to eliminate or confirm their cardiac origin. The patient should be encouraged to give a full and spontaneous description of his symptoms, with detailed questioning on the part of the examiner left until later.

### Dyspnoea (*see also* Respiratory System, p. 161)

The mechanism and physiology of this symptom have been more fully considered in Chapter 6.

As it is such a common symptom of heart disease, certain special points may be noted:

**Dyspnoea on effort** This generally precedes other forms of breathlessness, though there are exceptions to this rule. Serious cardiovascular disease, such as aortic incompetence or hypertension, may exist for many years without dyspnoea, yet in mitral stenosis dyspnoea is often an early feature.

The grade of the dyspnoea, provided that other causes mentioned in Chapter 6 are excluded, may give valuable information about the state of the cardiac reserve. For example, in valve disease for some years there may be no dyspnoea, then a patient becomes increasingly breathless with physical tasks of diminishing grade, until finally, when he reaches the stage of cardiac failure, dyspnoea will occur even on slight movement in bed.

**Paroxysmal dyspnoea at rest** These attacks generally occur in bed and may follow a period of dyspnoea on exertion, but occasionally they are the first indication of a rise in pulmonary venous pressure in many types of heart disease, notably left ventricular failure and mitral stenosis. They are associated with a rise in left atrial pressure of whatever cause, as this prevents an adequate return of blood from the lungs to the left side of the heart. The attacks are often called 'cardiac asthma', i.e. paroxysmal dyspnoea of cardiac origin to distinguish it from bronchial asthma. Sometimes both occur in the same patient.

**Orthopnoea** Orthopnoea is said to be a later feature of cardiac failure than paroxysmal dyspnoea, though the two conditions are often found in the same patient.

**Cheyne-Stokes breathing** (*see also* p. 169) In heart disease this type of respiration, also known as periodic breathing, is commonest in similar affections to those in which cardiac asthma occurs. The waxing and waning of the respiration, periods of hyperpnoea and apnoea, are particularly common during sleep, which they may interrupt.

Any or all of these types of dyspnoea may be found in the same patient.

### Palpitation

This term means that the patient is conscious of his heart-beats, which he may describe as 'bumping', 'throbbing', 'pounding' or 'fluttering' in the chest or peripheral vessels. Several factors may be responsible for the symptoms—namely, increased force, increased rate and irregularity of the heart—but unless the nervous system is unduly sensitive they may not result in palpitation. For this reason the symptom is more common in such conditions as hyperthyroidism and anxiety states than in organic heart disease. A placid patient with a heaving apical beat or with an abnormal rhythm or even tachycardia may be quite unaware of the heart's action.

If palpitation occurs in attacks careful attention must be paid to the patient's story. In simple sinus tachycardia, emotion or exercise generally causes the heart to beat faster, and as the precipitating cause diminishes so the heart rate and the palpitation lessen. By contrast, in abnormal rhythms, such as atrial flutter or paroxysmal tachycardia, the onset and offset of the attacks are instantaneous. The patient often states that he is conscious of the heart missing a beat or 'turning over' and then the palpitation is in full swing. Similarly, the attack passes away by a sudden consciousness of some alteration in the heartbeat. Short attacks of this character are suggestive of paroxysmal tachycardia; longer attacks, lasting many hours or days, suggest atrial flutter. Atrial fibrillation may also come in attacks, and the patient may be able to date the onset of the attack by the sudden appearance of palpitation having an irregular character. Extrasystoles are usually appreciated as occasional irregularities. The patient may be aware of a missed beat or an extra large bump corresponding with the next normal beat after the extrasystole. In most cases of palpitation the heart beats faster than normal, but occasionally, in heart block, the increased stroke volume may cause awareness of the heart's slow action.

### Cardiac pain

Pain as a symptom of heart disease is very important but sometimes difficult to evaluate. It occurs so frequently without gross evidence of cardiovascular disease that a diagnosis may have to rest on this symptom alone. For this reason an accurate and careful description of the site, character and duration of the pain is essential.

**Angina pectoris** This is merely a name for pain of a particular type, namely strangling, which is experienced in the chest, generally midsternal or transternal, and often spreading to one or both arms, less commonly to the neck or jaw, and sometimes to the epigastrium or back.

It occurs under the following circumstances:

*1. Angina of effort* In this the pain is provoked by varying degrees of physical exertion, especially walking quickly or uphill, or against a wind. It is usually worse in cold weather and on walking after a meal. Similar pain may result from emotion. The pain usually disappears within a few minutes of rest or freedom from emotion.

It may be described as like a tight band, a sense of crushing or pressure, or very commonly as 'indigestion', with which it is often confused.

Its severity varies, according to the degree of myocardial ischaemia, the patient's threshold of pain and whether the provoking factor is removed.

*2. Acute coronary insufficiency* (sometimes called 'herald angina', 'angina decubitus', 'ingravescent angina'). The pain has a similar character and distribution but may occur at rest and lasts longer than angina of effort. It occurs when there is impairment of coronary blood flow and usually indicates critical (more than 95 per cent) narrowing of a major coronary artery; hence it is now commonly described as 'pre-infarction angina'. It may also occur in aortic disease, in severe anaemia (in which there is inadequate oxygenation of the heart muscle) and occasionally during a rapid dysrhythmia of the heart.

*3. Cardiac infarction* This usually results from occlusion of a major coronary artery (*see* p. 252); pain may present and persist at rest.

**Other forms of precordial pain** It will be useful here to mention the frequency with which pain in the chest results from non-cardiac causes which must be carefully distinguished from the type of pain just described. Pain of aching character is common in an effort syndrome, especially associated with fatigue. Aching or sharp pains occur in various rheumatic, traumatic and neuralgic affections of the chest wall. These pains are usually worse on movement of the affected parts and are sometimes associated with localized tenderness. The pain of pleurisy is generally severe, cutting or burning in character, and constantly related to breathing. All these pains tend to be mammary, axillary or dorsal in position rather than substernal. Further, they are often of long duration—hours or days. Sometimes oesophageal lesions cause a centrally placed pain like angina, as in obstructive lesions and hiatus hernia. Such pains may be related to swallowing or posture, but only occasionally to physical effort.

**Aneurysm** Aneurysm by erosion (*Fig.* 7.22, p. 225) may produce severe pain in the precordium, in the back or in the upper abdomen according to the site of the aortic dilatation. The pain may be due to pressure effects on bony structures and nerves, but in dissecting aneurysm the pain is caused by the splitting of the aortic wall.

### Gastrointestinal symptoms

In cases of congestive heart failure where the viscera—liver and gastrointestinal tract—are engorged with blood, dyspeptic symptoms are common. Loss of appetite, nausea, fullness after meals and distension of the abdomen are the usual features. Vomiting occurs occasionally, and the bowels are usually constipated. Such symptoms may be the result of therapy (digitalis and diuretics). Pain over the liver is common, owing to congestion of the organ and stretching of its capsule, especially if this occurs rapidly. Jaundice is rare and only in advanced cases, but some impairment of liver function may precede it.

### Respiratory symptoms

With the onset of pulmonary venous hypertension, the lungs are usually congested, resulting in cough, dyspnoea and not uncommonly in haemoptysis. In long-standing cases altered blood may be found in the sputum. If there is oedema of the lungs, the sputum may be plentiful and frothy, sometimes tinged pink by blood.

### Urinary symptoms

Altered circulation through the kidneys leads to decrease in the secretion of urine, rarely to complete suppression. The urine passed is highly coloured owing to its great concentration, and frequently contains protein casts, and red cells. 'Oliguria', as this decrease in urinary output is called, is one of the most important symptoms of cardiac failure and is a useful guide to the grade of failure and its response to treatment.

### Cerebral symptoms

The most important of these is syncope, which is considered separately below. Dizziness, headache and psychological changes are not uncommon features in cerebral atherosclerosis and cardiac failure, but they also occur more commonly in effort syndrome in which no organic cardiovascular lesion can be found. An important cardiac cause for central nervous symptoms is embolism from the left side of the heart.

**Syncope** (*see also* Chapter 1) Transient loss of consciousness may result from inadequacy of the cerebral blood flow. This is known as syncope and has to be distinguished from epilepsy, coma and hysteria.

The symptoms are more fully described below.

A small, but important, group of cases can be classified as cardiac syncope. They include abnormalities of rhythm with very high rates, as in paroxysmal tachycardia. Unless the speed of the heart is abnormal on examination, a careful study will be necessary to avoid overlooking these possibilities. Stokes–Adams seizures in heart block depend upon the degree of bradycardia and may merely take the form of syncope, but in more prolonged cardiac standstill convulsions and coma occur.

Syncopal attacks in aortic valve diseases are associated with a low fixed output. Exercise results in blood being directed away from the brain to the muscles and other organs, and cerebral anoxia occurs. Effort syncope is an important symptom in aortic valve disease as an indication of its severity.

Sudden mechanical obstruction of the circulation is rare, e.g. a ball-valve thrombus or myxoma blocking the mitral orifice, but illustrates how immediate syncope may occur and often cause death.

Lastly, local cerebral vascular changes, as in hypertension and cerebral arteriosclerosis or occurring as a result of hyperventilation or anoxia, are occasional causes of syncope.

### Other symptoms

Finally, it should be noted that in serious heart disease a great variety of symptoms may arise owing to malnutrition of the body as a whole or of certain special organs. In children, wasting and lack of normal development are a common result, and even in adults some loss of weight is usual, though increase of weight may also occur from inactivity or as an early sign of oedema. Fatigue has been accepted as a symptom indicating a low fixed output, especially in tricuspid valve disease. (*See* Fatigue, p. 331).

■ ## PHYSICAL SIGNS: EXAMINATION OF THE CARDIOVASCULAR SYSTEM

The examination of the cardiovascular system comprises a study of the heart and blood vessels, but corroborative evidence of heart disease is so frequently present in other organs that certain signs should be looked for in every case. These may conveniently be discussed first.

### Oedema

The patient may complain of swelling of the ankles or feet, but if this symptom does not enter into the history, it should be sought purposely. The pathology of oedema is not discussed here, save certain mechanical factors of clinical importance. Gravity plays an important part, especially in cardiac oedema, and the swelling is found in the most dependent parts of the body—in the feet, ankles and legs when the patient is ambulatory, over the sacrum (sacral cushion—*Fig.* 7.1), lumbar region, genitalia, and backs of the ankles and thighs in patients who are sitting upright in bed. Looseness of the subcutaneous tissues also favours the accumulation of oedematous fluid, hence the occurrence of oedema in the genitalia and beneath the eyes in renal disease or extreme cardiac failure. Interference with the return of the blood to the heart also contributes to oedema. This is seen in cases of localized venous thrombosis, e.g. in patients with varicose veins, but there is little doubt that the more generalized obstruction to venous return which occurs in many types of heart disease acts in the same way. Much is ill-understood in the pathology of oedema and for fuller discussion textbooks of pathology and medicine should be consulted, with particular reference to the part played by sodium retention and the reduction of plasma-proteins.

Oedema is recognized by the characteristic 'pitting' on pressure and should be distinguished from the more solid swelling of myxoedema or lymphatic blockage. As a gauge of the disappearance of oedema the weight of the patient is generally reliable, for, with the dispersal of the fluid and its excretion through the kidneys, bowel and skin, there is a rapid reduction in weight; while, conversely, increase in weight suggests fluid retention. Oedema is not confined to the subcutaneous tissues, but may affect serous sacs, causing pleural and pericardial effusion and ascites.

### Cyanosis

This physical sign is fully discussed in Chapter 6, p. 164, and may be of considerable diagnostic value in certain forms of heart disease: It occurs in

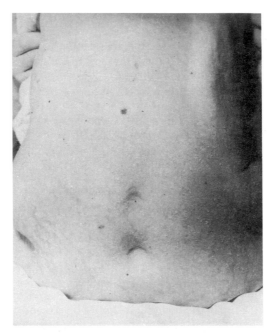

**Fig. 7.1** Sacral cushion of oedema. Pitting on pressure over the sacrum is common in patients who have been bedridden in the usual sitting posture adopted in heart failure.

mitral stenosis, but not always, and also in conditions where pulmonary arterial hypertension occurs together with a low cardiac output. It is seen whenever non-oxygenated blood reaches the systemic circulation, as in the reversed, or right-to-left, shunting of blood in some forms of congenital heart disease.

### Respiratory distress

While the patient is undressing, the physician will note the presence or absence of breathlessness and will compare this with the patient's subsequent statement. If there is no apparent breathlessness special exercises may be employed to demonstrate its presence or absence with a more severe degree of exertion. This may be accomplished by getting the patient to touch his toes a dozen times, or, while lying on a couch, to sit up and lie down quickly. Naturally such tests must be subject to the safety with which they can be employed. In all cases the lungs should be examined, for, apart from the congestion which occurs in cardiac failure, such abnormalities as chronic bronchitis or fibrosis may be responsible for the production or aggravation of the heart condition.

### Abdominal signs

The abdomen should be examined in all cases of heart disease, as there may be enlargement of the liver or ascites, suggestive of congestive failure, and enlargement of the spleen in cases of bacterial endocarditis. The hepato-megaly of congestive heart failure can be demonstrated best by palpation, which determines the presence of a firm tender enlargement between the costal margin and the umbilical level. This can be confirmed by percussion (*see also* p. 177). When ascites is present, an enlarged liver can often be determined easily by 'dipping' (*see also* p. 100, *Fig.* 4.21).

**Pulsation in the epigastrium**  Epigastric pulsation may be due to:

1. The contraction of the right ventricle; it is seen as a systolic retraction in the epigastrium, and may occur in normal persons; when the heart is hypertrophied it may be felt as a systolic thrust on palpation.

2. Aortic pulsation in nervous but otherwise normal persons, especially when the abdominal wall is thin; aortic pulsation follows the heartbeat by about 0·1 s.

3. Abdominal aortic aneurysm, in which an expansile swelling bigger than the normal aorta is present.

4. Pulsation of the liver; the area of pulsation extends more to the right than in the case of aortic or ventricular pulsation, and signs of congestive failure are usually present. It is generally due to tricuspid incompetence and is therefore systolic in time. It is to be noted that the enlarged liver may transmit pulsation from the heart or aorta.

Examination of the femoral pulses can be undertaken at this time (*see later*).

### Signs pointing to the aetiology

As the causes of cardiovascular disease are comparatively few, the examiner should be alert for evidence of arthritis, rheumatic nodules, chorea or tonsillitis which may suggest a *rheumatic* origin (or a history of these in the past), for evidence of *syphilis* particularly a positive Wassermann reaction, and for clubbing of the fingers, anaemia and petechiae suggestive of *bacterial endocarditis*. Cyanotic types of *congenital heart disease* are at once suggested by the colour of the skin and tongue, and by clubbing of the fingers, but acyanotic forms may be discovered only by accident on routine examination. Hyperthyroidism may explain cases of heart disease in which no other aetiological factors are found. Conversely, cardiac changes may result from hypothyroidism. In the cardiovascular diseases of older age-groups, notably hypertension, atheroma and coronary artery disease, a familial tendency to heart disease and also diabetes are of considerable importance. Xanthelasma (*Fig.* 7.2) and other evidence of hyperlipida-

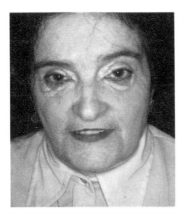

**Fig. 7.2**
Xanthelasma.

emia should also be sought. Chronic pulmonary disease is a not uncommon cause of cardiac failure and rarer causes include alcoholism, vitamin deficiencies and endocrine abnormalities.

We may now proceed to investigate the cardiovascular system proper. This involves examination of the peripheral vascular system (arterial and venous) and the heart.

The abnormalities to be found on examination of the cardiovascular system will be illustrated by actual recordings of *arterial and venous pulse waves*, the electrical activity of the heart (*electrocardiography*), heart sounds and murmurs (*phonocardiography*) and changes in structure and function of the heart as revealed by ultrasound (echocardiography). The reader will find descriptions of these recording methods on pp. 270, 273.

## ■ EXAMINATION OF THE PULSE

It is usual to examine the pulse before proceeding to the examination of the heart itself. This should include inspection, palpation and auscultation of important vessels, especially the radial, brachial and axillary arteries, the carotids, temporal and retinal vessels, and the femorals and their distal branches. Most information is derived from the radial artery, commonly called *the* pulse, though it should be checked by examination of the brachial artery. The most important method of examination is palpation, which will be considered first.

### PALPATION

The pulse should be felt in both wrists, as variations are sometimes found on the two sides both in health and disease. Inequality suggests: (1) Abnormally placed artery; (2) Abnormal aortic arch, due either to congenital malformation or acquired disease such as aneurysm with intravascular clotting; (3) Obstruction of brachial or subclavian arteries by atheroma, thrombosis or embolism. The femoral pulses should be routinely palpated to rule out aortic defects such as coarctation. Thereafter the following points should be noted in sequence.

### 1 Rate

The pulse rate normally averages about 72 per minute, but in children is more rapid (90–110), and in old age may become slow (55–65). Quite trivial disturbances are sufficient to cause an acceleration in the pulse rate—for example, the emotion roused by a medical examination, or the effort of climbing stairs or hurrying to the consulting room. Due allowance must be made for these factors before attaching too much importance to a rapid pulse rate, and it is useful to take the rate at the beginning of the consultation and again before the patient leaves. The heart rate should always be compared with the pulse rate, as in some cases there is a 'pulse deficit', i.e. the pulse rate is less than the ventricular rate.

### 2 Rhythm

The normal pulse waves succeed one another at regular intervals, but respiratory variations are common in health, the pulse quickening with inspiration and slowing with expiration. If this variation in rate is noticeable even with quiet breathing the term 'sinus arrhythmia' is applied (*Fig.* 7.3). If other forms of

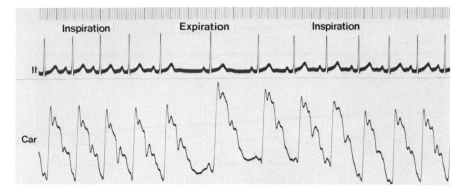

**Fig. 7.3** ECG and carotid pulse tracing of sinus arrhythmia. The record was taken from a healthy young woman. (Recording speed 25 mm/s.)

irregularity are present, the observer should note whether the pulse is irregular all the time or only occasionally. Finally, the effect of effort on the rhythm should be noted. Decisions as to rhythms should always be deferred until examination of the heart has been made, as the pulse alone may be deceptive (*see* pp. 262–267).

The commonest irregularities detectable in the pulse are extrasystoles (premature beats) and atrial fibrillation (*Figs.* 7.4, 7.5), though variable heart block and atrial flutter may be suspected if the rate changes abruptly. Extrasystoles usually produce an occasional irregularity where a beat appears to be missed or in which a small pulse wave occurs earlier than is expected. If the extrasystoles are numerous, the pulse may appear to be completely irregular. In atrial fibrillation the pulse is persistently irregular, and this is usually easily recognized, though it may not be observed if the heart rate is slow, so that exercise should be employed to

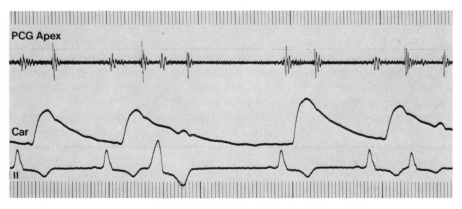

**Fig. 7.4** ECG, phonocardiogram (PCG) and carotid pulse of ventricular ectopic beats. The ECG is abnormal, showing a left bundle-branch block (LBBB) pattern (*see Fig.* 7.48). (Recording speed 50 mm/s.)

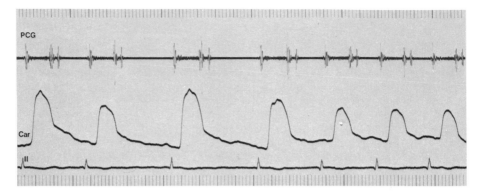

**Fig. 7.5** ECG, PCG and carotid pulse of atrial fibrillation; the pulse is irregular in spacing and form. The patient had mitral stenosis and regurgitation, the PCG showing a clear opening snap and systolic murmur. (Recording speed 50 mm/s.)

quicken the heart. Extrasystoles, on the other hand, often disappear with exercise though they may reappear with increased frequency shortly after the period of exertion.

### 3 Blood pressure

Only a very rough idea of the blood pressure can be achieved by estimating the degree of digital compression necessary to obliterate the artery, and hypertension can never be detected in this way.

**Instrumental estimation of blood pressure** This is accomplished by use of a sphygmomanometer. Many instruments are on the market, some with a mercury manometer and some of the aneroid type.

The inflatable bag should be about 10 cm in width (and 25 cm long), as narrower ones are known to give false readings.

The band is wrapped firmly and evenly around the arm about 8 cm above the elbow, which should be quite free to move, so that the bell of the stethoscope can be placed in the cubital fossa. The arm band contains a rubber bag which is blown up until the brachial artery is occluded. At this point the radial pulse disappears.

*The systolic pressure* The systolic pressure (i.e. the maximum pressure during the propagation of the pulse wave) may be estimated by:

1. *The palpatory method.* The armlet is pumped to a greater degree than is necessary to obliterate the radial pulse. The air is then slowly released until the pulse is once more palpable. The reading on the manometer at this point represents the systolic pressure.

2. *The auscultatory method.* The bell of the stethoscope is placed over the brachial artery (located first by palpation) at the bend of the elbow, and the armlet pumped up until all sounds disappear (*Fig. 7.6*). It is then gently released until a soft puffing noise is first heard. This point represents the systolic pressure (*Fig. 7.7*).

It is preferable to use the auscultatory method for the systolic as well as the

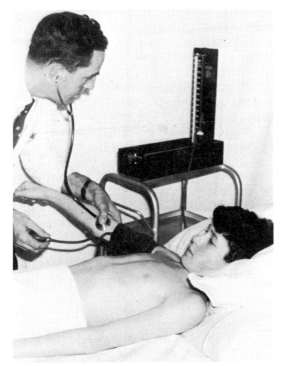

**Fig. 7.6**
Auscultatory method of
estimating blood
pressure.

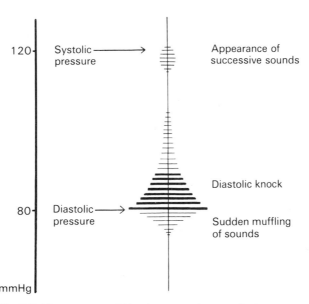

**Fig. 7.7** Measurement of blood pressure by auscultation.
Shows the sounds which may be audible over the brachial
artery.

diastolic pressure, but the systolic should be checked by the palpatory method, by which it may be found 5–10 mm lower. Further, in a few cases of hypertension, auscultation will show disappearance of the sounds, which reappear higher up the scale. This is known as the 'auscultatory silent gap' and will not be overlooked if the pressure is checked by palpation.

**The diastolic pressure** The diastolic pressure (i.e. the constant pressure in the artery between each systole) is only roughly measurable.

The auscultatory method is employed. The procedure is the same as for obtaining the systolic pressure; the observer listens for sounds over the brachial artery at the elbow. Following the puffing noise heard at and below the systolic reading, there occurs a knocking or thudding sound which increases in intensity and then passes suddenly into another softer sound. The sharp transition from the loud knocking to the soft blowing sound is taken as the diastolic pressure. Sometimes it is impossible to record the diastolic pressure owing to lack of any distinction between the knocking and soft sounds. In aortic incompetence the soft sounds may continue almost to zero and it is impossible to state the exact diastolic pressure.

A useful confirmation of the diastolic pressure is obtainable by noting that it corresponds with the sudden decrease of the maximum oscillation of the mercury column.

### 4 Form

Under this heading may be considered the volume and variations in the type of the pulse wave, which can really be best appreciated by graphic methods. Considerable experience is necessary before much information can be obtained by the use of the fingers alone, but by careful comparison of a series of normal (*Figs.* 7.8 and 7.12) and abnormal pulses the student will learn to distinguish a thin thready pulse (pulsus parvus) from a full bounding one, and with experience the slighter grades of these extremes. The pulsus parvus is found in conditions where there is a low stroke output, e.g. in mitral stenosis, and in shock, where vasoconstriction with pallor and sweating may also be present, as

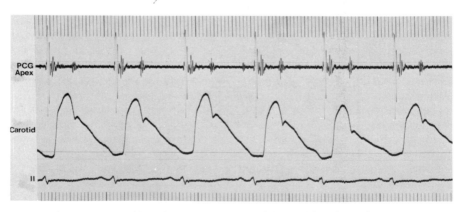

**Fig. 7.8** Normal carotid pulse. The PCG and ECG in this tracing are abnormal. (Recording speed 50 mm/s.)

occasionally happens with cardiac infarction. The bounding pulse on the other hand is found in hyperkinetic circulatory states where there is vasodilatation and increased stroke output, e.g. pregnancy, thyrotoxicosis, fevers and anaemias. Special varieties of pulse form are as follows:

1. The *plateau pulse* (*Figs. 7.9, 7.10, 7.15*) in which the summit of the pulse wave has a longer duration than normal.

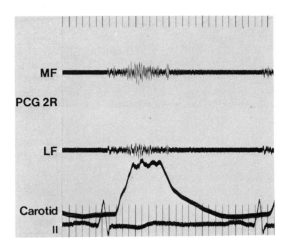

**Fig. 7.9** 'Plateau' pulse in aortic stenosis. The slow rising pulse has coarse summit vibrations which could be felt as a thrill. Note the crescendo–decrescendo 'diamond' shape of the systolic murmur in the accompanying PCG. The ECG also is abnormal, with a negative T wave and a bifid P. (Recording speed 100 mm/s.)

2. The *collapsing pulse*, in which the peak of the pulse wave occurs early and is of very brief duration, and from which there is an equally swift descent. It is the rapid fall in pulse pressure which gives the characteristic 'collapsing' sensation, but when the stroke output of the left ventricle is very large, as in aortic regurgitation of severe degree, the rapid ascent to a high systolic pressure level contributes to the typical pulse contour. The bisferiens pulse of aortic regurgitation and stenosis has a rapid rise, a double peak and a fall not quite so rapid as in a true collapsing pulse (*see Fig. 7.16*).

3. The *dicrotic* or *hyperdicrotic pulse* in which the dicrotic notch and wave are so pronounced as sometimes to give the impression of two separate pulse waves, the second being smaller then the first (*see Fig. 7.13*). It is present when a low stroke output is accompanied by peripheral vasodilatation.

The plateau pulse is found in aortic stenosis where the systole of the heart is more sustained than usual. The collapsing pulse, best elicited by placing the hand around the patient's wrist with his arm held vertically (*Fig. 7.11*), is found in conditions where the diastolic pressure is so low as to produce a relative emptiness of the arteries and a flaccidity of their walls, and occurs in aortic regurgitation,

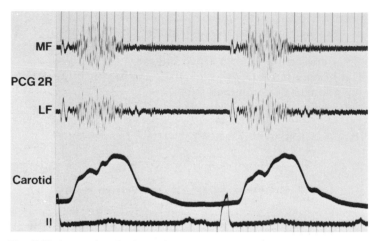

**Fig. 7.10** Anacrotic pulse in aortic stenosis. The slow rise of this pulse is of the same nature as the 'plateau' pulse shown in *Fig.* 7.9, showing a well-defined anacrotic notch on the upstroke of the pulse, and a sustained peak.

The PCG shows a typical 'ejection' systolic murmur, this time followed by a much less intense decrescendo diastolic murmur, produced by an insignificant degree of aortic regurgitation. (Recording speed 100 mm/s.)

arteriovenous fistula, especially patent ductus arteriosus, and to a lesser extent in hyperthyroidism and other conditions causing vasodilatation.

The patient may complain of throbbing headache or pulsation in the finger tips. The collapsing or 'water-hammer' pulse derives its name from the effect of concussion of moving water against the sides of a pipe on sudden stoppage of the flow. In studying the form of the pulse invaluable knowledge may be acquired by comparing pulse tracings (*Figs.* 7.12–7.16) with the results of palpation.

Alteration in the volume of the pulse may occur from beat to beat. In normal persons the volume was once thought to be greater with inspiration because of increased venous return to the heart. In fact this is not the case, but a fall in pulse volume during inspiration is still known as 'pulsus paradoxus'. This may be seen physiologically if the breathing is thoracic in type or if the chest is held rigidly with the shoulders braced backwards and also in severe asthma. If these conditions have been excluded, pulsus paradoxus suggests the presence of pericardial effusion or constrictive pericarditis—conditions which interfere with the normal return of blood to the heart and produce a diminished stroke output at the height of inspiration.

In *pulsus alternans* (*Fig.* 7.14) there is an alternate variation in the size of the pulse wave, said to be due to a defective myocardium in which not all the fibres are capable of contracting at each heartbeat. It is often found in serious myocardial disease and is a sign of grave omen when the cardiac rhythm is normal. It is important, however, to realize that pulsus alternans may occur without serious myocardial disease if the ventricular rate is rapid, as, for example, in paroxysmal tachycardia.

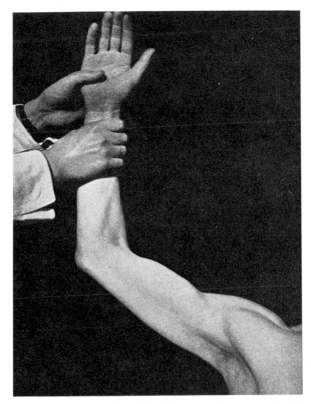

**Fig. 7.11** The collapsing pulse. (The water-hammer pulse.) To elicit the collapsing pulse the patient's arm should be raised well above the head and the wrist grasped so that the palm of the examiner's hand lies over its anterior aspect. This intensifies the collapsing sensation felt in the arteries after each systole of the heart.

The uncommon condition of hypertrophic obstructive cardiomyopathy (HOCM) produces a 'jerky' pulse with an initial sharp rise followed by prolongation, as in aortic stenosis. The shape of the recorded pulse wave is quite typical (*Fig.* 7.17).

### 5. Condition of the arterial wall

The examination of the pulse is completed by observations on the wall of the artery. An attempt should be made to roll the vessel under the index and second fingers. In many young persons the arterial wall is so compliant that with pressure of this kind it seems to merge into the surrounding tissues and to have no separate entity. In middle age it becomes distinctly palpable, and in the later decades can usually be felt as a cord-like structure. No hard-and-fast rule can be laid down as to what should be considered physiological and what pathological

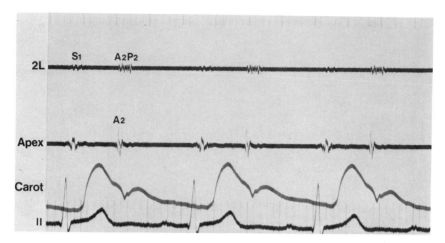

**Fig. 7.12** Normal carotid pulse. The ECG is normal, and the PCG, recorded by separate microphones at 2L (pulmonary area) and apex, shows normal splitting of the second sound at the pulmonary area, the aortic component first. The PCG recorded at the apex is also normal, showing a single (aortic) component of the second sound. (Recording speed 100 mm/s.)

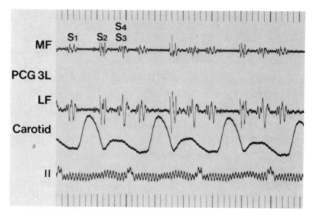

**Fig. 7.13** Dicrotic pulse. The ECG shows marked a.c. interference. The carotid pulse is typical of low stroke output, being an almost symmetric triangle in shape, followed by a large dicrotic wave. The PCG shows a summation gallop rhythm. The patient had congestive cardiomyopathy. (Recording speed 75 mm/s.)

arterial thickening. Again it is only by experience that the examiner can form suitable standards for comparison.

While palpating the arterial wall note should also be made of any irregularity in its surface and of any tortuosity in its course. Irregularities are chiefly associated with those types of arteriosclerosis where calcareous material is deposited in the

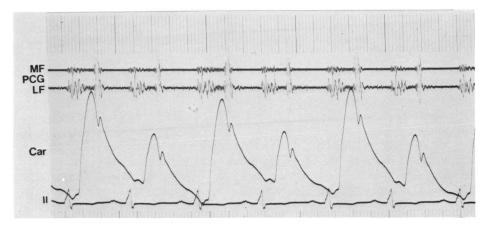

**Fig. 7.14** Pulsus alternans. This patient was recovering from open heart surgery, and aortic valve replacement. The alternating volume and duration of the pulse is well shown. There are abnormalities also in the ECG and PCG. (Recording speed 50 mm/s.)

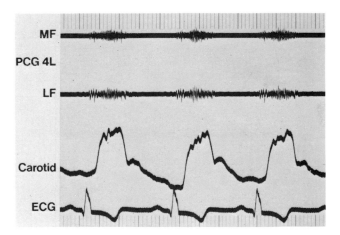

**Fig. 7.15** Plateau or anacrotic pulse. A patient with aortic stenosis. Compare this figure with 7.9 and 7.10. The ECG is also abnormal, and the PCG shows an ejection murmur. (Recording speed 50 mm/s.)

vessel wall, the 'pipe-stem' arteries of old age, and in certain cases hard ring-like structures can be felt along the course of the vessel, giving it a semblance to the trachea. Rarely, a localized aneurysm or inflammatory thickening of a peripheral artery may be found, as in giant-cell arteritis. Further consideration of the peripheral vessels now follows. (*See also* p. 282.)

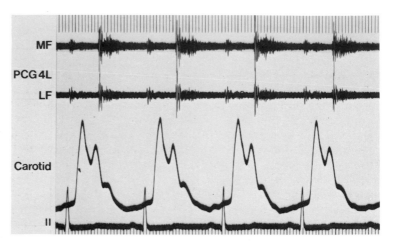

**Fig. 7.16** Bisferiens pulse. This pulse has a palpable dip, resembling in some ways the dicrotic pulse, but with distinguishing features on palpation. Present when there is a combination of aortic regurgitation and stenosis, the diastolic murmur of the regurgitation is particularly well seen here. *See Fig.* 7.36 for the pulse of aortic regurgitation without stenosis— the 'collapsing' pulse. (Recording speed 50 mm/s.)

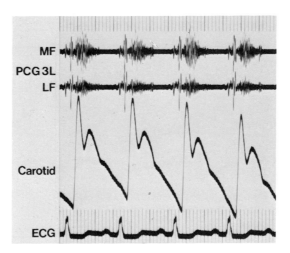

**Fig. 7.17** The sharp rise of the 'jerky' pulse of hypertrophic obstructive cardiomyopathy (HOCM) can be readily seen here. The initial sharp upstroke is followed by the much slower rise to the second peak. The PCG shows a fourth heart sound immediately before the first heart sound; no ejection sound, and no diastolic murmur. (Recording speed 50 mm/s.)

## INSPECTION AND AUSCULTATION OF THE PERIPHERAL VESSELS

### Inspection

Although the principal examination of the pulse is by palpation, useful information may be derived from inspection and auscultation. All the important peripheral vessels should be inspected. In those conditions in which a collapsing pulse is found, notably aortic regurgitation, the arteries pulsate vigorously and in a jerky manner (Corrigan's sign). This is well seen in the carotids, causing the head to nod or the ears to move with each systole of the heart.

Arteriosclerosis may often be recognized by the tortuosity of the superficial vessels (e.g. superficial temporal and brachial arteries) due to their lengthening while remaining more or less fixed at their proximal and distal points. In particular when the arm is flexed at the elbow to about 110°, the tortuosity of the brachial artery becomes most noticeable, and the snake-like movements of the tortuous vessel with each systole have earned for this phenomenon the name of 'locomotor brachial'. It is important that the elbow shall not be flexed beyond a right-angle, otherwise spurious tortuosity may be apparent.

The *retinal vessels* should be specially examined (*see* p. 344).

*Capillary pulsation* is found where there is marked vasodilatation, particularly if there is also a big pulse pressure. It is therefore most frequently seen in aortic regurgitation but may be found in normal persons if the skin is warm and in hyperthyroidism in which the skin is usually warm. It may be observed by pressing with a glass slide on the fingernail or lip sufficiently heavily to cause partial blanching (*Fig.* 7.18). The blanched area becomes pink with each systole of the heart.

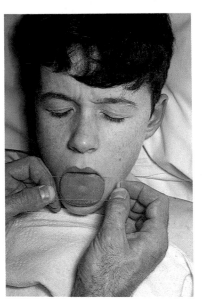

**Fig. 7.18**
Capillary pulsation (aortic regurgitation). Pressure may be made on the tongue or everted lower lip and the glass slide pressed on the mucous membrane sufficiently firmly to produce an area of blanching. With each systole of the heart the blanched area becomes pink. This can be seen particularly at the junction of the blanched area with the normal mucous membrane.

It can also be demonstrated by shining a pen torch through the pad of the thumb and watching the pulsations in the nail bed. When there is a very big pulse pressure as in severe aortic regurgitation, capillary pulsation may be seen in the patient's forehead and face, when the alternate blanching and flushing is known as the 'lighthouse sign' for obvious reasons.

### Auscultation

Murmurs are not uncommonly propagated into the great vessels. The harsh systolic murmur of aortic stenosis is usually transmitted into the carotids. A systolic murmur is heard on pressure of the stethoscope over the great vessels (especially the femorals) in aortic regurgitation. Similarly, in this disease, the sudden output of a large quantity of blood from the left ventricle into the relatively empty arteries causes the 'pistol shot' sound to be heard. This has the same significance as the water-hammer pulse.

A systolic murmur may be heard over a stenosed peripheral artery, e.g. over the kidneys in renal artery stenosis and in the neck in carotid or vertebral stenosis.

## EXAMINATION OF THE VEINS

This should include inspection and palpation of the superficial veins for evidence of engorgement, varicosity, and the presence of thombi or evidence of inflammation.

### Venous engorgement

Venous engorgement is most easily observed in the neck (*Fig.* 7.19), though other veins than the jugulars may exhibit evidence of it. In judging whether veins are over-distended, it is necessary to fix a zero level. This is taken to be the sternal angle, i.e. the junction of the manubrium with the body of the sternum, for in whatever position the patient may be, sitting, standing, lying or in intermediate postures, it represents the zero position in the venous system, the level, in other words, of the blood in the mid-right atrium. Veins above this level are collapsed; veins below filled to varying degrees.

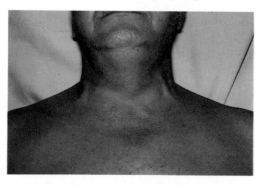

**Fig. 7.19** Over-filled jugular vein in a case of constrictive pericarditus. A similar appearance is seen in congestive cardiac failure, in which, however, the veins are pulsatile. (Cf. *Fig.* 6.4, p. 167.)

Judgement as to whether a vein is pathologically over-filled, therefore, will depend upon the height above the sternal angle at which the distension can be recognized. Normally, when the patient is supine with the head on pillows, the level of the blood in the jugular veins reaches about one-third of the way up the neck. This level will be found to coincide with the level of the sternal angle. In early cases of congestive failure in the same position, the jugular column rises half-way to the jaw, and, in more severe cases, right to the jaw. Now if the patient sits gradually more upright, the column of blood will fall, in normal subjects, to such an extent that it can no longer be seen (it has sunk to the level of the sternal angle and is no longer filling the jugular veins). In cases of congestive failure, however, the column may still be visible above the clavicle for several centimetres or even throughout the course of the veins. Before assuming that a rise in venous pressure is due to cardiac failure (the commonest and most important cause), it must be recognized that a rise may also occur from increased intrathoracic pressure, but in this case the venous engorgement will usually disappear on deep inspiration. Obstruction to the superior vena cava is also a cause, but errors will be uncommon if search is made for supporting signs of congestive cardiac failure. (Cf. also Mediastinal Obstruction, p. 193.)

The filling of the veins should be bilateral and roughly equal, though the right side is more reliable as it is unaffected by aortic unfolding. A local obstruction may cause unilateral distension, often removed by turning the head. The venous engorgement should be accompanied by pulsation even when it is due to constrictive pericarditis or tamponade, but the venous pressure in these patients may be so high as to make the pulsation difficult to observe.

When more precise information about the venous pressure is required these simple clinical procedures can be checked by direct measurements. The height above the sternal angle can be recorded in a vertical saline-filled tube connected to a catheter introduced into the superior vena cava or right atrium, a method of measuring the central venous pressure used in intensive care wards.

### Pulsation of the veins

This should be noted carefully. It often helps to localize the upper limit of jugular engorgement. In itself it is not pathological but may indicate that the level of venous distension is above the sternal angle. It must be distinguished from arterial pulsation, which is more obvious in the erect posture, while venous pulsation will diminish or disappear as the venous column falls with the assumption of an erect posture, unless the pressure is raised. It is difficult to feel normal venous pulsation, and then only with lightly placed fingers, but arterial pulsation pushes the fingers away forcibly. None the less, the distinction between the two is sometimes difficult, and when the jugular venous pressure is raised, it is readily palpable deep to the clavicular head of the sternomastoid, a fact well known to cardiographers who use very firm pressure in this area in recording the jugular pulse. It may be helpful to note that two positive waves may be identified in jugular pulsation but only one in carotid pulsation, though venous and arterial pulsations are often visible together. These two venous waves are the 'a' and 'v' waves identifiable graphically (*see below*).

Pulsation in the jugular veins (*Fig.* 7.20) affects both external and internal vessels. The former is more easily recognized in the normal person, but the latter

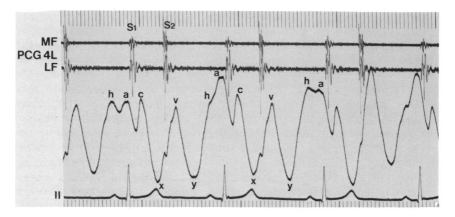

**Fig. 7.20** Normal jugular pulse. Shown with a normal ECG and PCG. 'a' occurs with atrial systole, 'c' as the tricuspid valve moves into the atrial cavity with ventricular systole. Note the second, tricuspid component of the first heart sound occurs at the notch between the 'a' and 'c' waves. The 'x' descent occurs with atrial relaxation, and the rise to the 'v' peak (interrupted by a small notch coincident with the second heart sound) occurs with the passive filling of the right atrium from the great veins.

After the tricupid valve opens, the passage of blood into the relaxing ventricle corresponds with the descent of the pulse wave form from the 'v' peak to the 'y' trough, at which point the ventricle becomes more resistant to filling, the pressure in the atrium rises again, and when the heart rate is sufficiently slow, the wave form levels out at a point designated 'h'. This latter point is often summated with the next 'a' wave, as shown in the second complex here. (Recording speed 50 mm/s.)

is more often found in congestive failure. When venous pulsation is not easy to identify, it may help to observe the patient in a good light, looking obliquely across the root of the neck from the front. Inspiration, by increasing venous return to the thorax, may make the venous pulse more obvious.

When the engorgement is due to non-cardiac causes such as mediastinal tumours, there is often no pulsation, as the pressure of the tumour interferes with the movement of blood between the jugular veins and right atrium. This is made more obvious by compression of the abdomen, which still further increases the jugular over-filling and pulsation in cases of congestive failure, but not when the veins are obstructed. The test also has the advantage of distinguishing carotid pulsation which is uninfluenced by abdominal pressure.

The pulsation observed in the jugular veins reflects the pressure changes in the right atrium, provided no obstruction of the vein exists. As the atrium contracts, so the pressure in the atrium rises, to force blood into the right ventricle, at the end of ventricular diastole. This rise in atrial pressure shows in the jugular veins as the 'a' wave, which begins at the peak of the 'P' wave of the ECG, immediately before the onset of the first heart sound and the carotid pulse.

As the atrium relaxes, the intra-atrial pressure falls, represented by the down-stroke from the peak of the 'a' wave, but at the same time ventricular systole begins and the intraventricular pressure rises above that in the atrium, resulting in closure of the tricuspid valve. As the valve cusps balloon into the atrial cavity, there is a temporary halt in the falling intra-atrial pressure and a transient rise, shown as the 'c' wave. The onset of the 'c' wave corresponds with the incidence of the tricuspid component of the first heart-sound.

As atrial relaxation continues after the 'c' wave, the pressure also fall until at the 'x' trough it reaches its lowest point, when with the inflow of blood from the great veins pressure begins to rise again to the second peak of the venous pulse, the 'v' wave. At this point, ventricular diastole has proceeded far enough for the intra-atrial pressure to exceed that in the ventricle, and the tricuspid valve opens. The intraventricular pressure is still falling and blood flows through the valve into the ventricle, with a resultant fall in the intra-atrial pressure also, until at the 'y' trough the ventricle is filled, and the pressure in ventricle and atrium begins to rise again, to even out until the onset of the next 'a' wave (*Fig. 7.20*).

Any rise in right atrial pressure will cause an increase in the height of the 'a' wave. Thus, if tricuspid stenosis is present, very large 'a' waves are seen in the neck. If the intraventricular pressure is high at the end of diastole, as will occur in pulmonary arterial hypertension and pulmonary stenosis, and in other conditions where there is right ventricle hypertrophy and loss of compliance, the right atrial contraction must be correspondingly more vigorous if it is to force blood into the ventricle, and the 'a' wave will again be high (*Fig. 7.21*).

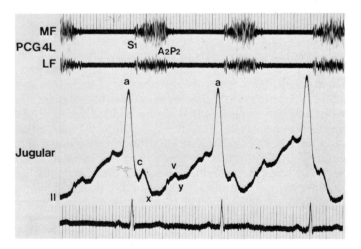

**Fig. 7.21** Tall jugular 'a' waves in pulmonary stenosis. The PCG shows a characteristic systolic murmur extending through the position of the aortic component of the second sound, to end before the small pulmonary component of this sound. The tall 'a' wave occurs because of right ventricle hypertrophy, making a rise in right atrial pressure necessary to produce late diastolic ventricular filling properly. The 'a' wave begins at about the peak of the P wave in the ECG, is followed by a normal 'c' wave and 'x' descent, but the descent to the 'y' trough after the 'v' peak is slow. (Recording speed 50 mm/s.)

If the ventricle contracts before or at the same time as the atrium because of premature beats, nodal rhythm or other disturbances of conduction, then the atrium will contract on to a closed tricuspid valve, resulting in a very high intra-atrial pressure, reflected in the jugular pulse as 'cannon' waves.

Rapid regular atrial contraction in atrial flutter can be seen in the jugular pulse, as 'a' waves interspersed with 'cannon' waves.

When atrial fibrillation is present, the 'a' wave disappears, and the 'x' descent is also obliterated as no significant atrial relaxation occurs, so that the jugular pulse is seen as a single positive wave, the 'v' wave.

With tricuspid incompetence, it is unusual for sinus rhythm to be present. Since the intraventricular pressure is transmitted to the atrium, the jugular pulse in these circumstances shows a tall systolic wave only, the 'x' descent being totally obliterated. With the cessation of ventricular contraction, the pressure quickly falls and blood flows rapidly back through the tricuspid valve, shown in the jugular pulse as a rapid descent to the 'y' trough. In these circumstances the 'y' collapse after the tall 'v' wave is easily seen.

The clinical analysis of jugular pulsations needs some practice and skill, and rapid action of the heart tends to fusion of the waves. Graphic methods of recording these pulsations can be of great value.

# ■ EXAMINATION OF THE HEART

The examination of the heart should follow the usual routine of inspection, palpation, percussion and auscultation.

*Inspection* enables the examiner to see the position and extent of the cardiac impulse and its rhythm. The presence of abnormal pulsation is noted over the precordium, over the great vessels in the neck and in the epigastrium. Some of these points have been considered under the Examination of the Pulse, p. 208.

*Palpation* confirms the position of the apex beat and gives more information about the force, duration and character of the cardiac impulse. Thrills, a special form of vibration, are communicated to the hand. Expansile pulsation may be detected in cases of aneurysm.

*Percussion* has been discredited as a method of examining the heart because of the greater accuracy of radiology and will not be considered in detail. It may have some value when the patient is too ill to move by showing the increased dullness due to pericardial effusion. Occasionally it may demonstrate the basal dullness, especially to the right of the sternum, in cases of aortic aneurysm.

*Auscultation* is of great value in the detection of abnormalities of the valves which commonly produce both changes in the heart-sounds and added sounds called *murmurs*. It is also of importance in other diseases which alter the character of the heart sounds, and in pericarditis where a friction sound is present. The rhythm of the heart is determined by examination of the pulse and auscultation of the heart.

These points will now be considered more fully.

## INSPECTION

This method of examination is of greatest value in studying the position, character and rhythm of the cardiac impulse (p. 226). Abnormal pul-

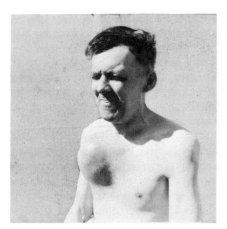

**Fig. 7.22**
Aortic aneurysm bulging
through chest.

sations especially of cardiac hypertrophy and aneurysms, may also be visible (*Fig.* 7.22). The patient should be in a good light, and the cardiac and other pulsations examined both in the erect and recumbent posture.

### PALPATION

Palpation also should be carried out with the patient first in the recumbent and then in the erect posture. The flat of the hand should be placed systematically over the apex beat and over the base of the heart. The extent of the cardiac impulse already defined by inspection should be confirmed; the force and character of the cardiac thrust can also be appreciated. The hand should then be placed on all areas of the precordium in order to detect any abnormal pulsations or vibrations.

As the cardiac impulse is normally circumscribed at the apex beat, the palm of the hand is too large for accurate palpation, and the information gained by it should be supplemented by the use of two fingers allowed to rest lightly over the cardiac thrust (*see Fig.* 7.28, p. 236). In this way the area of the cardiac impulse and its quality can be defined more carefully.

Apart from radiology, palpation is the most reliable method of estimating the size of the heart. It is essential, however, that the position of the apex beat should be measured from the mid-sternum to the farthest point towards the axilla at which the palpating fingers are actually lifted. With a normal heart this distance varies from 7·5 to 10·5 cm (3–4 in) according to the patient's stature or build.

It should be noted that in the normal adult little or no pulsation is communicated to the hand from the heart base or great vessels. Undue pulsation in this region is suggestive of aneurysmal enlargement of the great vessels, especially of the ascending part or arch of the aorta, more rarely of the pulmonary artery. Pulsation in the second left intercostal space may, however, be seen normally in children. Left parasternal pulsation may be caused by right ventricle hypertrophy, but it may also be the result of transmitted pulsation from an enlarged left atrium due to severe mitral regurgitation (*see also* p. 257).

The student should make it a practice to place the hand on each side of the chest in turn, especially when the apex beat is not easily palpated in its normal position on the left side. In this way he will avoid overlooking *dextrocardia*.

### The cardiac impulse

The cardiac thrust is maximal normally at the apex beat and can be examined by inspection and palpation. Two separate aspects must receive attention, the position and the character.

**Position** The normal impulse (apex beat) is usually visible and distinctly palpable 7·5–10·5 cm (3–4 in) from the midline and generally in the fifth intercostal space. It is circumscribed and can usually be covered by a 10p piece. It is almost invariably within the nipple line except occasionally in children and adolescents. In women this landmark for obvious reasons is of no value, but in men it is useful, as the nipple is generally further from the midline in sthenic individuals whose hearts are also proportionately larger. The systolic thrust is caused by the contracting left ventricle lifting the chest-wall. Internal to the thrust may be seen an area of systolic retraction caused by movements of the right ventricle, and it is necessary that this systolic retraction should not be confused with that of pathological origin. With changes of posture (lying on one side) the apex beat may move as much as 1·5–2 cm. If the impulse is abnormal in position, particular care should be taken to look for causes of cardiac displacement such as scoliosis and funnel sternum; also pleural and pulmonary diseases (e.g. pleural effusion and pulmonary fibrosis). When these causes have been eliminated, an abnormal position generally signifies cardiac enlargement.

*Left ventricular hypertrophy* results in downward (sixth space) and outward displacement of the apex beat.

*Right ventricular hypertrophy* causes strong pulsation in the left parasternal region and often movement of the sternum and ribs (*see above*).

**Character** In normal persons the apex beat gently raises the palpating fingers. The strength of this thrust can only be judged by experience. It is diminished in health by a thick chest wall (muscle or fat) or by emphysema, and is more noticeable in thin persons.

If the impulse is feeble, less significance can be attached to it, unless it has been watched from day to day and is known to have changed. In this case a feeble diffuse impulse, combined with change in position towards the axilla, may suggest dilatation. Diffuseness alone or sometimes with temporary increased forcibility often results from simple overaction of the heart as in nervous persons, after exercise or in hyperthyroidism. Certain special types of cardiac impulse are recognizable to the experienced fingers, such as the tap or shock of mitral stenosis. If the thrust is forcible, hypertrophy is suggested. When great cardiac enlargement is present there may be a diffuse heave.

The position and character of the cardiac impulse thus give valuable information as to the presence of cardiac enlargement and whether this is due to hypertrophy or dilatation. It will be convenient here to consider briefly the clinical significance of these phenomena.

### Hypertrophy

The presence of hypertrophy indicates that the heart is working under an extra load. The clinical examination is therefore directed primarily to the discovery of this load, which may include hypertension, valve disease, pulmonary diseases and others. The degree of the hypertrophy is also a rough indication of the extent of the load, i.e. the seriousness of the condition causing hypertrophy. Left and right ventricular hypertrophy can generally be recognized clinically, but enlargement of the atria cannot easily be detected except radiologically, although left atrial enlargement may be suspected when there is systolic pulsation in the left parasternal area in patients with mitral regurgitation.

### Dilatation

This may be physiological as in exercise, when the cardiac output increases with increased venous input because of the stretch on the ventricular muscle fibres at the end of diastole.

Pathological changes in the heart muscle may alter the response to the stretch, so that although the heart dilates, its output falls.

This may be seen in various cardiac muscle disorders, in cardiac infarction and as a temporary response when the ventricles beat at a high speed as in atrial flutter.

Dilatation is not easy to recognize, though in acute cases displacement of the apex beat may be apparent, and radiology will demonstrate enlargement of the cardiac shadow.

It is often accompanied by hypertrophy as in mixed aortic valve disease, heart block and sometimes in athletes, where the stroke output of the ventricle is increased.

Atrial dilatation, usually with hypertrophy, is seen in some types of valvular and congenital heart disease. A good example is the enlargement of the left atrium in mitral stenosis.

### Thrills

When vibrations are communicated to the palpating hand from the heart or its great vessels, they are spoken of as thrills. They are usually detected best when the breath is held in expiration. A thrill is a palpable murmur and is produced in the same way, though as a rule the conditions necessary for its production must be more exaggerated than in the case of a murmur. Of these conditions the main ones are obstruction to the passage of blood from the chambers of the heart though a narrowed valve, and the abnormal blood flow in certain congenital defects, but the thrill will be more readily palpable if the chest wall is thin, if the blood flow is rapid, and if the site of production is comparatively near the surface. Like murmurs, thrills may be systolic or diastolic in time, or, more rarely, may occur continuously throughout the cardiac cycle. For the novice it is often difficult to time a thrill accurately, and it is justifiable to consider the timing in conjunction with that of the murmur which always accompanies it. The presence of a thrill is more certain evidence of organic disease of the heart than the presence of a murmur.

At the base of the heart thrills are more commonly systolic. In aortic stenosis and in aneurysm of the great vessels at the root of the neck a powerful systolic thrill may be palpable over the second right interspace, usually spreading upwards towards the neck. To the left of the sternum in the second interspace pulmonary stenosis gives rise to a similar type of thrill. Lower down the sternum, usually in the second interspace, systolic thrills are occasionally felt due to congenital lesions of the heart, particularly patency of the interventricular septum. Occasionally systolic thrills are found at the apex alone, due to mitral regurgitation, but it is not uncommon for a thrill arising at the other areas mentioned to extend into the region of the apex.

By contrast, diastolic thrills at the apex are relatively common and usually due to mitral stenosis. They correspond in time with the murmur, and if this is presytolic, the thrill may end with a systolic shock at the apex synchronizing with an abrupt first sound. Because diastolic murmurs with mitral stenosis are of very low pitch, they are often easily palpable although not so easily heard.

The combination of a systolic and diastolic thrill is rare. It sometimes occurs over the base of the heart in patients with patent ductus arteriosus. If such a thrill exists care should be taken not to overlook the possibility of other vascular abnormalities, such as an enlarged overactive thyroid gland, a vascular mediastinal tumour, or still more rarely an arteriovenous aneurysm.

## AUSCULTATION

Auscultation ranks with inspection and palpation as a most important method of examining the cardiovascular system. A suitable stethoscope is one that has a bell chest piece for low-pitched sounds, e.g. the diastolic murmur of mitral stenosis, and a flat diaphragm-like chest piece which is more suitable for high-pitched sounds such as the murmur of aortic regurgitation. By means of auscultation the rate and rhythm of the heart may be confirmed and compared with those of the pulse, but its main value is in the information it yields concerning the functions of the heart valves and to a lesser extent of the state of the myocardium and pericardium. The student should learn to concentrate first on the auscultation of the heart sounds before turning his attention to any additional sounds, called *murmurs*, which may be present. He should also pay attention to each heart sound separately, ignoring the others for a while, and at each separate area ask himself the following questions:

1. Can I hear the first sound, and is it normal? If it is not normal, how does it differ from the usual?

2. Can I hear the second sound, and is it normal? Can I hear splitting of the second sound, and if so, does it vary normally with respiration?

3. Can I hear any added sounds? If so, where in the cardiac cycle do they occur, and what character do they have?

4. Are any murmurs present? If so, where in the cardiac cycle do they occur, what relationship do they have to the sounds and added sounds, what is their character and to where are they propagated?

## THE HEART SOUNDS

Even in perfect health considerable differences exist in the intensity and character of the heart sounds in different individuals. To form some idea of the limits of these variations the beginner should examine as many normal hearts as possible. In obese persons, in emphysema or in those with well-developed musculature, the sounds are diminished in intensity. Conversely, thin coverings of muscle or fat on the chest wall allow the sounds to be conducted more clearly and loudly to the stethoscope. Therefore, it is usually easy to define the heart sounds at all areas of the precordium in children.

Auscultation of the heart should be made over a large area of the precordium, but especially over the apex and base of the heart, i.e. a little distance from the anatomical position of the valves. The apex is sometimes called the 'mitral' area, and the base is divided into 'aortic' and 'pulmonary' areas. The 'tricuspid' area at the lower end of the sternum is of less importance. These areas are chosen for auscultation because of the variability of the heart sounds over them and also because murmurs associated with valve disease may be heard most commonly at one of them, e.g. the diastolic murmur of mitral stenosis at the mitral area. However, auscultation must not be confined to these named areas, and the site of any abnormality heard should be recorded in terms of intercostal level and distance from the sternum (to left or right). It must be clearly understood that sounds produced in the heart have a common origin, though their component elements may be heard with a different intensity over different parts of the chest. The first sound, associated with closure of the mitral and tricuspid valves, is heard best at the apex, and as the mitral element is louder than the tricuspid, this is the most easily heard component of the first sound. The second sound is associated with closure of the aortic and pulmonary valves. Normally the aortic component of the second sound is best heard over the aortic area and is transmitted to the apex. The pulmonary component, on the other hand, is generally heard best over the pulmonary area and in the region of the second and third left interspaces. Both components of the second sound may normally be heard, the aortic component preceding the pulmonary. The intensity of the components varies with age, the aortic element dominating in the older age groups and the pulmonary element in the young.

A third sound is sometimes heard, particularly in childhood and adolescence, and may cause confusion in deciding whether or not a mitral diastolic murmur is present. It is associated with rapid distension of the ventricle in early diastole, although its exact mode of production is not clear. It occurs at the nadir of the trough in the appropriate venous pulse, shortly after the second heart sound, and is best heard at the apex and left sternal border, with the patient recumbent.

If atrial systole is abnormally vigorous it may produce a fourth heart sound, occurring before the first sound. This occurs when atrial augmentation of ventricular filling in late diastole take place with a 'non-compliant' ventricle, i.e. one not easily distended.

The heart sounds are often likened to the syllables 'lub-dup' and have definition which helps to distinguish them from additional sounds such as murmurs. It is important to be aware of the notable variation of the heart sounds in health which makes difficult any precise imitation of the sounds.

Just as the pulse rate and the blood pressure should be examined at the end of the consultation as well as at the beginning, in order to exclude the effects of emotion or exercise, so the heart sounds should be compared at the beginning and end of the examination. If this is done systematically the student will learn that a considerable modification of the sounds may take place as the result of excitement or physical effort—both of which tend to make the heart sounds sharper and louder than normal, though the relative intensity of the sounds remains the same, the first sound being louder at the apex and the second sound at the base.

## Normal rhythm of the heart sounds (*Fig.* 7.23)

In a normal heart the first and second sounds are quite close together, but the interval following the second sound is relatively long. The sequence is thus lub-dup-pause, lub-dup-pause.

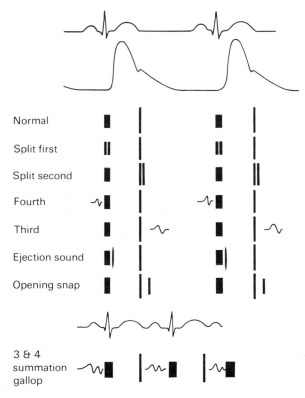

**Fig. 7.23** Diagram of heart sounds *Note*: the diagrammatic representation of the fourth and third heart sounds is to indicate that they have a lower frequency than the first and second sounds.

## Exaggeration of the Sounds

The heart sounds become louder in conditions which increase the activity of the heart, e.g. nervousness, exercise and hyperthyroidism. The increase is most obvious in the first sound at the apex and to a lesser extent in the second sound at the base. The first sound is also louder and abrupt in mitral stenosis, particularly at the apex. The second sound (aortic component) is increased at the aortic area in systemic hypertension. At the pulmonary area the pulmonary component of the second sound is increased when the pulmonary arterial pressure rises, as may occur in mitral stenosis, in certain forms of congenital heart disease and in some pulmonary diseases.

### Diminution of the sounds

Diminution in the heart sounds is more often due to extracardiac than to cardiac causes. Of these, emphysema is one of the most important, as the air-containing lung spreads over the area where the heart normally comes in contact with the chest wall. Similarly, fluid or air in the pleural or pericardial cavities may form a layer preventing the heart sounds from reaching the surface normally. Until these causes and the physiological ones mentioned earlier have been considered, feebleness of the heart sounds does not rank as an important sign; but if the patient has been examined previously and was known to have well-defined heart sounds which have become feeble, the sign is of more significance and may suggest cardiac failure.

### Splitting of sounds

Splitting of the first or second sound may be audible, the two elements being very close together. This closeness is an essential character of splitting, and distinguishes it from various forms of gallop rhythm in which three sounds are present but at considerable intervals one from the other. Splitting may be imitated by the syllables 'l-lub' and 'd-dub'. When affecting the *first sound* it is usually heard best at the apex, and is probably due to an asynchronous closure of the mitral and tricuspid valves. It is not pathological but the inexperienced may confuse it with an ejection click or even a short presystolic murmur.

Splitting of the second sound due to asynchronous closure of the aortic and pulmonary valves varies with respiration, is common and is often physiological. When the splitting is wide and fixed, i.e. not varying with respiration, it is more likely to be pathological. Normal splitting of the second sound is recognized by a widening of the interval between the aortic and pulmonary components during normal inspiration, and narrowing with expiration. This is caused by a temporary increase in venous return to the right heart, with prolongation of right ventricular systole, and consequent delay in pulmonary valve closure. Abnormalities of conduction, e.g. bundle-branch block, will alter the normal pattern of ventricle contraction, and in the case of left bundle-branch block may so delay left ventricle contraction as to cause the aortic component of the second sound to follow the pulmonary, when normal inspiration will then cause the splitting of the sound to narrow—the phenomenon of 'reversed splitting' of the second sound.

### The opening snap (*Fig.* 7.24)

This has considerable importance in the clinical appraisal of mitral stenosis. It is associated with the sudden movement of the valve as it opens in early diastole and is of a relatively sharp character. Its intensity probably depends upon the mobility of the mitral valve and the severity of the stenosis, but when it is present it should indicate that at least part of the valve is still mobile.

With lessening mobility of the valve, as happens commonly in mitral incompetence, the opening snap is less well heard, and, of course, calcification and fibrosis may make it totally inaudible.

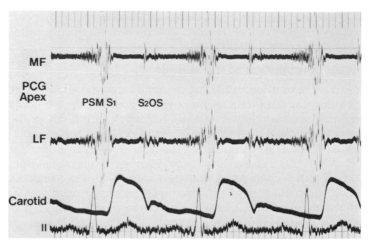

**Fig. 7.24** The sound records show a presystolic murmur (PSM) rising to a crescendo to meet the loud first heart sound (S1). S2 (the second heart sound) is followed by a clear opening snap (OS). The S2–OS interval is about 0·06 s. The carotid pulse is normal. (Recording speed 100 mm/s.)

It is often heard over a wide area of the precordium, but usually best over an area from the apex to the left sternal edge.

### Ejection clicks

These are sharp sounds, and occur coincidentally with the onset of the arterial pulse tracing, immediately after the first heart sound. They occur with the sudden opening of the appropriate semilunar valves, in conditions where this opening is delayed, e.g. in aortic valve stenosis, hypertension, pulmonary valve stenosis, or where the opening of the valve is abnormally rapid. In a similar way to the opening snap of the mitral valve, the ejection sound is an indication of the mobility of the appropriate semilunar valve.

Thus if aortic valvular stenosis is congenital with no calcification, an ejection click will be present. When the valve becomes calcified and immobile, the ejection click is absent or very much diminished.

It is often difficult to distinguish the first sound from an ejection sound, but phonocardiography will be of help in this distinction (*See Fig. 7.35, p. 244*).

### Gallop rhythm

This term is applied to *triple rhythms* produced by the addition of the third or fourth heart sounds to the normal first and second. As mentioned before, a normal third sound is often heard in youth, but over the age of 40 years any triple rhythm should be regarded with suspicion.

The *third sound gallop rhythm* (formerly called *protodiastolic*) is a sign of serious myocardial disease, and is thought to be produced by distension of a diseased myocardium in early diastole after the atrioventricular valves open. Arising from the right ventricle, it is best heard parasternally or in the epigastrium. From the left ventricle it is loudest at and internal to the apex.

The *fourth sound* or *'atrial' gallop* is produced by an abnormally loud fourth sound, which occurs when atrial contraction is forcing blood into a ventricle where the end diastolic pressure is abnormally high. This may occur in the early stages of ventricular failure but also when the ventricle is 'non-compliant', e.g. with severe ventricular hypertrophy, as in aortic stenosis, when the cavity of the ventricle is small, and atrial contraction has to produce a considerable pressure rise to augment ventricular filling.

The fourth sound disappears, of course, in atrial fibrillation. Its areas of maximal intensity are similar to those of the third sound.

True gallop rhythm has a fancied resemblance to the noise of a galloping horse and only occurs with a rapid heart rate, arbitrarily stated to be 100 per minute or over. In these cases the third and fourth sounds occur together and are said to be 'summated'. This summation gallop rhythm is of even greater seriousness than the third or fourth sound triple rhythm alone (*Fig.* 7.25).

### Midsystolic clicks

These sounds were thought to be of no significance, produced by pericardial adhesions, but recent studies have shown them to be produced by abnormalities of the atrioventricular valve mechanism, usually the mitral valve. They are caused by abnormal prolapse of the valve into the atrial cavity and are often accompanied by a systolic murmur of mitral regurgitation. They are readily identified by phonocardiography and demonstrated as being associated with valve prolapse by echocardiography (*Fig.* 7.26).

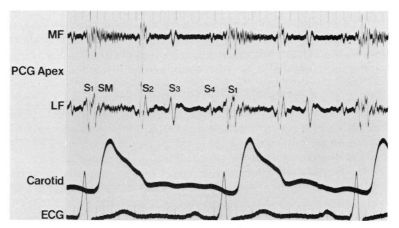

**Fig. 7.25** Illustrates the third (S3) and fourth (S4) heart sounds, in a patient with myocardial pathology of unknown aetiology. The carotid pulse and ECG are normal. Also present is wide splitting of the first heart sound (S1) and an early systolic murmur (SM). The second heart sound (S2) is normal. When S1, S2, S3 and S4 are audible it represents an unusual quadruple rhythm, a variety of so-called 'gallop' rhythm. *See Fig.* 7.23. (Recording speed 100 mm/s.)

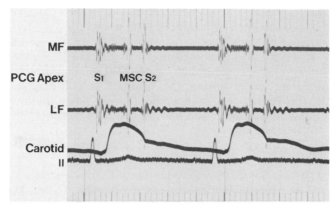

**Fig. 7.26** The ECG and carotid pulses are normal, but the sound records show a clear midsystolic click (MSC) between a normal S1 and S2, and after a low intensity short systolic murmur. This is an unusual variety of triple rhythm, most often associated with an abnormal mitral subvalvar mechanism. (Recording speed 75 mm/s.)

## ADDITIONAL SOUNDS

These include the class of sounds known as murmurs, originating at the valves or in the great vessels, and friction sounds produced in the pericardial layers and in the pleura which lies in close contact with the heart. Peculiar sounds are also heard occasionally due to impact of the heart against surrounding tissues—for example, against fluid or air in the pleural cavity, or through the diaphragm against the air- and fluid-containing viscera. These sounds have little importance, and, although their origin is often uncertain, they are rarely confused with the murmurs and pericardial sounds to be described.

### Pericardial friction sounds (*Fig.* 7.27)

A friction sound or rub is heard in cases of acute pericarditis and is comparable with a pleural rub. It is produced by the movement of the two layers of pericardium over one another in the presence of an exudate. The sound may be heard over any part of the precordium, and sometimes over so small an area as to be overlooked, while at other times it is so extensive as to be present over every part of the heart. The rub has a peculiar superficial quality and is sometimes rough and grating in character, sometimes scratchy, and at other times soft and blowing, so that it may be confused with the to-and-fro murmur so frequently heard in aortic regurgitation. Its intensity may be increased by heavier pressure with the stethoscope. Not uncommonly pericarditis is associated with pleurisy, and the pericardial friction rub may become continuous with the pleural rub and extend outside the limits of the precordium. Classically 'tripartite', the friction over the ventricle is heard during ventricular systole; in diastole when early filling of the ventricle is happening, and in late diastole when atrial augmentation of ventricular filling occurs.

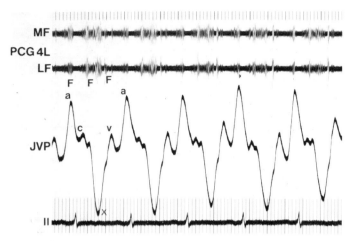

**Fig. 7.27** Pericardial friction occurring where tuberculous pericarditis was later shown to be present. The high-frequency friction sounds (F) have been recorded at the left sternal edge and, by comparing with the simultaneous carotid, jugular and ECG traces, can be seen to be present when there is movement associated with atrial contraction (and ventricular filling), with ventricular contraction during systole, and, during ventricular relaxation and rapid passive filling of the ventricle in early diastole. The friction noise is recorded at times when there is rapid movement of the cardiac chambers, with changes in volume. (Recording speed 50 mm/s.)

## Murmurs

When the position and character of the heart sounds have been determined, the student is in a position to pay attention to any murmurs which may be present.

### GENERAL POINTS FOR CONSIDERATION

The following points should be ascertained whenever a murmur is present:

**1. The time relationship** This implies not only whether the murmur occurs in systole or diastole but also whether it occupies a part or the whole of these. Great care is often necessary to time a murmur successfully. If the cardiac impulse is sufficiently great to lift the stethoscope during systole, or to be palpable with the finger, this forms an easy way of timing the first sound of the heart and thus of the murmur (*Fig. 7.28*). If the impulse is feeble, reliance must be placed on the pulsation of the carotid artery and allowance made for the fact that this occurs about one-tenth of a second later than the actual contraction of the ventricles. Many systolic murmurs follow the first sound immediately, although some are mid or late systolic. Diastolic murmurs may appear immediately after the second sound or only after an appreciable interval and, in case of presystolic murmurs, just precede the first sound. It is sometimes very difficult to time a murmur with certainty, and its position in the cardiac cycle may then be suggested by its

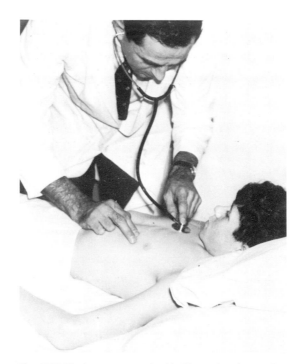

**Fig. 7.28** Timing murmurs. In this illustration the stethoscope is placed so as to time an aortic murmur. The fingers are lifted with each systole of the heart corresponding with the first heart sound. When the apex beat cannot be felt reliance must be placed on palpation of the carotid artery in which the palpation follows that of the apex beat by 0·1 s.

character, to which close attention should be paid. Phonocardiography may be needed, but even without this aid identification of the second heart sound should have been decisive in showing the division between systole and diastole.

**2. The character of the murmur** Murmurs may vary from a soft blowing sound to a harsh rasping one. Loud and especially rough murmurs are more commonly associated with organic valvular and congenital lesions. Soft murmurs are often harmless, though some, e.g. that of aortic incompetence, may be conclusive of pathological changes. It should be emphasized, however, that there is no correlation between the loudness of a murmur and the haemodynamic severity of the lesion producing the noise.

**3. Distribution** A careful record should be made, preferably in the form of a diagram, of the area over which the murmur is heard and of the point of maximum intensity. A record of this kind constitutes a valuable method of assessing the significance of a murmur and its place of production. Associated with this observation there should be noted:

**4. Direction of spread** When the maximum intensity of the murmur has been noted, the stethoscope should be moved radially from this point in different directions to observe whether the murmur is circumscribed or conducted to other parts of the chest wall. The direction of conduction, or, on the contrary, the absence of conduction, is characteristic of certain murmurs.

**5. Relation to respiration, posture and exercise** Many murmurs, especially innocent ones, are modified by respiration, often disappearing at the height of inspiration. This is particularly true of pulmonary systolic murmurs, but may occur in the case of mitral systolic murmurs. Aortic diastolic murmurs can best be heard on expiration, tricuspid murmurs on inspiration.

The effect of posture should be observed, as some murmurs—e.g. an aortic diastolic—are best heard in the erect posture with the patient leaning forwards, while others—e.g. a mitral diastolic—are heard most clearly when the patient is recumbent, especially in the left lateral position.

Again, exercise modifies murmurs, and when there is no contra-indication (e.g. active carditis or heart failure) the patient should be exercised to increase the cardiac output and hence the rate of flow across the valves. Presystolic mitral murmurs are often intensified by such exercise.

### Causes of murmurs

The ultimate cause of many murmurs is uncertain and our views are changing in the light of the information now available from operations on the heart and from direct sound recordings via a cardiac catheter. In general, the factors which are responsible include turbulence and eddy currents resulting from modification in the size of the valve opening, irregularities and deformities in the valve itself and in surrounding parts, such as the chordae tendineae. In many cases, especially where there is obstruction at a valve, the production of the murmur depends upon the relative disproportion of the orifice, which is narrowed, and the chamber beyond.

The velocity of the blood flow also plays a considerable part, and this is well seen in the increase of the diastolic murmur of mitral stenosis by exercise. Increased velocity of the blood flow may also be responsible for murmurs which occur even when the valves and their rings are normal, e.g. in thyrotoxicosis and anaemia. The regurgitant murmur in aortic incompetence is again due to the blood passing through a relatively narrow orifice at high velocity and possibly setting up vibration in structures upon which it impinges.

From a clinical point of view it is useful to divide murmurs into *innocent* or *insignificant* on the one hand, and *organic* or *significant* on the other. From the brief description of the causation it will be appreciated that very minor variations in the anatomical proportions of the valve orifices and the heart chambers may give rise to insignificant murmurs. These are always systolic in time, usually faint in character, though increased by exercise, and quite commonly found over the pulmonary area and to a lesser extent over the cardiac apex. These characteristics, together with the complete absence of any other signs of cardiac disease (in particular any abnormal heart sounds) or of any past aetiological factors which might produce such disease, will often justify the dismissal of the murmur as of no moment. These murmurs are commonly 'ejection' in type, i.e. occurring only at an interval after the first sound and ceasing before the second sound. There are, however, certain systolic murmurs which, while they do not indicate permanent valve or congenital heart disease, may be significant. Such is the murmur of mitral incompetence due to papillary muscle–chordal dysfunction produced by dilatation of the left ventricle from causes such as hypertension or aortic disease without any involvement of the mitral valve. It is possible for such a murmur to disappear, though this is uncommon, but when the murmur results from deformed cusps it will remain permanent. The murmur equally persists when it is due to obstruction or a congenital lesion which remains stationary, though alteration in the dynamics of the heart may modify the murmur from time to time.

Careful judgement is necessary to determine the significance of many murmurs. This is particularly so in the case of systolic murmurs, which are often harmless, but may raise suspicion of organic disease when there is a history of rheumatic fever or associated signs of heart disease.

The decision as to the seriousness of these murmurs is important, for on the one hand the patient may be unnecessarily alarmed, or on the other an early valve lesion may be overlooked, and the patient will go untreated.

Diastolic murmurs are more simple. Sometimes, as in the case of mitral stenosis, the murmur alone suffices to make the diagnosis probable. Similarly the diastolic murmur of aortic incompetence is rare except in that disease, though corroborative vascular phenomena help to complete the picture. The signs which support a diagnosis of valve disease are considered elsewhere.

Special details relating to murmurs may now be discussed under the headings of the areas of the heart where they are found, again remembering that loudness does not necessarily correlate with severity.

### Murmurs at the cardiac apex

**Systolic murmurs** Systolic murmurs at the cardiac apex are common, and may be difficult to evaluate as indications of organic disease. The murmurs are often soft in character, but if sufficiently loud and caused by a posteriorly directed flow of regurgitant blood through the mitral valve, they are conducted in a characteristic manner towards the axilla and often through to the back at the inferior angle of the left scapula (*Fig.* 7.29). The murmur alone gives limited indication of the degree of leakage.

Some of the conditions which produce papillary muscle–chordal dysfunction to a greater or lesser degree are susceptible of improvement, with a corresponding disappearance of the mitral regurgitation and the systolic murmur. The murmur therefore may be described as 'functional'. The diagnosis of the true value of the murmur is made by looking for the causal disease, and by watching the patient to see if the murmur disappears or changes. If the murmur does not disappear, as may happen for example in dilatation of the left ventricle due to hypertension, the mitral regurgitation remains as a permanent feature of the illness, and the murmur may then be regarded as no less important than if there were damage to the valve cusps.

Systolic murmurs dependent on abnormality of the cusps of the mitral valve from rheumatic or other causes may be similar to the so-called innocent or insignificant murmurs. In assigning to them their correct importance, attention should be paid to a history of rheumatic illness, the size of the heart and the presence of any other valve lesion; but it must be admitted that it is sometimes impossible to decide whether or not a systolic apical murmur indicates the presence of organic disease of the mitral valve cusps, though the course of the disease and the subsequent development of other evidence of rheumatic damage to the myocardium

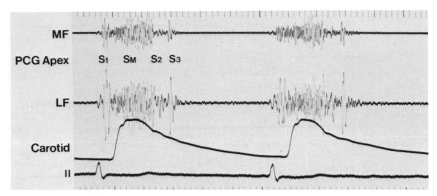

**Fig. 7.29** Mitral regurgitation. The carotid pulse is normal, the ECG shows no atrial activity, i.e. atrial fibrillation is probably present. The murmur is pansystolic (SM) extending from S1 to S2. A short diastolic murmur envelops a loud third sound (S3). The pansystolic murmur should be compared with the midsystolic murmur of aortic stenosis (cf *Figs.* 7.9, 7.10, 7.15, 7.35). (Recording speed 100 mm/s.)

or valves may establish a correct diagnosis. When it is suspected that a systolic murmur indicates rheumatic mitral regurgitation, a persistent search must be made for the diastolic murmur of mitral stenosis which so commonly accompanies the disease in this form.

Since rheumatic fever has become a much less common disease from the year 1950 and onwards, so the incidence of rheumatic valve disease has decreased, at least in Western Europe and North America. Rheumatic mitral regurgitation is still a common cause of an incompetent mitral valve, but other abnormalities of the mitral valve mechanism producing regurgitation are now more easily recognized, and in particular the prolapsing cusp in the midsystolic click—late systolic murmur syndrome—has been shown to be relatively common by phono- and echocardiography. The stream of regurgitant blood through the valve may be directed other than posteriorly, and if this direction is superior and medial, the systolic murmur may be propagated in the same direction and be best heard parasternally rather than in the axilla, and thus be easily confused with the murmur of aortic stenosis (*Fig.* 7.30).

It only remains to add that murmurs originating at other areas of the heart may be conducted to the apex and imitate those due to mitral insufficiency. An example of this is sometimes seen in aortic stenosis. In determining the origin of the murmur it is helpful if a distinction can be made between a pansystolic murmur, usual in mitral incompetence and ventricular septal defects, and the midsystolic murmur which characterizes aortic and pulmonary stenosis (*Figs.* 7.29, 7.35).

Correct timing is of great importance, though sometimes difficult without a phonocardiogram. Pansystolic murmurs in mitral incompetence and ventricular septal defects start with the first sound and continue to, or even through, the second sound, whereas ejection murmurs, as in aortic stenosis and pulmonary stenosis, cannot be heard immediately after the first sound but are easier to time as ending before the second sound. Timing of the murmur can only be achieved by recognition of the heart sounds, hence the emphasis on these signs.

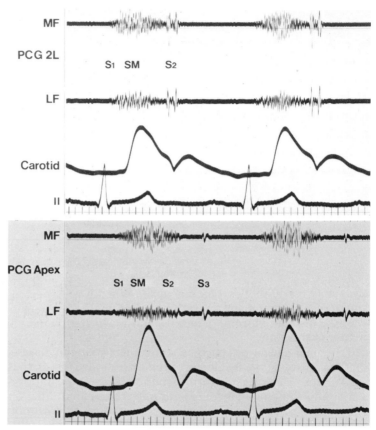

**Fig. 7.30** Mitral regurgitation. These phonocardiograms from 2L (pulmonary area) and apex were recorded from a man with mitral regurgitation in sinus rhythm, and no aortic valve disease. Both illustrations show the pansystolic murmur starting with a low intensity S1, and passing up to S2—the latter being widely split in the 2L position. A third sound (S3) is recorded at the apex. The systolic murmur is crescendo–decrescendo in shape, as in aortic stenosis, but is shown to be pansystolic in timing and position. Compare with *Fig.* 7.29, where atrial fibrillation is present. (Recording speed 100 mm/s.)

**Diastolic murmurs** When a diastolic murmur is heard only at the mitral area it is nearly always due to mitral stenosis, in which the valve cusps are fused together and the orifice from the left atrium into the ventricle is narrowed. Only rarely is a diastolic murmur heard when the mitral valve is normal, and in such cases there is increased velocity and volume of the blood flow across the mitral valve, as in ventricular septal defects and other types of left-to-right shunting 'downstream' from the mitral valve. The same cause may be at work in mitral and aortic regurgitation, though in the latter it is possible that the diastolic and presystolic murmur, called, after its describer, the 'Austin Flint', is due to impingement of the regurgitation stream on the aortic cusp of the mitral valve. This causes a functional partial

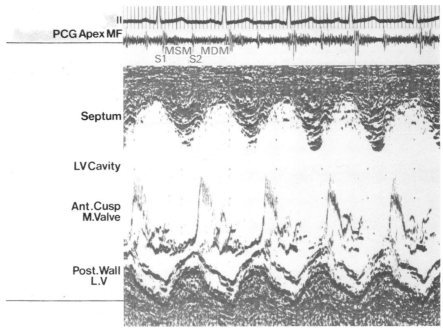

**Fig. 7.31** This combined ECG, PCG and echocardiogram shows the diastolic murmur (MDM) at the apex, with an appearance similar to that of mitral stenosis (cf *Figs.* 7.23, 7.33, 7.34). The echocardiogram of the mitral valve shows the vibration of the anterior cusp associated with an Austin Flint murmur, and the valve movement is otherwise normal.

The left ventricle wall movement and that of the interventricular septum is in excess of normal, as is the left ventricular cavity size (cf *Fig.* 7.32). (Recording speed 50 mm/s.)

obstruction at the mitral orifice, and the regurgitant stream may also cause the aortic cusp of the mitral valve to vibrate (*Figs.* 7.31, 7.32).

The mitral diastolic murmur of mitral stenosis is nearly always of low pitch and rumbling in character. It is often appreciated with difficulty by the unpractised ear, and to avoid overlooking it the student should examine the patient in the recumbent posture, when it may easily be audible in cases in which it was not apparent with the patient erect. The murmur is often intensified when the patient lies on the left side so that the cardiac apex is brought into closer contact with the chest wall. Exercise may also bring out a murmur which is otherwise difficult to hear, and the stethoscope should be applied immediately the patient lies down after the effort, so that the first few heart-beats will not be missed, for it is in these, when the blood velocity is high, that the murmur is generally heard. Diastolic murmurs, in contrast with systolic, are circumscribed and often localized to an area of a few square centimetres around the apex beat. The murmur is separated from the second sound by a short pause, but may then fill the remainder of diastole (*Figs.* 7.33, 7.34). If it is chiefly late diastolic and becomes continuous with an accentuated first sound, it has an apparently crescendo character and is

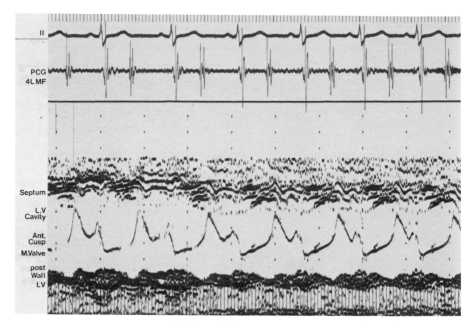

**Fig. 7.32** Normal ECG, PCG and echocardiogram of a patient aged 26 without heart disease. Note the normal second sound splitting on the PCG. Movement of the anterior cusp of the mitral valve is normal, in diastole and systole (cf Fig. 7.31). Ventricular cavity size is normal, as is movement of the interventricular septum and left ventricle posterior wall. (Recording speed 50 mm/s.)

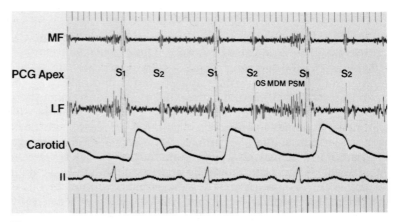

**Fig. 7.33** The long diastolic murmur of mitral stenosis, ending before the accentuated S1 with presystolic accentuation (MDM and PSM). S2 is the position of the second sound, and OS the opening snap. The carotid pulse and ECG are both normal. (Recording speed 75 mm/s.)

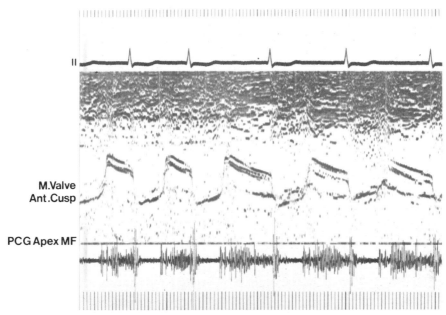

**Fig. 7.34** Echocardiogram, ECG and PCG of mitral stenosis with atrial fibrillation. The echogram shows thickening of the cusp, but normal early diastolic movement coincident with the opening snap (OS) of the PCG. The long diastolic murmur is shown in conjunction with the shallow diastolic (E–F) slope of the anterior cusp of the mitral valve, demonstrating how the valve is held down into the ventricular cavity. (Recording speed 50 mm/s.) (*See Fig. 7.32 for comparison.*)

often called a *presystolic murmur*, though in reality it is usually only a part of a longer diastolic murmur. Before making a diagnosis of mitral stenosis on the presence of a presystolic murmur the observer should listen most carefully for the low-toned rumble which is generally present in other parts of diastole, and for the characteristic abnormalities of the heart sounds.

### Murmurs at the aortic area

**Systolic murmurs** Systolic murmurs are very common at the aortic area and may be associated with increased cardiac output as in anaemias or with increased stroke output as in aortic incompetence. The murmur of increased output is often soft and blowing, but where stroke output is increased in aortic incompetence there is also valve deformity and the murmur may be very loud.

A similar murmur may be heard with dilatation of the aorta and calcification at the root of the aorta, but its loudness is not an indication of valve narrowing.

The systolic murmur of *aortic stenosis* (*Fig.* 7.35) is harsh in character, conducted upwards into the carotid arteries, and usually accompanied by a thrill. The position of the murmur, as mentioned, is roughly midsystolic, but being often preceded by an ejection click this latter may be mistaken for a first heart sound, and the murmur for one of pansystolic timing. The murmur may also be heard at the

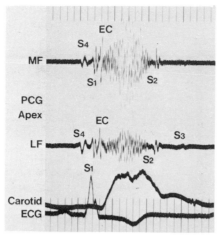

**Fig. 7.35**
Aortic stenosis. The murmur
is recorded as having a
characteristic diamond-shape,
crescendo–decrescendo,
starting with the ejection click
(EC) and ending before the
second sound (S2). Both 3rd
and 4th sounds are present,
there is a plateau or anacrotic
pulse, and the ECG (lead II) is
abnormal. (Recording speed
100 mm/s.)

apex and the student should be cautious in making a diagnosis of aortic stenosis unless other evidence of obstruction is present, as systolic murmurs at the aortic area may be due to the alternative causes mentioned. If the stenosis produces much narrowing of the valve opening, a plateau type of pulse will be present (*Fig. 7.35*), an important confirmatory sign in diagnosis.

**Diastolic murmurs** These are rarely found at the aortic area except in *aortic regurgitation*. The murmur is usually soft and blowing in character and is heard over a large area of the chest wall. It is propagated characteristically down the sternum and towards the apex beat. In the aortic area itself it is often faint and difficult to hear, and it reaches its maximum intensity about the middle of the sternum at its left border. It may be well heard over the apex or even in the axilla but can generally be distinguished from a diastolic murmur of mitral origin by its higher pitch and by the fact that it follows immediately after the second sound, except when it is faint. In listening for this murmur the student should have the patient in an erect posture, leaning forwards and holding his breath in expiration, and should auscultate systematically from the second right costal cartilage down the sternum and towards the apex beat (*see also Fig. 7.36*).

### Murmurs at the pulmonary area

**Systolic murmurs** Systolic murmurs over the pulmonary area may be soft and blowing like those sometimes found over the aortic zone. They occur with great frequency in perfectly healthy individuals, and are probably due to turbulence being produced by rapid blood flow through a normal valve (*Fig. 7.37*). The murmur of *congenital pulmonary stenosis* (*Fig. 7.38*) is comparable with the murmur of aortic stenosis, as it is loud, rasping and usually accompanied by a thrill, with the difference that in the more severe grades of pulmonary valve stenosis the crescendo part of the murmur is later than is the case in aortic stenosis. There is delay in the appearance of the soft pulmonary component of the second sound (*Fig. 7.38*).

**Diastolic murmurs** At the pulmonary area diastolic murmurs are uncommon

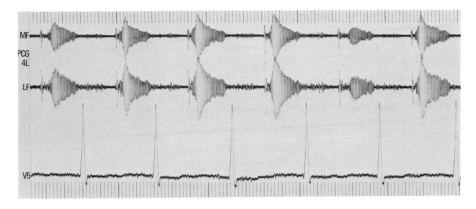

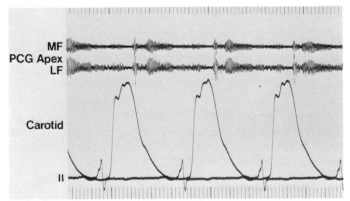

**Fig. 7.36** Aortic regurgitation. The murmur in this patient is intense, and the regularity of the vibrations is unusual. When this characteristic is recorded the sound has a musical quality when heard with a stethoscope. This patient has a valve cusp perforated by infective endocarditis. The carotid pulse is abnormal, showing the characteristic 'collapsing' quality of aortic regurgitation. (Both illustrations, recording speeds 50 mm/s.) (cf *Figs.* 7.10, 7.14, 7.15).

and in many cases sound exactly the same as those of aortic regurgitation. A pulmonary diastolic murmur due to regurgitation will occasionally occur in pulmonary arterial hypertension, or dilatation of the pulmonary artery (Graham Steell murmur); this is most commonly due to mitral valve disease or congenital lesions with an Eisenmenger reaction.

### Murmurs at the tricuspid area

Murmurs at the tricuspid area are commonly associated and confused with those arising from mitral disease. Systolic murmurs may be present at the lower end of the sternum in tricuspid regurgitation, and diastolic murmurs of a low rumbling type may occur in tricuspid stenosis, but diagnosis is always difficult, although both these murmurs are increased by deep inspiration, sometimes a

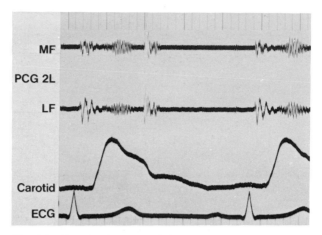

**Fig. 7.37** Functional or innocent systolic murmur. The ECG and carotid pulse are normal. The heart sounds are normal, with no added sounds. The murmur is midsystolic, seen to be of low frequency and, when heard, has a 'buzzing' quality, most easily detected along the left sternal border. (Recording speed 100 mm/s.)

useful manoeuvre in distinguishing them from murmurs arising at the mitral valve. Examination of the venous pulse may reveal other clues in the diagnosis of tricuspid valve disease (*Figs*. 7.39, 7.40).

### Other murmurs

Sometimes murmurs are found which do not correspond with any of the 'valvular' areas. In these cases the possibility of congenital heart disease always arises. Systolic murmurs midway between the pulmonary and mitral areas, i.e. over third and fourth left interspaces, may be present in cases of pulmonary stenosis when the obstruction is near the origin of the artery from the right ventricle, infundibular stenosis, and in cases of patency of the interventricular septum (*Figs*. 7.41, 7.42). These murmurs are nearly always rough, and generally accompanied by a thrill. A murmur occupying both systole and diastole, present over the base of the heart, and maximal over the pulmonary area, is characteristic of a *patent ductus arteriosus* (*Fig*. 7.43). Usually the murmur has a characteristic quality described by Gibson as 'machinery-like'. It is almost continuous but waxes and wanes and is most pronounced in late systole. Similar murmurs may be heard in various forms of arteriovenous fistula, but these are rare.

Systolic murmurs may also be found over the base of the heart in coarctation of the aorta and atrial septal defects, but the murmur is not the main feature in the diagnosis.

Murmurs which have a vascular as opposed to a cardiac origin are usually systolic in time and blowing in character and may be heard over an engorged thyroid gland, over vascular tumours in the thorax and over aneurysm of the aorta or other large vessels. The *bruit de diable* is the name given to a continuous venous hum sometimes heard over the neck in profound anaemias and is thought to be

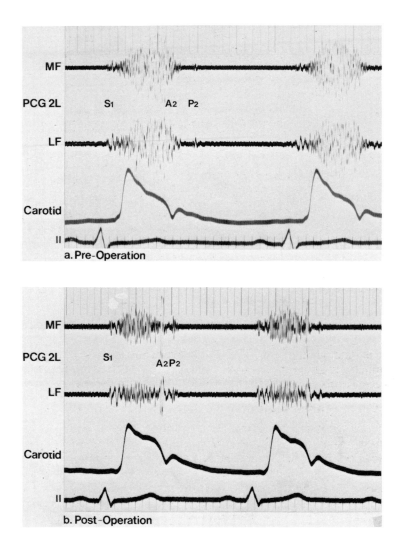

**Fig. 7.38** Congenital pulmonary valve stenosis. The systolic murmur is similar in shape to that of aortic stenosis, but reaches the crescendo later in systole, to end before the delayed pulmonary component (P2) of the second sound. The distance from the aortic second sound (A2) to P2 is a measure of the severity of the obstruction at the pulmonary valve, and the shortening of this interval after surgery (compare the preoperation with the postoperation records) is a measure of the success of the operation.

caused by the associated hyperdynamic circulatory state with blood flowing very rapidly through the great veins to the heart. A venous hum is occasionally heard over the jugular veins or even over the chest, in health, but disappears in recumbency or pressure over the neck veins (*Fig.* 7.44).

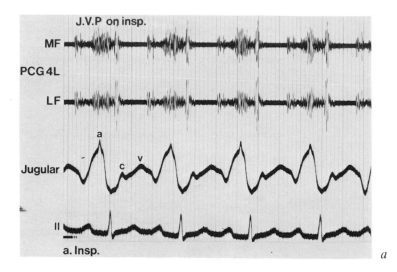

*a*

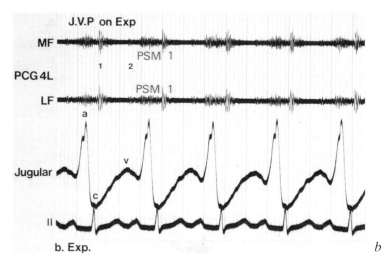

*b*

**Fig. 7.39** Tricuspid stenosis with jugular pulse recordings. Record *a* is taken during inspiration, *b* during expiration. Both records show prolongation of the P–R interval on the ECG, and both show a presystolic murmur of crescendo–decrescendo shape, ending before the first heart sound. This is a true atrial systolic ejection murmur, ending before S1 because of the early atrial contraction. The increased venous return produced by inspiration raises the right atrial–right ventricle pressure gradient in diastole, flow across the stenosed valve increases and the murmur is louder. The jugular pulse, recorded most easily in expiration, shows a tall 'a' wave, small delayed 'c' wave and marked delay in descent from the 'v' wave. These findings are typical of tricuspid stenosis. The smaller 'a' during inspiration is artefactual, caused by difficulty in recording the pulse beyond a tense sternomastoid muscle.

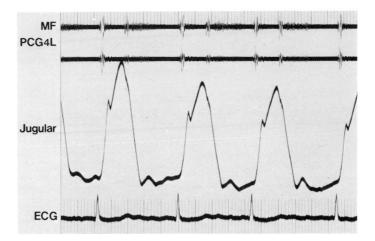

**Fig. 7.40** Tricuspid regurgitation with jugular pulse recording. The phonocardiogram shows little systolic murmur, and a short diastolic murmur. The jugular pulse has almost the appearance of a collapsing arterial pulse, and indeed the pressure was high enough to move the earlobes. The patient had gross tricuspid regurgitation, with a pulsatile liver also.

Atrial fibrillation is present, so that no 'a' wave is recorded. The 'c' notch is followed by a huge 'v' wave which is followed by a precipitate fall to the 'y' trough, both the rise to the 'v' peak and the fall to the 'y' trough being typical of this condition.

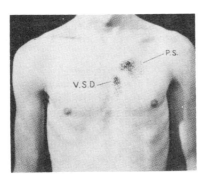

**Fig. 7.41** Murmurs of congenital heart disease. PS, Pulmonary stenosis; VSD, Ventricular septal defect. These murmurs are systolic in time.

# THE DIAGNOSIS OF HEART DISEASES

It is convenient to deal with the diagnosis of heart disease under two headings: (1) Structural defects; (2) Derangements of function. These are commonly found together, but one may occur without the other.

## STRUCTURAL DEFECTS

Diseases of the heart resulting from anatomical changes may involve the pericardium, the heart muscle and the endocardium and valves. Con-

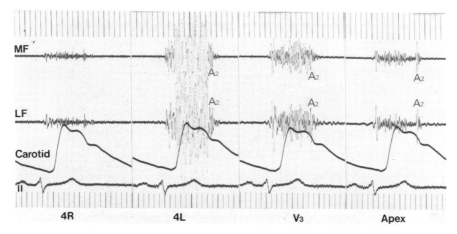

**Fig. 7.42** Ventricular septal defect. PCG recorded across 4R, 4L, V3 and apex position, with the carotid pulse. This shows the murmur to be loudest at the left sternal edge, to begin with the first sound and extend throughout systole, to 'spill over' the position of A2, and end before or with P2.

The murmur is very loud, but it should be remembered that loudness does not equate with severity of the left-to-right shunt.

genital defects may affect any or all of these structures. The majority of diseases result from inflammatory or degenerative processes, and the signs by which they may be recognized overlap to a considerable extent.

### The pericardium

**Pericarditis** Inflammation of the pericardium is recognized in its acute stage by the friction rub (*see* p. 234). This may appear during the course of an acute illness, especially rheumatic fever, but also in pneumonia, tuberculosis and virus infections. It is a common feature of cardiac infarction and of uraemia. The rub is usually discovered as a result of routine examination in these conditions, rather than by any special complaint of the patient, though in some cases there may be pain. The electrocardiogram characteristically shows RS–T segment arching, with inversion of the T waves.

**Pericardial effusion** Some increase in pericardial fluid occurs in most cases of acute pericarditis but may only be discovered on routine examination and may not cause symptoms. If the intrapericardial tension is high, resulting in restricted venous return and lowered cardiac output (tamponade), severe dyspnoea may occur, but the usual pattern is one of a lowered blood pressure with cyanosis, sweating and signs of right-heart failure, depending upon the acuteness with which the effusion occurs.

The most important signs are:

1. Feebleness of the cardiac impulse and faintness of the heart sounds because of the separation of the impulse from the chest wall by the fluid.

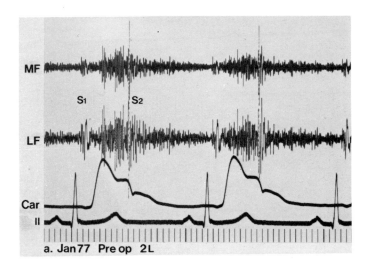

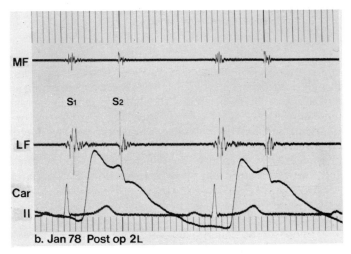

**Fig. 7.43** Patent ductus arteriosus. Pre- and postoperation records from the same patient, after surgical obliteration of the ductus. The typical murmur rises to a crescendo just before the position of the second sound, but is seen to be continuous throughout systole and diastole.

2. The first heart sound may be soft because of reduced late diastolic filling and the second sound because the blood pressure is low.

3. An early diastolic added sound, dull in character, representing restriction of ventricular filling.

4. Pulsus paradoxus (*see* p. 214).

5. Persistence of pericardial friction.

Radiology confirms the heart and fluid outlines (*Fig.* 7.45) and the layer of

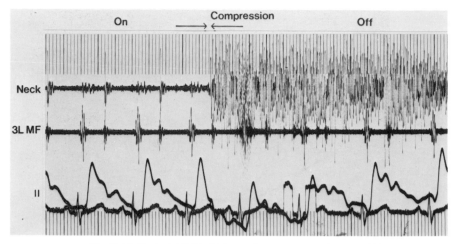

**Fig. 7.44** *Bruit de diable*. This continuous venous hum could be heard over both internal jugular veins, in a healthy girl. Compression of the veins readily abolished the hum.

fluid can also be shown by echocardiography. Special techniques with cardiac catheterization are occasionally necessary. Paracentesis may be justifiable.

**Constrictive pericarditis** This is generally tuberculous in origin and insidious in development and may be associated with pleurisy. On rare occasions it follows other infections.

The most important signs are elevated venous pressure with liver enlargement and ascites, in a patient in whom no valve disease or other cause of cardiac failure is found. The degree of dyspnoea may be relatively slight. The heart is often not enlarged, but radioscopy may show calcification. Pulsus paradoxus may be present.

### The myocardium

There are no conclusive symptoms or signs of myocardial disease, though the electrocardiogram may reveal evidence of this (*Fig.* 7.46–7.48), especially when conduction disorders of any kind are present. It is possible, however, to suspect that the myocardium is involved when there is cardiac enlargement due to unexplained hypertrophy or dilatation or both, or when the heart shows signs of failure which cannot easily be attributed to any extra burden it is carrying. Suggestions of myocardial weakness (whether due to myocardial disease or increased load) are to be found in the presence of pulsus alternans and gallop rhythm, which sooner or later are associated with clear evidence of heart failure.

Echocardiography (*see Fig.* 7.32) is of great value in assessment of myocardial contractility and shows particularly well the impaired movements of the ventricle in cardiomyopathies (*Fig.* 7.47).

*Myocardial ischaemia* and *cardiac infarction* are the commonest disorders affecting the cardiac muscle and the cardinal symptom of this condition—anginal pain—has already been considered (p. 203). It only remains to add that while the

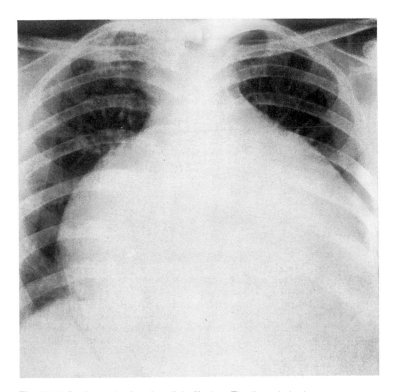

**Fig. 7.45** Radiograph of pericardial effusion. The 'heart' shadow is enlarged, the enlargement being greater in the transverse diameter than the longitudinal. There is obliteration of the normal notches on the heart's outline so that the shadow becomes globular or pear-shaped with a short vascular pedicle, but these minor changes in the shape of the cardiac outline should not be overstressed.

pain is usually severe, it may be slight. It is of variable duration but, when infarction is present, the pain lasts generally a number of hours and nearly always is longer than in other forms of angina. It may be accompanied by collapse, shown by pallor, sweating, faintness, a feeble pulse, and falling blood pressure, and commonly by vomiting. (*See* Shock, p. 16.) Disorders of conduction and of rhythm may occur.

The infarct in contact with the pericardium may result in an area of pericarditis with its sign – a friction rub – and the necrotic processes in the myocardium may be evidenced by pyrexia and leucocytosis, and by a rise in sedimentation rate and serum transaminase level. These signs are usually maximal 2–3 days after cardiac infarction. If the infarct involves the endocardium, a mural thrombus may form and result in systemic embolism, usually a week or two later.

In some instances cardiac failure, especially of the left ventricular type, results, and sometimes a papillary muscle ruptures or the weakened area of heart muscle bulges to form an aneurysm which can be recognized by observation and palpation

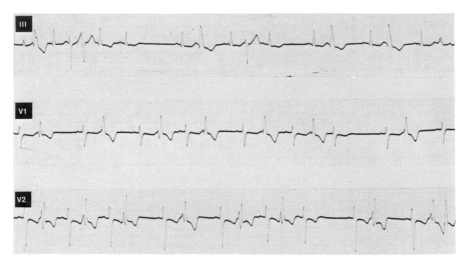

**Fig. 7.46** Electrocardiographic evidence of myocardial disease. The three leads shown were taken from a patient with evidence of myocardial disease of uncertain aetiology and where there was a family history of myocardial failure and sudden death.
The ECG picture is dominated by multiple ventricular ectopic beats of bizarre pattern, some coupled, others interpolated.

and confirmed radiologically. The diagnosis of cardiac infarction is usually established by characteristic ECG changes (*Figs.* 7.50–7.52).

**Acute cardiomyopathy** During the course of rheumatic fever and certain infections, viral or bacterial, involvement of the myocardium may be suspected by the onset of precordial oppression, a rapid feeble pulse with a fall of blood pressure, and cardiac dilatation. When the conducting system is involved in the myopathic process, bradycardia can occur, and the ECG may show evidence of heart block. Other disturbances of cardiac rhythm may happen.

A number of rare diseases of the myocardium, including endomyocardial fibrosis, various collagen diseases and the toxic effect of drugs or alcohol may give a similar picture. Diagnosis, which is difficult, may be made more certain by the development of signs of cardiac failure.

In *rheumatic carditis*, a term used to emphasize that any or all of the heart structures may be involved, it may be difficult to recognize the signs of myocardial affection because they are masked by pericardial or valvular signs. This disease, once very common, is now seen much less frequently.

### The Valves

Endocarditis, or inflammation of the endocardium, results in deformities of the valves, causing incompetence of the valve or narrowing (stenosis) of the orifice guarded by the valve. Incompetence causes regurgitation of blood through an orifice which should be closed. Stenosis impedes the passage of blood through the affected valve. Any of the valves may become incompetent or stenosed, but especially the mitral and aortic valves.

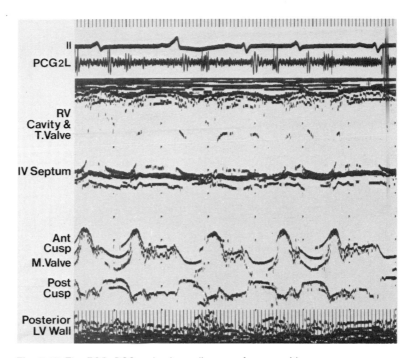

**Fig. 7.47** The ECG, PCG and echocardiogram of a man with congestive cardiomyopathy. The ECG is abnormal, with low voltage complexes and ventricular ectopic beats. The echocardiogram shows a dilated right ventricle, with an occasional echo from the tricuspid valve. The septum, of normal thickness, is immobile, and is separated from an almost immobile left ventricle posterior wall, by a large left ventricle cavity, in which the mitral valve is of normal thickness, but with diminished movement, and it can be seen that the anterior and posterior cusps do not meet in systole. (*For comparison, see normal echo and PCG in Fig.* 7.32.)

The diagnosis of valve diseases depends above all on auscultation, which reveals the characteristic murmurs and alteration of sounds already described.

Confirmatory evidence is furnished by enlargement of the heart caused by the extra work put upon it by the valve defect, and it may be possible to suspect which valve is involved from the type of cardiac enlargement. Disease of the aortic valve imposes more load on the left ventricle, disease of the mitral valve more on the left atrium and right ventricle, and some information on the type of enlargement may be gained by careful inspection and palpation, but in particular by radiology.

Supplementary evidence of valve disease is found in the character of the pulse— for example, the collapsing pulse and capillary pulsation of aortic regurgitation, the plateau pulse of aortic stenosis, and the small, thin pulse of mitral stenosis.

The most important valve lesions are: (1) Mitral stenosis; (2) Mitral incompetence; (3) Aortic incompetence; (4) Aortic stenosis.

**Mitral stenosis** (*Fig.* 7.24, 7.33, 7.34) Diagnosed by the presence of a mitral

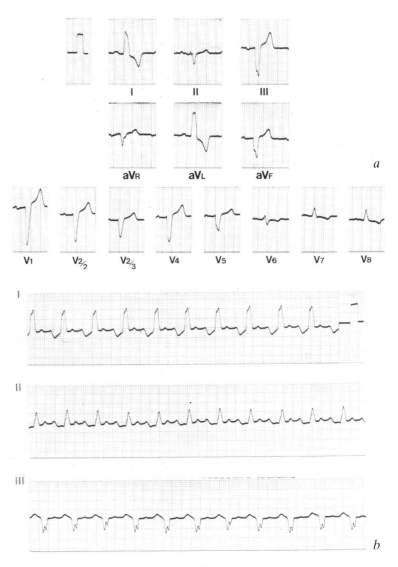

**Fig. 7.48** Left bundle-branch block (LBBB). *a*, This patient had aortic stenosis, with extensive calcification extending from the valve into the interventricular septum. Note QRS spread with dominant positive QRS defection in lead I, negative in lead III. The left axis deviation is pathological, and represents a conduction defect in the left anterior division of the left bundle, in addition to the main left bundle. This ECG therefore represents LBBB and left anterior hemiblock. *b*, This patient had ischaemic heart disease. The QRS spread again shows LBBB, but without the same degree of left axis deviation—the main defection being positive in lead II, there being no conduction defect in the left anterior division, i.e. there is no left anterior hemiblock.

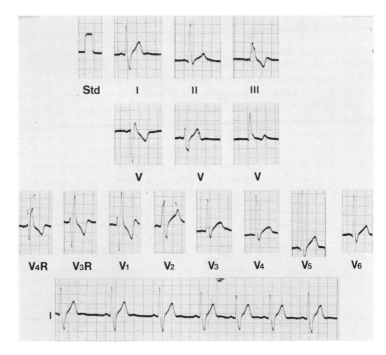

**Fig. 7.49** Right bundle-branch block. This patient had an atrial septal defect. The deep S waves in leads I, aVL, and the left chest leads are well shown, as is the QRS spreading, and the RSR complexes in V4R, V3R and V1. The continuous recording of lead I shows sinus arrhythmia.

diastolic murmur with accentuation of the mitral first sound and an opening snap. Confirmatory signs are the enlargement of the right ventricle, and, when there is pulmonary arterial hypertension, the pulmonary second sound is accentuated. The radiograph may show enlargement of the left atrium, and prominence of the pulmonary arc if there is pulmonary arterial hypertension, when recognizable changes in the vascular pattern of the lungs will also be present.

The commonest ECG change is an alteration in the P waves (*Fig.* 7.53). They are often bifid because of left atrial hypertrophy, though sometimes tall and sharp, because of right atrial hypertrophy when there is high pulmonary vascular resistance, and when there will also be evidence of right ventricular hypertrophy.

These graphic signs may be helpful when present, but the diastolic murmur remains the most certain diagnostic sign, though alone it does not indicate the severity of the stenosis.

**Mitral incompetence** (*Figs.* 7.29, 7.30) Often accompanies mitral stenosis; diagnosed by the presence of a mitral pansystolic murmur conducted to the axilla and enlargement of the left ventricle. The difficulties of diagnosis between mitral regurgitation due to disease of the valve cusps and to relative incompetence from papillary muscle–chordal dysfunction have been discussed under systolic

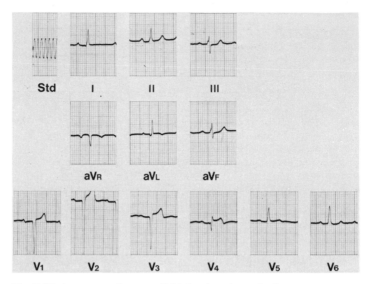

**Fig. 7.50** Anteroseptal myocardial infarction shown in the precordial leads and aVL only. The P–R interval is at the upper limits of normal, the Q wave in aVL is abnormal, as it is in leads V1 to V4, with RS–T segment elevation in V3, V4 and inversion of the T wave in aVL.

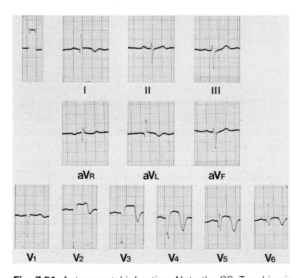

**Fig. 7.51** Anteroseptal infarction. Note the RS–T arching in leads I, aVL, V2 to V6. Abnormal Q waves are present in I, aVL, V2 to V5, and T wave inversion is present in the same leads.

Abnormal left axis deviation, with S greater than R in lead II, indicates the presence of conduction deficiency in the left anterior division of the left bundle-branch.

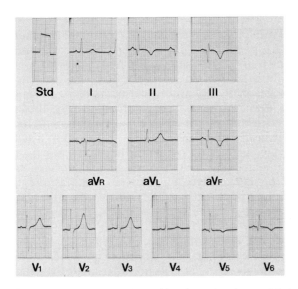

**Fig. 7.52** Inferolateral infarct. Note here the abnormal Q waves in leads II, III, aVF and V5 and V6 with RS–T arching and negative T waves in the same leads.

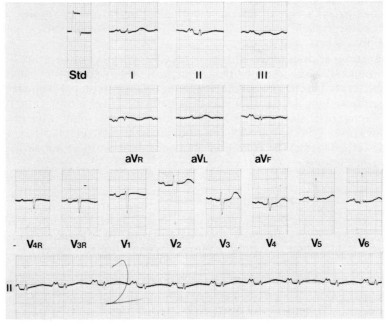

**Fig. 7.53** Bifid P waves, left atrial hypertrophy. This ECG also shows a long P–R interval; and is the record from a patient with severe mitral stenosis. The long recording of lead II shows the bifid P waves particularly well.

murmurs. Unusual cases of rupture of the mitral cusps, chordae tendineae or papillary muscle may result in severe and sudden mitral incompetence, when the picture is dominated by the presence of pulmonary oedema of acute onset.

**Aortic incompetence** (*Figs.* 7.16, 7.31, 7.36) Characterized by an aortic diastolic murmur of classic distribution. The corroborative signs in aortic regurgitation are of great value, especially the collapsing pulse, capillary pulsation and undue pulsation of the large arteries. The heart is enlarged, principally downwards and to the left. The enlargement is confirmed by a chest radiograph, in which the left ventricle is characteristically rounded. Electrocardiography usually shows left ventricular hypertrophy, phonocardiography the characteristic murmurs and echocardiography the dilated left ventricular cavity and perhaps the vibration of the anterior cusp of the mitral valve. The low-pitched diastolic murmur at the apex—the Austin Flint murmur—may make difficult the differentiation from a coincidental mitral stenosis, but the above-mentioned investigations should be decisive.

**Aortic stenosis** (*Figs.* 7.9, 7.10, 7.15, 7.35) This was a less common lesion than the other valve diseases described until the declining incidence of rheumatic heart disease, but now increasingly recognized as non-rheumatic. The diagnosis should not be made without the presence of the rough systolic murmur conducted into the neck and the characteristic anacrotic arterial pulse. Sometimes the murmur is transmitted to the apex (*see* p. 244), and if there is a sufficiently severe degree of left ventricle hypertrophy, this ought to be recognized, often also with an audible and palpable fourth sound. Aortic regurgitation of some degree often accompanies stenosis. Special radiological and catheter studies, especially the pressure gradient across the aortic valve, may be necessary to establish the degree of obstruction, and its site.

**Bacterial endocarditis** This must receive special consideration if a valve lesion is found. It is suggested by the association of valve murmurs usually regurgitant with signs of septicaemia, notably splenic enlargement, pyrexia, anaemia, embolic manifestations and the discovery of organisms in the bloodstream (blood culture). Characteristic signs in the fingers include clubbing, splinter haemorrhages in the nails (*Fig.* 7.54) and tender red nodules in the finger pulp due to tiny emboli (Osler's nodes). The condition may complicate congenital as well as acquired cardiac lesions.

### Congenital lesions

These have assumed a much more important role in diagnosis because of the possibility of surgical treatment. They are dealt with here in a very brief fashion, but constitute a most important part of paediatric medicine (*see* Chapter 14).

History-taking is often unhelpful, but respiratory distress, cyanosis and signs of cardiac failure will have been noted. Failure to gain weight may be present, partly because of dyspnoea and distress during feeding.

Occasionally, the congenital abnormality is found by routine medical examination, but it should be remembered that auscultation is not easy in small children, and not all murmurs indicate serious underlying disease. Cardiac diagnosis in the seriously ill infant is a highly specialized practice, and depends to a very large

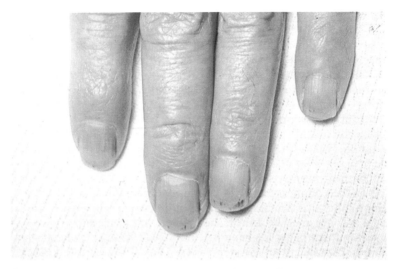

**Fig. 7.54** Polyarteritis nodosa: splinter haemorrhages in the nails. These may also occur in cases of bacterial endocarditis.

extent upon a detailed knowledge of applied embryologic anatomy and the interpretation of angiocardiograms.

As the child grows older, history-taking becomes less of a problem, signs correspond to those found in adults and problems of diagnosis which are non-urgent are dealt with in a way similar to the routine used in adults.

**Atrial septal defect** Often asymptomatic until middle age, and found as an abnormality of the cardiac outline on routine chest radiograph, the signs depend upon the size of the left-to-right shunt at atrial level. The shunt itself is silent, but increased flow across the tricuspid valve may reveal itself as a mid-diastolic low-pitched murmur at the tricuspid area. The prolongation of right ventricular systole, together with the usually present right bundle-branch block (*Fig.* 7.49) causes wide fixed splitting of the second sound because of delay in pulmonary valve closure. The large stroke volume from the right ventricle may produce an ejection sound from the pulmonary valve with an ejection systolic murmur in the pulmonary area.

On X-ray examination the right heart chambers are enlarged and the pulmonary artery and its branches are both enlarged and unduly pulsatile. Cardiac catheterization will confirm the diagnosis.

**Ventricular septal defect** (*Fig.* 7.42) Like atrial septal defect, ventricular septal defect may be found on routine examination of a symptomless patient, but here the loud pansystolic murmur audible in the left parasternal region, and often accompanied by a thrill, has long been recognized as typical. A very small defect may produce a lot of noise, while a large defect, with equal pressures in the left and right ventricles and thus unaccompanied by left-to-right shunting, may be silent. There may be evidence of increased flow across the mitral valve shown by the presence of a diastolic murmur at the apex. The increased load placed on the left ventricle produces evidence of left ventricular hypertrophy, shown by ECG and radiology, while the increased blood flow through the lungs shows as an increase in size of the pulmonary artery and its branches, although this is rarely so marked as in atrial septal defect. Cardiac catheterization and angiocardiography will reveal the site and severity of the lesion.

**Patent ductus arteriosus** (*Fig.* 7.43) The murmur is characteristically continuous in systole and diastole, as shunting from the aorta to the pulmonary artery is continuous also. If the shunt is sufficiently large, the load upon the left ventricle may cause left ventricular hypertrophy. There may be an audible 'flow' murmur across the mitral valve, the pulmonary artery and its branches enlarge and are pulsatile, while the pulse pressure widens in the systemic circulation because of the 'run off' from the aorta to the pulmonary artery during diastole.

**Pulmonary stenosis** (*Fig.* 7.41) When part of Fallot's tetralogy, it becomes one of the common causes of cyanotic congenital heart disease. As an isolated abnormality it is characterized by a midsystolic murmur, often sufficiently loud to be accompanied by a thrill, heard best in the second and third left intercostal spaces parasternally. Right ventricular hypertrophy is present, to a degree dependent on the severity of the stenosis (*see Fig.* 7.67), and radiology will show post-stenotic dilatation of the pulmonary artery, if the obstruction is at valve level.

**Coarctation of the aorta** This is a common cause of cardiac failure in infancy. Often present with other congenital abnormalities, both cardiac and non-cardiac, it should not be missed if physical examination is properly performed with palpation of both femoral arteries. This should be an invariable routine in any patient presenting with systemic hypertension.

The signs include absent or delayed femoral pulses, collateral vessels palpable around the shoulder girdle, and there may be a late systolic murmur present over these vessels and audible over the precordium also. The radiological finding of rib-notching is diagnostic.

Very complicated combinations of congenital malformations may occur, not only affecting the cardiovascular system but the other main systems also. In particular, the association of the skeletal deformities of Marfan's syndrome with septal and valve defects is well known (*Fig.* 7.55).

## DISORDERS OF HEART FUNCTION

The heart may be subject to disturbance of function with little or no anatomical change. This is seen in the *dysrhythmias*, or abnormal rhythms, which, although commonly associated with pathological changes in the heart muscle, may occur quite independently. *Cardiac failure* is also a disturbance of function, but is almost invariably dependent upon structural defects. Apparent alteration of function is also observed in psychoneuroses and is referred to as effort syndrome.

### Abnormal rhythms

Many abnormal rhythms can be identified with reasonable certainty by skilful examination of the pulse, but some are very confusing and require not only examination of the pulse and heart, but graphic methods, for their elucidation. The more important disturbances of the heart rhythm and rate are:

**Extrasystoles (premature or ectopic beats)** These are extra contractions of the heart arising away from the normal pacemaker (sino-atrial node) and inter-

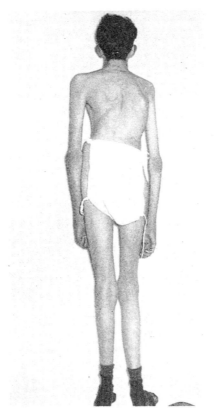

**Fig. 7.55**
Marfan's syndrome: tall, thin
build, long arms, scoliosis.
(*See also Fig.* 3.35, p. 59.)

rupting the normal, regular rhythm. As they occur prematurely, before the ventricles have been properly filled, the beats are small. They are generally followed by a long pause until the next normal beat which may be obviously of bigger volume than normal, as the ventricle has had a longer filling time. These points are appreciated by feeling the pulse, but sometimes even if the beat is not sufficiently strong to produce a pulse wave, yet the heart sounds corresponding with it may be heard (*Figs.* 7.56, 7.57).

The most characteristic feature of extrasystoles is that they are not present all the time, though if very numerous they may appear to be, and may then imitate other irregularities, especially atrial fibrillation. They usually have no serious significance unless associated with known myocardial disease such as infarction, and tend to disappear when the heart-rate is increased by suitable exercise.

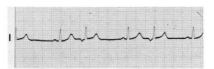

**Fig. 7.56**
Atrial extrasystoles. The P
wave, arising from an ectopic
focus, is inverted, but the
following QRST complex is of
of normal form.

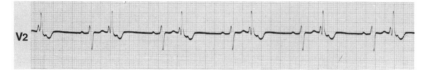

**Fig. 7.57** Ventricular extrasystoles. These are 'coupled' to the preceding normal complex, but themselves are of abnormal form. The coupling interval, from normal to ectopic beat, is fixed, and the extra beats look like complexes with the form of a right bundle-branch block. This is because the ectopic focus from which they arise is part of, or close to, the left-sided conducting system. (*See Fig.* 7.8.)

**Atrial fibrillation**   In this condition the atria cease to beat properly, individual areas of atrial muscle producing minute contractions or 'fibrillations' at a rate of 400–600 per minute which are conducted in an irregular pattern through the AV node. In its turn this causes irregular action of the ventricles. The results are shown in a complete irregularity of the pulse and apex beat, manifested by a variation in the size of the beats and in the interval between them (*Figs.* 7.58, 7.59). Atrial fibrillation generally occurs with other serious heart disease, e.g.

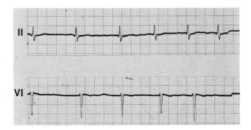

**Fig. 7.58** Atrial fibrillation (*see Fig.* 7.9). Leads II and V1 show complete irregularity of the QRST complexes, and absent P waves. This is the 'fine' type of atrial fibrillation.

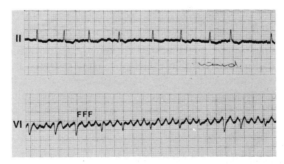

**Fig. 7.59** Atrial fibrillation, coarse (*see Fig.* 7.58). Leads II and V1 show total irregularity of the QRST complexes, with irregularly shaped and timed fibrillation, or 'f' waves.

valve or myocardial affections, but may occur alone. It is most commonly associated with mitral stenosis, thyrotoxicosis and ischaemic heart disease.

The rate is generally rapid, and the force of some of the ventricular contractions may not be strong enough to open the aortic valves and allow transmission to the pulse. In such cases the ventricular rate will be greater than the pulse rate, and in fibrillation reliance should be placed on the heart rate rather than the pulse rate, both when making the diagnosis and in assessing the effect of treatment.

**Atrial flutter** Comparable in many ways with atrial fibrillation, flutter may exist along with other forms of heart disease, or be an isolated phenomenon.

The atria beat at a great rate (200–400), but owing to refractory properties of the AV bundle, the ventricles usually respond to a smaller number of these contractions (2:1, 3:1, 4:1) depending upon the number of atrial impulses which 'penetrate' the AV node to cause ventricular action (*Fig.* 7.60). Flutter may be suspected clinically when a high regular ventricular rate (120–200) persists for a long time (days to weeks). The usual ventricular rate is 160 or less. The tachycardia can sometimes be reduced temporarily by pressure over the carotid sinus (bifurcation of the common carotid artery below the angle of the jaw at the level of the upper border of the cricoid cartilage), causing vagal inhibition of conduction through the AV node.

Occasionally the rapid contractions of the atria communicate a pulsation to the jugular veins at a greater rate (usually twice) than that at which the ventricles are beating, and cannon waves appear when the atrium contracts on to a closed AV valve.

Sudden doubling or halving of the ventricular rate strongly suggests atrial flutter, with a varying degree of AV block.

**Paroxysmal tachycardia** The heart beats regularly at a high rate (150–200, commonly over 160), and the condition may be mistaken for atrial flutter, but apart from the higher ventricular rate the condition is of much shorter duration than flutter. Its duration is usually minutes to hours, and attacks may be stopped by simple measures such as a change of posture, or pressure over the carotid sinus. The pressure should be exerted firmly below the angle of the jaw on one

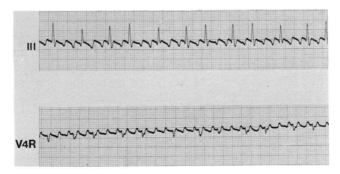

**Fig. 7.60** Atrial flutter. The flutter waves are regular in form and shape, representing atrial activity, with a rate of 300 per minute. There is a varying 2:1 and 3:1 atrioventricular block.

The regular inverted 'P' waves in lead II give a characteristic regular 'saw-tooth' pattern.

side only for a period of about 1 min, but only with ECG monitoring, and with resuscitation services at hand.

One of the most important signs is the characteristic sudden onset and offset, a sign which also applies in the case of flutter.

When the patient is not seen during an attack, great attention should be paid to the story of the mode of onset and offset and the circumstances under which the attacks appear. Abnormal rhythms (paroxysmal tachycardia and flutter) are unexpected and unexplained, whereas simple tachycardia is often expected and provoked by emotion or exercise. Polyuria may occur after high heart rates, especially in paroxysmal tachycardia.

One of the most important developments in cardiac investigation has been the use of long-term monitoring of cardiac rhythm, using tape recordings over many hours. In this way, transient changes of rhythm, of great importance, may be successfully detected.

**Simple tachycardia** It has already been observed that tachycardia may be produced in normal individuals by emotion, exercise, fevers, toxaemias—especially thyrotoxicosis—and other causes, and the pulse rate may be as high as is found in paroxysmal tachycardia or atrial flutter but rarely remains more than 140 when the patient is at rest.

In distinguishing simple tachycardia from abnormal rhythms, such as flutter or paroxysmal tachycardia, the student should note that exercise, emotion and other causes influencing a simple tachycardia do not alter the heart rate in abnormal rhythms.

**Bradycardia** A slow heart rate—simple bradycardia—like tachycardia, may occur in perfect health, especially in athletes, and is common in old people. Rates of 60 are common, and may even be lower than 50.

Various non-cardiac conditions may be responsible for temporary bradycardia, notably the after-effects of febrile illnesses such as influenza and pneumonia; jaundice; increased intracranial pressure such as occurs in cerebral tumour; and hypothyroidism.

The most important cardiac condition in which bradycardia occurs is heart block, a condition in which the ventricles do not respond, in the normal way, to the impulses reaching the AV node. This may be the result of diminished conduction through the node itself, or through the more peripheral parts of the conducting system. When the ventricle fails to respond to the impulses reaching the AV node, the condition is known as 'heart block'; 'partial' when the ventricles respond to some but not all the impulses, 'total' when all the impulses are without effect (*Fig.* 7.61, 7.62). The result is a higher atrial than ventricular rate, the latter usually varying between 30 and 50 according to the degree of block and to where the subsidiary pacemaking focus is situated. The intrinsic rate of the AV node

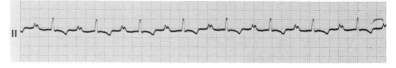

**Fig. 7.61** First degree heart block, P–R interval prolonged to 0.36 s. There is right and left atrial hypertrophy also.

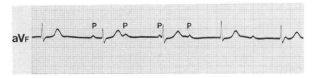

**Fig. 7.62** Complete heart block. The QRST complexes occur independently, at a rate of 47 per minute, from the P waves which are occurring at a rate of 88 per minute. The narrow QRS suggests this block is of congenital origin.

itself is about 60 per min, and that of the peripheral parts of the conducting system is about 20, so that the more peripheral the subsidiary pacemaker the slower the ventricular rhythm, and this rhythm is not usually influenced by exercise or emotion.

In partial heart block irregular action may be present, and the rate may be suddenly increased (generally doubled) by exercise. The earliest stage of heart block may only be recognizable by electrocardiography, which shows prolongation of the P–R interval (*Fig.* 7.61). At the other extreme, periods of ventricular standstill may occur in Stokes–Adams attacks (*Fig.* 7.63).

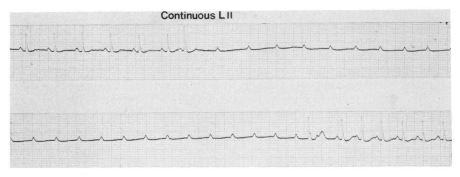

**Fig. 7.63** Ventricular standstill. Normal atrial activity persists, but there is no ventricular activity for a period of 13 s. This is a continuous strip of electrocardiographic tracing, lead II.

From this description of cardiac dysrhythmias the student will appreciate that in every case where the heart rate or rhythm appears abnormal it is essential to observe carefully

1. The rate at the pulse and apex beat.
2. The variation of these with exercise and excitement.
3. The mode of onset and offset of the attacks, preferably by observation; if not, from the history.
4. The presence of any jugular pulsations and their rate.
5. The electrocardiogram without which the diagnosis of dysrhythmias is not complete. It may be necessary to undertake long-term ECG monitoring.

## HEART FAILURE

The examination of the heart is not complete when a diagnosis of valve, myocardial, or other disease has been made. The most important question still remains to be answered, namely—What is the heart's capacity for work? This question has been partially discussed in describing the symptoms of heart disease, especially breathlessness, which, when it occurs without the customary degree of effort, is the earliest indication of cardiac failure. Later, objective signs appear which are usually of serious import. They result from failure of the ventricles to discharge their contents adequately into the systemic and pulmonary circulations. As a result the heart is unable to receive back from the systemic and pulmonary veins the optimum amount of blood.

In general the heart fails as a whole, i.e. both left and right ventricles, but in many cases the burden is laid on one ventricle more than the other, at least for a time. It is thus customary to speak of left and right heart failure.

### Left ventricular failure

This is liable to occur from the increased load which the ventricle must bear in hypertension or aortic valve disease. Similarly the damaged muscle in myocardial infarction and certain types of cardiomyopathy may be incapable of meeting the normal demands upon the heart. The left ventricle fails to discharge its contents successfully and the end diastolic pressure in the ventricle rises, causing a rise in the left atrial pressure, and hence in the pulmonary veins, resulting in pulmonary congestion and in more severe cases in pulmonary oedema.

The failure is often relatively sudden. Paroxysmal dyspnoea (p. 201) and clinical signs of pulmonary congestion and oedema, cough, laboured breathing and crepitations at the base appear. There is little or no systemic venous congestion. Death may occur rapidly in severe cases when there may be the sudden onset of acute pulmonary oedema, with flooding of the alveoli resulting in asphyxiation because no transfer of oxygen is possible. Copious frothy sputum accompanies the dyspnoea, the froth being pink with bloodstaining, and later may become more fluid, literally pouring from mouth and nose.

### Right ventricular failure

This form of failure is usually produced more gradually and occurs especially in mitral stenosis (because of pulmonary arterial hypertension), in congenital lesions such as pulmonary stenosis and in respiratory diseases (e.g. chronic bronchitis and pulmonary fibrosis) which cause extra work for the right ventricle, which hypertrophies before it fails.

It is this form of failure which is chiefly responsible for the common *congestive heart failure*, which is a later feature of so many types of heart disease. Atrial fibrillation is often the precipitating factor of the actual failure, since ventricular function depends to a critical degree on atrial augmentation of filling.

Congestion is apparent in several ways. It is seen in the engorged external veins (*Fig.* 7.19, p. 220), in the enlarged and tender liver, in impairment of renal function shown by oliguria and concentrated urine; and in oedema.

These two types of failure, as previously mentioned, are commonly found together, but in varying degrees, and any attempt to separate them strictly would be artificial.

Both types of failure may disappear with treatment, leaving the causal state behind, but the failure may be repeated from time to time.

An acute form of right ventricular failure results from massive *pulmonary embolism* (*Fig.* 7.64). There is usually a sudden onset of dyspnoea, retrosternal discomfort and faintness, accompanied by venous engorgement and peripheral circulatory failure with a right ventricular gallop rhythm produced by an early diastolic filling sound and accentuation of the pulmonary second sound. Multiple small emboli cause a more insidious form of congestive heart failure, consequent upon the development of pulmonary arterial hypertension.

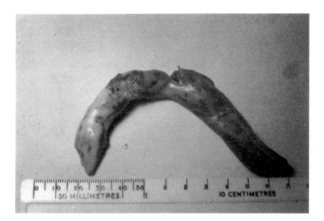

**Fig. 7.64** Pulmonary embolus successfully removed at operation from a 'saddle' position in the bifurcation of the pulmonary artery trunk.

### Effort syndrome

This condition, historically called 'da Costa's syndrome', is an expression of a psychoneurosis, usually an anxiety state. Although there is no organic heart disease, the patient complains of apparent cardiac symptoms such as dyspnoea on slight exertion, palpitation or inframammary pain. There are often other symptoms arising from disturbance of the autonomic system, e.g. sweating, dizziness and syncope. It has no specific physical signs, the diagnosis being dependent on a properly taken history of the disorder, and the absence of any signs of organic cardiovascular disease.

### ■ SPECIAL INVESTIGATIONS

The special investigations include instrumental examination by means of the electrocardiograph, the phonocardiograph, the echocardiograph and also the radiograph. Cardiac catheterization is a more specialized procedure but necessary in certain heart conditions.

## ELECTROCARDIOGRAPHY

The electrocardiogram (ECG) yields valuable data about electrical events occurring with cardiac muscle activity. Alteration of this activity results in departure from the normal pattern of the electrocardiogram and gives important information about the integrity of the heart muscle and the type of cardiac rhythm. For many years electrocardiograms were taken chiefly from what were known as the three standard leads. In lead I the patient is connected to the instrument by electrodes applied to his right and left arms; in lead II the electrodes are from the right arm and left leg; in lead III from the left arm and left leg. Later it was found that further information could be obtained by the use of a precordial lead, in which one electrode was placed on the right arm or left leg and the other in various positions upon the chest (CR and CF leads). These leads were bipolar, and there was a considerable difference in voltage between them. In an attempt to establish a commonly accepted practice unipolar leads are now commonly used. In these, the three limbs are connected to a single terminal forming one electrode; the other electrode is in contact with the chest at various points from the right of the sternum to the axilla or back (V or Voltage leads). Similarly, unipolar limb leads are derived from a single electrode joining the three limbs and a second electrode connected with one limb only (aVR, aVL, aVF). Fuller details of the relative value of these various methods of electrocardiography should be sought in specialized textbooks.

The excursion of the various waves is standardized by passing a current of known intensity through the instrument causing a deflection of 1 cm for 1 mV on the recording paper. Each record shows the method of time marking, vertical lines of 0·20 s (thick) and 0·04 s (thin) and horizontal lines of 1 mm with which the amplitude of the various waves and their distances apart can be measured.

### The interpretation of the electrocardiograph

The waves produced by the cardiac cycle are commonly named P, Q, R, S and T (*Fig.* 7.65). The following description applies to these in the standard leads:

**The P wave** P represents the spreading of electrical activity through the atria. It is absent in atrial fibrillation, when atrial activity is rapid, inco-ordinate and continuous. Abnormal P waves occur more frequently than the ventricular waves in atrial flutter with heart-block, in which the atrial rate is greater than the ventricular. Normally the P wave is upright, but it is inverted in lead I in true dextrocardia and may invert in conditions in which the cardiac pacemaker is not in the sino-atrial node (e.g. paroxysmal atrial or nodal tachycardia and atrial flutter), but isolated inverted P waves may have no pathological significance.

P is followed by the ventricular events Q, R, S and T. The P–R interval is normally 0·14–0·18 s and represents the time taken by the excitatory process to pass from the atrium to the ventricle. It is measured from the beginning of the P to the beginning of the R waves. The P–R interval is increased (more than 0·22 s is generally considered pathological) when the conduction through the atrioventricular bundle (of His) is decreased. This may merely indicate some temporary effect, e.g. digitalis poisoning, or may be a permanent condition in heart block, in which all grades of defective conductivity are found from slight prolongation

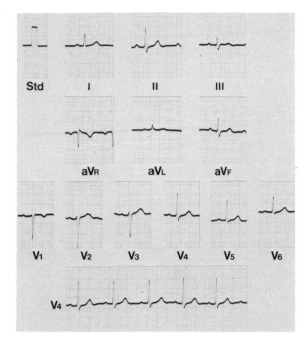

**Fig. 7.65** Normal electrocardiogram. The continuous record at the bottom of the trace shows normal sinus rhythm, with normal sequence of PQRS and T.

of the P–R interval to complete atrioventricular dissociation. In the last case the atrial P waves bear no relationship to the ventricular events Q, R, S and T: the P waves occur at a normal rate of 72 (approximately) per minute; the QRST only at about 30 per minute, when the pacemaking focus is situated in the periphery of the conducting system.

**The QRS complex** Q is the usually small initial downward deflection of the QRS complex, which corresponds with the initial part of ventricular septal activity. A deep or broad Q is abnormal and is often found over an area of cardiac infarction. R occurs next and is often the main deflection in the QRS complex. It is upright in all leads, and may be slightly notched even in health. S follows R and is normally a relatively small wave directed downwards. QRS together normally occupy no more than 0·1 s and QRS 'spread'—i.e. when the deflections occupy more than 0·1 s—indicates some impairment in conductivity through the branches of the atrioventricular bundle of His or their final arborization in the ventricular muscle. It is thus seen in bundle-branch block, and in these cases the QRS is usually notched and bizarre in shape.

Ventricular extrasystoles produce a large QRS complex, with the final deflection in an opposite direction to the initial. Axis deviation of the heart, which can be physiological, varying with the body build and the phase of respiration, may be shown by alteration in the amplitude of the R and S waves in leads I and III. In right-axis deviation S is prominent in lead I and R in lead III. The signs are

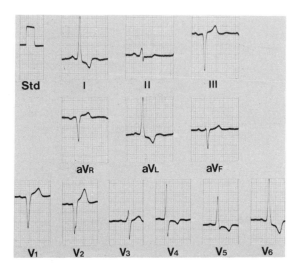

**Fig. 7.66** Left ventricle hypertrophy. This record is from a patient with severe aortic stenosis. The leads VI–V5 are recorded at half sensitivity. There is left axis deviation, deep Q–S waves in leads V1 and V2, tall R waves in leads V5 and V6, and negative T waves in leads I, aVL, V4, V5 and V6.

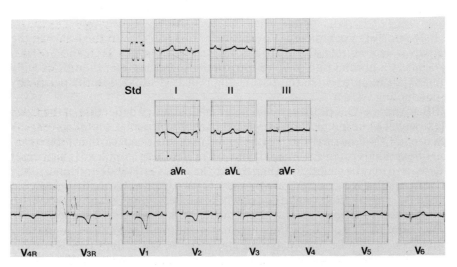

**Fig. 7.67** Right ventricle hypertrophy. This patient had severe pulmonary valve stenosis. Leads V4R and V3R are recorded from right chest positions similar to V3 and V4 on the left. Right-axis deviation is present, with tall R waves in leads V4R, V3R (over the right ventricle), V1 and V2, with negative T waves in the same leads.

opposite in left-axis deviation. More pronounced changes of this kind, sometimes with T wave inversion, are seen in left and right ventricular hypertrophy (*Figs.* 7.66, 7.67). Unipolar limb leads help in difficult cases, but care must be shown before pronouncing axis deviation as normal or abnormal.

**The T wave** T represents the final electrical change coincident with ventricular contraction. It is upright and slightly rounded in lead I but frequently inverted (negative) in lead III in normal subjects as a part of left-axis deviation. Persistent negativity of the T wave in leads I and II is found in myocardial diseases, especially ischaemic, and may occur temporarily in toxaemias (e.g. digitalis poisoning and fevers).

Sometimes the S–T interval is modified. Instead of a flat portion, it may become curved, elevated or depressed. Such changes in the S–T interval occur with cardiac ischaemia.

### PHONOCARDIOGRAPHY

This is used to record heart sounds and murmurs, and relate them to haemodynamic events, using a simultaneous tracing of carotid, jugular or apex pulse.

Cardiac muscle activity is associated with low-frequency vibrations of considerable amplitude, much greater than that of heart sounds and murmurs, which have a frequency within the audible range. Since it is the latter that have to be recorded in phonocardiography, a filtering mechanism is used to remove high-amplitude, low-frequency vibrations and allow amplification of those in the higher-frequency, lower-amplitude range.

The terms, HF, MF and LF refer to the three frequency recordings found most satisfactory in clinical use—HF or high frequency being where most of the low-frequency vibrations have been filtered out to allow amplification of low-intensity, high-frequency vibrations, e.g. the decrescendo diastolic murmurs of aortic incompetence. LF or low frequency corresponds to what is heard when using the bell end of a stethoscope, e.g. for the detection of a mitral diastolic murmur. MF is between HF and LF, and corresponds to what is heard with the diaphragm end of a stethoscope.

Phonocardiographs are obtained from crystal microphones applied to the chest wall and connected to a suitable recording apparatus through a series of amplifiers. The pattern commonly used is to record from the second and fourth right intercostal spaces by the sternal edge (2R and 4R), from the second, third and fourth left interspaces by the sternal edge (2L, 3L, 4L) from the position of the apex, both with the patient on his left side, and on his back, and from Erbs point—between the left sternal edge and the apex, corresponding to the V3 position in electrocardiography.

Together with the recording of heart sounds and murmurs, it is essential to record the lower-frequency events, i.e. the arterial pulse (usually carotid), the jugular venous pulse (JVP) and the movement of the apex beat (ACG). These recordings are needed for timing events in the cardiac cycle, but also have their own diagnostic value, e.g. in the recording of the arterial pulse in aortic stenosis (*Figs.* 7.9, 7.10). Several examples of normal and abnormal arterial and venous pulses have been illustrated in this chapter (*Figs.* 7.8, 7.9, 7.20). For recordings of apex cardiograms the reader is referred to more advanced books of cardiology, but the examples and descriptive legends included here give an indication of the usefulness of this technique.

### ECHOCARDIOGRAPHY

Echocardiography is a non-invasive method of investigation used particularly for the demonstration of congenital cardiac abnormalities, the diagnosis of pericardial effusion and certain types of valve disease and the assessment of cardiac chamber size and function.

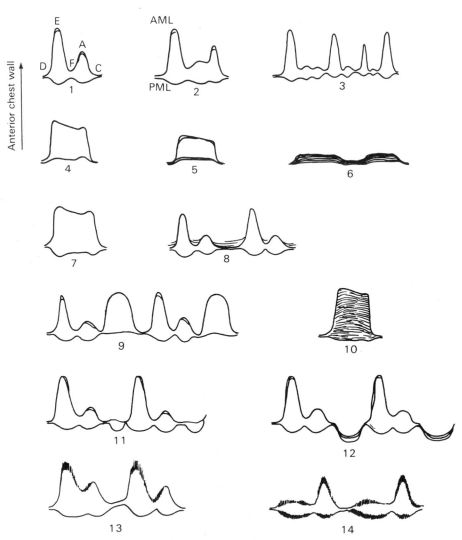

**Fig. 7.68** Common patterns of mitral valve movement shown by M-mode echocardiography. For explanations of nos. 1–14, *see text.*

Echocardiography represents a development of naval sonar used for the location and detection of underwater objects and the mapping of the sea bed. In principle, it depends upon the emission and reflection of a beam of pulsed high-frequency sound, generated by a piezo-electric crystal, which acts as transmitter and receiver. The delay that occurs between the emission and return of the ultra-sound is a measure of the depth of the reflecting surface, away from the energy source. Ultrasonic reflection occurs whenever there is a difference in the acoustic impedance of adjacent tissues. (Acoustic impedance is the product of the speed of sound in tissue and the density of the tissue.) Certain tissues are good reflectors, and send back narrow beams of high intensity—the heart valves are good examples, but when the valves become irregular and thicker, the beams reflected are wider and more diffuse. A change of impedance, say from fluid to denser tissue, as in a pericardial effusion, produces a reflecting layer which is clearly defined, and of great diagnostic value, but air-containing lung is a great absorber of ultrasound energy, and the interposition of lung between the heart and the transducer will make it very difficult to conduct this examination.

Display and recording of ultrasound has been developed into a method whereby the intensity of the reflected sound, shown as the brightness of a dot on an oscilloscope, at a calibrated distance from the ultrasound source, can be converted into a series of lines by sweeping the dots across the screen and record-ing the pattern produced. This is M-mode (or motion) echocardiography. The illustrations used here are mostly of M-mode echo traces.

A more recent extension of echocardiography is the 2-D (two-dimensional) echo, which is so arranged that a series of echo signals is produced and recorded, in real time, so that in effect a moving picture of a cross-section of the heart can be obtained and recorded. Of great value in the diagnosis of congenital cardiac malformations, it is likely to be an area where considerable advances in technique

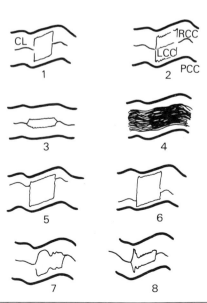

**Fig. 7.69**
Common patterns of aortic valve movement in M-mode echocardiography. For explanations of nos. 1–8, *see text.*

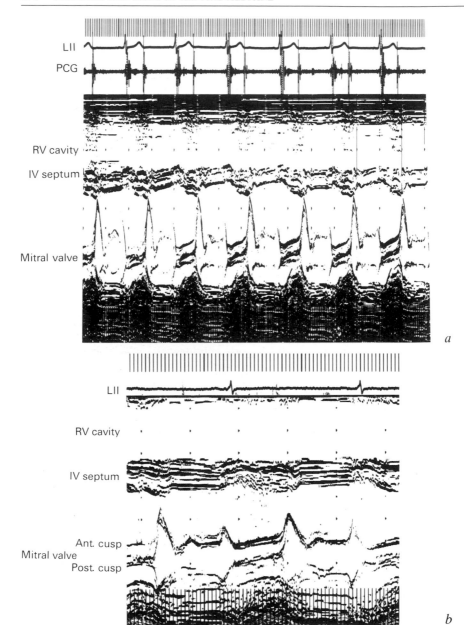

**Fig. 7.70** *a*, Normal mitral valve movement. This figure corresponds with pattern no. 2 in *Fig.* 7.68, but also shows a normal PCG, normal right ventricle, interventricular septum and normal left ventricle cavity size and movement. Note particularly the normal posterior cusp, moving away from the anterior cusp, during diastole. *b*, Normal mitral valve movement. No PCG is shown here, and note the recording paper speed is faster than in *a*. The normal E and F waves are shown, with the divergent movement of the posterior cusp of the mitral valve.

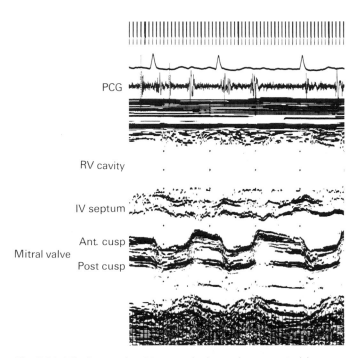

**Fig. 7.71** Mitral stenosis with regurgitation, pulmonary arterial hypertension. The ECG shows the pattern of atrial fibrillation, the PCG is not helpful. From above downwards, the echogram shows a dilated right ventricle, normal thickness of the interventricular septum, a normal sized left ventricle cavity, but the mitral valve is restricted in movement, the amplitude of which is low, the valves are slow to open and close, show dense echo shadowing, which represents calcification. The posterior cusp moves anteriorly, towards the anterior cusp, in diastole.

will be made in the near future. Still frames, as in *Figs*. 7.74 and 7.75 are not easy to produce and even less easy to interpret.

It is not possible here to illustrate many echocardiographic patterns, but the diagrams in *Figs*. 7.68 and 7.69 show some of the normal and abnormal patterns of the mitral and aortic valves.

In *Fig*. 7.68, no. 1 shows the pattern of mitral valve movement, in the normal heart, in sinus rhythm. At point D the anterior and posterior leaflets commence to separate. The larger excursion of the anterior leaflet can be measured and is the vertical distance between D and E. At the E point the two cusps are separated by their maximum amount, and the anterior cusp is almost in contact with the interventricular septum. Note that the posterior cusp is moving away from the anterior cusp.

After point E, the mitral valve moves into a more closed position as the ventricle fills, and the E to F slope represents the rate at which the closure movement

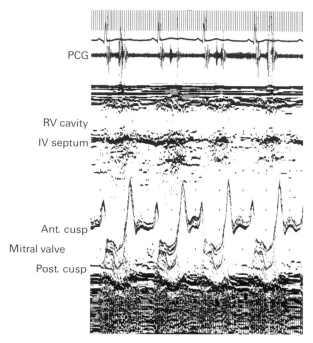

PCG

RV cavity

IV septum

Ant. cusp

Mitral valve

Post. cusp

**Fig. 7.72** Mitral valve prolapse. The PCG shows the mid-systolic click and variable late systolic murmur present in this case. The echo from above downwards shows a normal right ventricle and IV septum. The mitral valve echo shows a sudden backwards prolapse of the posterior cusp, 1 ss of the anterior cusp, in late systole. The start of this sudden prolapse is coincident with the mid-systolic click. Compare with no. 12 in *Fig.* 7.69.

occurs, the rate being markedly reduced in mitral stenosis. When atrial contraction occurs, the valve leaflets separate again to the A point, and the leaflets close at the point C when ventricular systole begins.

The excursion of the posterior leaflet is considerably less than the anterior and it should be emphasized that in the normal valve the movement in diastole is away from the anterior cusp, as the valve opens. The movement of the posterior cusp is less easy to record than the anterior, but is shown quite well in *Fig.* 7.70.

No. 2 in *Fig.* 7.68 is the normal valve in sinus rhythm, but with a slower rate, the extra separation of the cusps after F representing mid diastolic flow into the LV.

No. 3 shows the result of atrial fibrillation, the valve movement being normal. The A point has disappeared, the excursion to E shows a varying amplitude, and if coarse atrial fibrillation is present, small separations of the cusps can be seen.

No. 4 shows the effects of mitral stenosis, in sinus rhythm, and with a mobile valve. The total excursion is limited only slightly, but the E to F slope is greatly reduced. A small A wave can be seen, but the posterior cusp moves anteriorly, in the same direction as the anterior cusps.

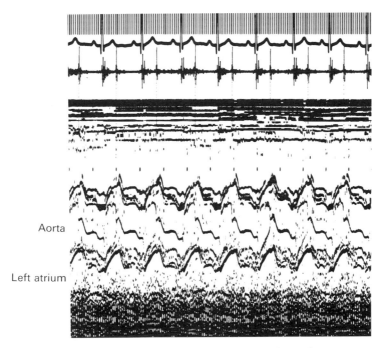

**Fig. 7.73** Normal aortic valve. The diastolic closure line of the valve is very clearly seen. The 'box' or parallelogram of the opened valve is best seen in the fifth and sixth complete complexes in the figure. Note the closure line is central. The left atrial size is normal.

No. 5 shows more severe mitral stenosis, the A wave has disappeared and the cusps are thicker. *Fig.* 7.34 (p. 243) demonstrates this well, where the posterior cusp is also shown, moving anteriorly.

No. 6 shows a calcified immobile mitral valve, the echoes from the anterior and posterior cusps being very limited in amplitude and very dense in appearance. An example of this is shown in *Fig.* 7.71.

No. 7 demonstrates the picture of a stiff left ventricle, as occurs in advanced systemic hypertension, or aortic stenosis. The amplitude of excursion may be slightly reduced, but of great importance is the fact that the posterior leaflet moves posteriorly, away from the anterior leaflet in diastole. This appearance closely mimics mitral stenosis, as in no. 4, but the direction of movement of the posterior leaflet is the differentiating point.

No. 8 shows a normal valve, the chordae appearing as parallel lines best seen in diastole.

No. 9 is the appearance in hypertrophic obstructive cardiomyopathy (HOCM), where the valve movement is normal in diastole, but in systole the valve mechanism moves anteriorly, approaching the septum (systolic anterior motion, or SAM), producing obstruction in the left ventricular outflow tract.

No. 10 shows the characteristic appearance of a left atrial myxoma, when the echoes from the tumour fill the space behind the anterior cusps of the mitral

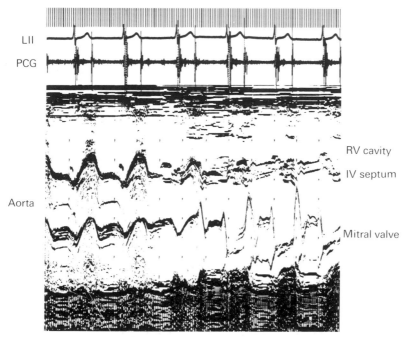

**Fig. 7.74** Normal echo scan, from the same person as *Fig. 7.70a*. From left to right, the scan passes from aorta to the mitral valve, showing aortic continuity with the IV septum anteriorly, and with the anterior cusp of the mitral valve more posteriorly. The chamber sizes, valve movements and septal thickness are all normal.

valve as the mass descends into the valve opening. Differentiation from valve vegetations and left atrial thrombus may be difficult.

Nos. 11 and 12 show two varieties of mitral valve prolapse. No. 11 demonstrates late systolic prolapse of the posterior cusp, the start of the prolapse being simultaneous with the mid-systolic click, followed by the systolic murmur, as in *Fig*. 7.26. No. 12 is the echo picture of pansystolic prolapse of both leaflets, and is usually associated with symptomatic mitral regurgitation.

Nos. 13 and 14 show the mitral valve in aortic regurgitation. No. 13 diagrammatically is a reproduction of *Fig*. 7.40, and represents a moderate grade of aortic regurgitation, with diastolic vibrations of a normally mobile anterior cusp of the mitral valve. The more severe grade of aortic regurgitation in no. 14 shows fluttering of both cusps, with a reduced excursion of the valve opening.

In *Fig*. 7.69 the common patterns of aortic valve movement are shown. No. 1 is normal. CL shows the closure line in diastole, central in position, ending with abrupt valve opening at the start of ejection, the cusps moving to the edge of the aortic wall. The right cusp (RCC) is anterior, the non-coronary, posterior cusps (PCC) being posterior. The resulting shape is a parallelogram, the cusps closing as abruptly as they open. Cusp opening corresponds to the position of the ejection click on the PCG; cusp closure corresponds to the position of the aortic component of the second sound.

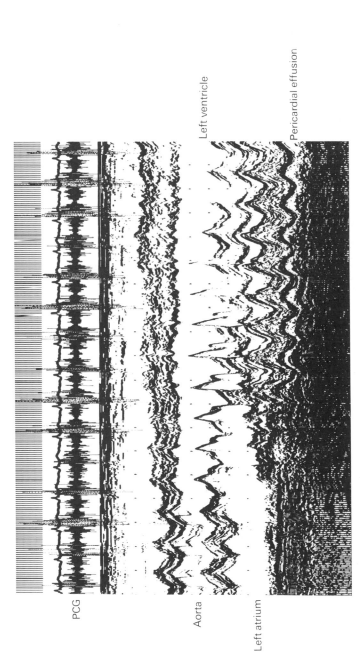

**Fig. 7.75** Echo scan, in a patient with uraemic pericarditis. The PCG reveals the very loud pericardial friction noise. The right ventricle cavity size is normal, but the interventricular septum and the left ventricle posterior wall are thicker than normal. The aortic and mitral valves are normal. Where the echo of the mitral valve becomes apparent, moving from left to right (from aorta to left ventricle), an echo-free space widens as the pericardial effusion becomes apparent. The pericardium is reflected from visceral to parietal layers at this point, hence the effusion is behind the ventricle only, and not behind the atrium.

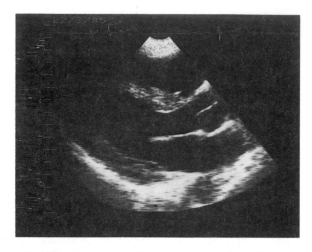

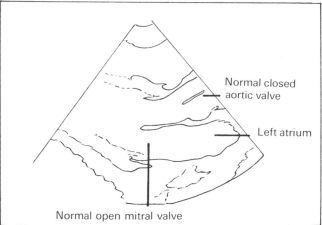

**Fig. 7.76** Two dimensional (2-D) echo of a normal heart, long axis view. The single line of aortic valve closure probably represents the central coaption of the valve cusps, but the widely open mitral valve is well seen.

No. 2 is also normal, but shows the rare appearance of the left coronary cusp. The fine vibrations are not abnormal.

No. 3 shows a relatively immobile aorta, and limited separation of otherwise normal valve cusps in a low cardiac output state.

No. 4 demonstrates the dense echoes appearing when the aortic valve is heavily calcified, where no discrete cusp movements can be seen, as in calcific aortic stenosis.

Nos. 5 and 6 show the eccentric closure line seen in a bicuspid aortic valve, where the cusps open normally, and are not yet stenosed. This pattern is suggestive, but not diagnostic, of a bicuspid valve.

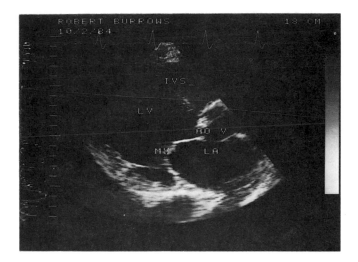

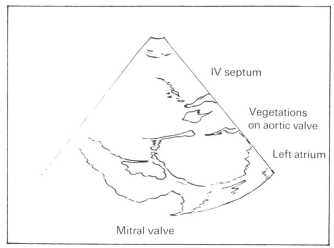

**Fig. 7.77** Two dimensional (2-D) echo of vegetations on an aortic valve in a 72-year-old man with infective endocarditis. The diagnosis was confirmed at surgery. The normal closed mitral valve is well seen.

No. 7 shows the ortic valve movement in HOCM (*see Fig.* 7.68 for mitral valve movement). The aortic valve shows premature closure in mid-systole. The pattern, however, is not diagnostic, and may occur in other conditions.

No. 8 is the echo pattern of discrete sub-aortic stenosis, showing early systolic closure, particularly of the right coronary cusp. The premature closure is much earlier than in HOCM.

The tricuspid and pulmonary valves are difficult to demonstrate echocardiographically unless the right ventricle and pulmonary artery are dilated. Wall movement and ventricular function can be assessed by echocardiography. The

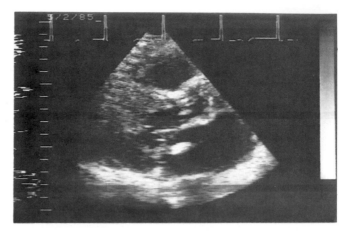

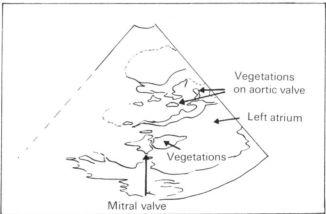

**Fig. 7.78** Two dimensional (2-D) echo of vegetations on the aortic and mitral valves in a 76-year-old woman with infective endocarditis. The vegetations on the mitral valve are particularly large.

internal measurements of the ventricle at end-systole and diastole can be measured, and stroke volume assessed. The immobile wall and interventricular septum in congestive cardiomyopathy, with the small mitral valve excursion in the dilated left ventricle, are shown in *Fig.* 7.47.

Left atrial size can be shown quite accurately, as can a dilated aorta, for example in dissecting aneurysm. By gradual movement of the transducer so that the exploring beam of ultrasound passes from the apex of the ventricle upwards towards the aortic valve, it is possible to do an echo 'sweep' of the underlying structures, as in *Fig.* 7.72. This technique can be used to visualize the left ventricle outflow tract, to show the presence of aortic–mitral continuity, aortic–septal continuity and, perhaps most important, in adult cardiology it helps to show the presence of a posterior pericardial effusion. The echo-free space of the effusion behind the ventricle disappears behind the left atrium where the pericardium is reflected off the wall of that chamber. This is well shown in *Fig*. 7.73.

Some final examples of echocardiography are given in *Figs*. 7.74 and 7.75, with 'static' frames of 2-D echocardiography in *Figs*. 7.76, 7.77 and 7.78.

### CARDIAC CATHETERIZATION

Catheterization of the right heart chambers is performed by the venous route, either through a femoral or an arm vein. The left heart chambers are approached retrogradely through the brachial or femoral artery, passing from aorta to left ventricle through the aortic valve. The left atrium is approached

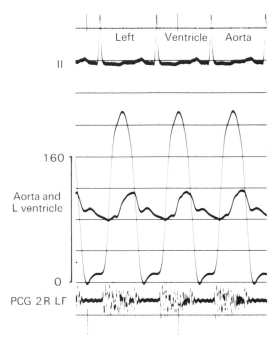

**Fig. 7.79** Cardiac catheter and PCG findings in aortic stenosis. The PCG shows the systolic murmur, but the pressure tracings show a left ventricle pressure of 220 systolic, and an aortic pressure of about 115 systolic. The aortic pressure pulse is of small amplitude and is anacrotic. This patient had aortic valve stenosis of a severe degree.

either through a patent foramen ovale, from right atrium to left, or by trans-atrial septal puncture, the catheter being introduced from the right atrium. All these manoeuvres, except in children, should be done using local anaesthesia only, since patient co-operation is needed for various movements and recordings.

Using a suitably designed cardiac catheter, it is possible with this method to:

1. Record intracardiac pressures and wave forms. With two or more catheters inserted, simultaneous pressure records from different sites can be recorded, e.g. left ventricle and aorta, in aortic stenosis (*Fig*. 7.79).

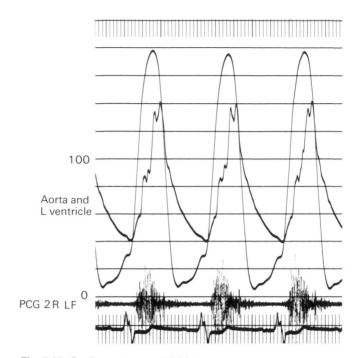

**Fig. 7.80** Cardiac catheter and PCG findings in aortic stenosis and regurgitation. The PCG shows the systolic and diastolic murmurs, the pressure tracings a left ventricle systolic pressure of 180, with an aortic systolic pressure of 140. The aortic pressure pulse is of high amplitude, and although there is some delay in its upstroke, the diastolic fall to 40, almost equalling the ventricular end-diastolic pressure, is typical of severe aortic regurgitation.

2. Because of the ability to take blood samples from the catheter tip, arterio-venous oxygen differences can be determined in cardiac output studies, and blood sampling throughout the cardiac chambers will help to determine the site and severity of left-to-right shunting.

3. Injection of indicator solution and sampling downstream from the injection site, enables curves to be drawn of indicator dilution and these are of assistance in calculating cardiac output and in determining site and size of left-to-right and right-to-left shunting.

4. Injection of radiographic contrast material selectively into cardiac chambers or vessels is used, for example, in the quantification of mitral regurgitation, when contrast material is injected into the left ventricle and a film recording made of the subsequent cardiac cycles. Injection into the aorta will help to identify and quantitate aortic regurgitation and injections into the left and right ventricles will show the interventricular septum and any defects therein. Coarctation of the aorta is readily shown by angiographic methods.

5. Left ventricular angiography, used to determine left ventricular function and morphology, is an important part of the now very common procedure of coronary arteriography. In this investigation, a special catheter is manipulated either by the femoral or brachial route to the left and right coronary orifice, and small volumes of contrast material are injected into the vessel, taking cine film in different views so as to build up a three-dimensional picture of the coronary arterial tree. This is a very important investigation, first to demonstrate the presence or absence of coronary arterial pathology and secondly to show the precise anatomy of any obstructed lesions, a necessity if coronary artery bypass surgery is to be performed. Postoperatively, the integrity of the newly established bypass vessels can be confirmed.

6. Finally, it is possible, using a wide-bore catheter as a protective sheath, to insert biopsy forceps into left and right ventricles, and remove pieces of myocardium for histological examination.

---

■ **PERIPHERAL VASCULAR DISEASES**

---

Examination of the peripheral arteries and veins has already been described in relation to disorders of the heart (p. 219 *et seq.*). Diseases of these vessels themselves may, as in the case of the heart, be functional or structural in origin.

*Functional* disorders of the arteries consist of changes in vasomotor tone which may be diffuse or focal. A diffuse increase in arteriolar tone gives rise to hypertension which, though functional in origin, may have serious structural effects upon the arteries and left ventricle. Examples of focal disorders of arterial tone are Raynaud's phenomenon (*Fig.* 7.81), in which there is cold-induced spasm of the digital arteries, and migraine characterized by constriction followed by dilatation of the cranial arteries (*see* p. 433). Erythrocyanosis frigidum (chilblains) also arises

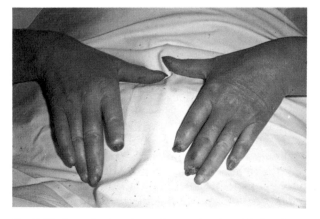

**Fig. 7.81** Case of scleroderma (systemic sclerosis) showing atrophy of terminal phalanges and early gangrene. Similar appearances may be seen in other types of Raynaud's phenomena.

from an instability of vasomotor tone. Prolonged exposure to cold may induce gangrene from intense vasoconstriction (*Fig*. 7.82).

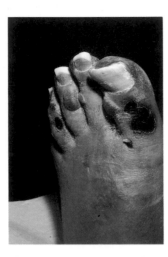

**Fig. 7.82**
Cold injury to the feet: frostbite.

*Structural* arterial disease is usually metabolic, degenerative or inflammatory in origin. The most important cause is *atheroma* in which arteries are damaged by the deposition of a lipoid material beneath the intima. This occurs most often in middle-aged men, especially those with disordered fat metabolism, as in diabetes and familial hyperlipidaemia. The degenerative process in the arteries is accelerated by hypertension and heavy smoking. Atheroma may be complicated by thrombosis, sometimes with embolism to more distal parts of the artery, and also by aneurysmal dilatation or rupture of the vessel. The aorta and its main branches and the coronary and cerebral arteries are most commonly affected.

*Thrombosis and embolism* may also lead to arterial occlusion in the absence of any primary disease of the artery. Thrombosis can occur in certain blood disorders (*see* Chapter 8), and emboli may arise from intracardiac thrombus, as in mitral disease or after myocardial infarction.

Inflammatory vascular disease or *vasculitis* is usually the result of an auto-immune process which may occur at any age and, unlike atheroma, favours the smaller peripheral vessels. The disease is often widespread and lesions in the kidneys, heart and lungs are of special importance. Infective forms of arteritis are now rare but two are worthy of mention: (1) Syphilitic aortitis causing dilatation of the proximal aorta leading to aneurysm and regurgitation (*see* p. 292). (2) Mycotic aneurysm due to infection of the arterial wall by an embolus from the aortic or mitral valve in patients with bacterial endocarditis.

*The symptoms and signs* of arterial disease are due either to narrowing of the lumen or to inflammation, distension or rupture of the wall. Luminal narrowing affects parts supplied by the diseased artery while changes in the vessel wall may also involve the structures surrounding it. The clinical features of some common arterial diseases will now be described.

### Obliterative arterial disease

The effects of coronary and cerebral arterial insufficiency are described elsewhere. The symptoms and signs of obstructed limb arteries depend upon the site and nature of the stenosis. The legs are much more commonly affected than the arms because the lower part of the aorta and its branches are more prone to atheroma. The ischaemic changes in the limb are sudden and profound when occlusion is by embolism. Narrowing by atheroma or thrombus is usually more gradual, allowing time for the development of a collateral circulation.

The commonest symptom of obliterative arterial disease is ischaemic muscle pain on effort ('intermittent claudication'). The level of the lesion determines the site of the pain which is most often in the calf but may occur in the buttock, thigh or sole of the foot. The pain resembles angina in that it is aching or cramping in character, regularly occurs after walking a certain distance, compels the patient to stop and disappears when he does so. Effort tolerance may progressively diminish until pain occurs even at rest and disturbs sleep. The patient may also complain that the foot on the affected side feels cold or numb and he may notice paraesthesiae or colour changes.

Inspection of the ischaemic limb may reveal cyanosis, pallor or trophic lesions in the skin, especially in the more peripheral parts. If the limbs are elevated and then quickly lowered to a dependent position, the veins re-fill and the colour returns more slowly on the side most severely affected. Trophic lesions include loss of hair, ulcers and gangrene (*see Fig.* 3.37, p. 60), seen first on he toes sand later more proximally. The temperature of the skin will vary with the ambient temperature, but a difference between the two limbs, best detected with the dorsum or ulnar border of the hand, is significant. In patients complaining of effort pain, the dorsalis pedis and posterior tibial pulses are usually absent. The popliteal and femoral pulses may also be absent or diminished and a bruit may be audible over them.

### Systemic hypertension

Although an abnormally high systemic blood pressure is rarely due to primary arterial disease, it is usually mediated by increased arteriolar tone. In most cases, a cause for this cannot be found though a family history is common, and to these the term 'essential' hypertension is applied. The majority of the remainder will be suffering from some form of chronic renal disease (*see* Chapter 5). Rarer causes include coarctation of the aorta and endocrine disorders such as phaeochromocytoma and Cushing's syndrome (*see* Chapter 11).

There is no evidence that hypertension of itself causes symptoms and indeed the majority of cases are discovered at a routine medical examination. Symptoms such as headache and dizziness are often due to the patients' anxiety about their blood pressure. Symptoms and signs are otherwise attributable either to the cause or to cardiac and arterial complications such as left ventricular failure and degenerative changes in the cerebral and coronary circulations.

The diagnosis is established by finding a persistent or recurrent elevation of the systemic blood pressure above 140 mmHg systolic and 90 mm diastolic even after a period of rest. An index of the severity of the hypertension is given by retinoscopy (*Fig.* 7.83; *see also* p. 344). The term 'accelerated (or malignant) hyper-

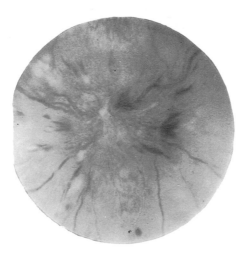

**Fig. 7.83** Malignant or accelerated hypertension: retinal haemorrhages, exudates and papilloedema.

tension' is applied to a severe rapidly progressive form of the disease associated with papilloedema and renal failure.

### Raynaud phenomenon

This condition is characterized by intermittent spasm of digital arteries induced by cold and relieved by heat. Young women are most often affected and usually no underlying cause can be found (Raynaud's disease), but some cases are associated with occlusive arterial disease, arteritis, blood disorders, neurogenic lesions or repeated trauma to the hands.

The patient complains that, when exposed to cold, the fingers and less commonly the toes go numb and white, sometimes with patchy cyanosis. This is followed by redness, throbbing and tingling due to a reactive hyperaemia occurring either spontaneously or on re-warming. The hands may appear normal between attacks but trophic lesions develop in long-standing cases, especially those associated with organic disease. The fingers may then become thin and tapered with tight shiny skin ('scleroderma'), telangiectasia, deformed atrophic nails and infarcts causing painful ulcers at the fingertips (*see Fig.* 7.81).

### Vasculitis ('connective tissue diseases')

It is appropriate here to consider a group of disorders characterized by inflammatory changes in connective tissues and in the walls of small peripheral vessels (necrotizing vasculitis). The cause is unknown but an auto-immune process, sometimes drug-induced, may be responsible in certain cases. These conditions are therefore distinguished by the clinical syndromes with which they present rather than by specific aetiological tests.

**1. Polyarteritis nodosa** The manifestations are so diverse that a purely clinical diagnosis may be impossible until several systems have been involved. The most characteristic features are renal failure, multiple organ infarction, asymmetrical peripheral neuropathy, intractable bronchial asthma and polymorph leucocytosis with eosinophilia. Splinter haemorrhages in the nails (*see Fig.* 7.54) and small infarcts in the finger tips (*Fig.* 7.84) may be seen in this and other vasculitic disorders.

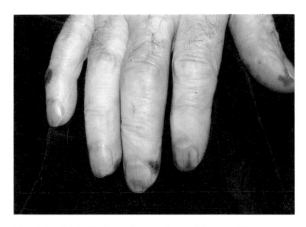

**Fig. 7.84** Digital infarcts in a patient with vasculitis.

**2. Giant-cell arteritis** The inflammatory process mainly affects the cranial vessels of elderly subjects and tends towards spontaneous recovery. The temporal and occipital arteries may be tender, inflamed and pulseless. Sudden blindness can result from retinal artery occlusion. The condition is often associated with painful stiffness of the proximal limb muscles (*polymyalgia rheumatica*).

**3. Systemic sclerosis** This condition usually presents with a Raynaud phenomenon and the typical changes of scleroderma in the hands and face (*see Fig.* 3.29, p. 56 and *Fig.* 7.81). Dysphagia and malabsorption from alimentary tract involvement, myocardial ischaemia and dyspnoea due to fibrosing alveolitis are other typical features of this disease.

**4. Systemic lupus erythematosus** The name of this syndrome is derived from the red 'butterfly' rash which affects the nose, cheeks and other parts exposed to light (*see Fig.* 3.10, p. 42). Another cutaneous manifestation of connective tissue disease is livido reticularis (*Fig.* 7.85). Many organs may be involved including the joints, lung, heart, liver, kidneys, haemopoietic and nervous systems. As distinct from polyarteritis, systemic lupus is more common among women than men and is more often associated with leucopenia and thrombocytopenia than with leucocytosis.

**5. Rheumatoid disease (***see also*** Chapter 9)** A rheumatoid form of arthritis is a common feature of the vasculitic or connective tissue group of diseases and

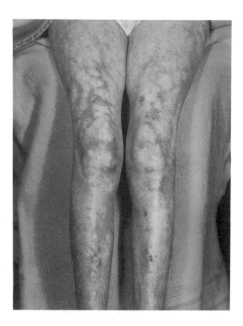

**Fig. 7.85**
Livido reticularis.

vasculitic lesions in the skin, eyes and elsewhere may be found in patients presenting with classic rheumatoid arthritis.

An inflammatory cause for a peripheral vascular disorder should always be considered when the patient has fever or a raised ESR.

### Aneurysm

Congenital, inflammatory or degenerative changes in the arterial wall may lead to focal or diffuse dilatation and eventually rupture of the vessel. The cerebral arteries and the aorta are most commonly affected.

Aneurysm of a cerebral artery, whether congenital ('berry' aneurysm), infective ('mycotic' aneurysm) or atheromatous, usually presents with subarachnoid or intracerebral haemorrhage (*see* Chapter 10). Aneurysm of the aorta may be of two kinds: (1) Saccular or fusiform and (2) Dissecting. Saccular or fusiform aneurysms of the thoracic aorta are either syphilitic or degenerative in origin and usually manifest as mediastinal tumours with pressure effects upon surrounding structures (*see* Chapter 6). More common today is atheromatous aneurysm of the abdominal aorta. This causes a persistent aching or throbbing pain in the abdomen or back but may leak and simulate a perforated viscus with severe pain, circulatory collapse and abdominal rigidity. A tender fusiform pulsating mass may be palpable in the abdomen to the left of the midline and a bruit may be audible over it.

Dissecting aneurysm results from degenerative changes in the medial coat of the aorta. These changes are either congenital, as in Marfan's syndrome (*see* Fig. 7.55), or acquired when they may be associated with hypertension. Blood penetrates the intima, tracks through the media and may then either rupture the outer coat of the aorta or re-enter the lumen lower down. The process usually starts in the upper thoracic aorta giving rise to intense retrosternal pain simulating myocardial infarction or pulmonary embolism. Pain radiates to the back and, as the dissection proceeds, may descend towards the abdomen and the loins. The origins of the carotid and subclavian vessels may be affected to cause cerebral signs and absent radial pulses. Signs may also result from leakage of blood into the pericardial, pleural or peritoneal cavities.

### Venous disorders

The three most important abnormalities of veins are dilatation and tortuosity with incompetent valves (*varicose veins*), inflammation (*phlebitis*) and *thrombosis*. These three conditions may coexist or follow one upon the other. Each may both cause and result from impaired venous drainage and, because of gravity, the legs are affected more often than the arms. Predisposing causes include obesity, prolonged standing, pregnancy, pelvic tumours and chronic congestive cardiac failure. They also include conditions favouring thrombosis such as the postoperative state, immobilization, certain oral contraceptive agents and blood disorders (e.g. polycythaemia). Venous thrombosis may complicate malignant disease and give rise to the syndrome of *thrombophlebitis migrans* in which there are flitting episodes of inflammation in superficial veins as well as deep vein thrombosis.

The symptoms and signs of a venous disorder depend upon its duration and speed of onset. In cases of deep vein thrombosis (e.g. postoperative) the onset may be sudden with pain and discomfort in the leg. Physical signs include low grade fever, deep tenderness in the calf or thigh, increased girth of the affected limb and pitting oedema. Dorsiflexion of the foot may cause pain in the calf (Homans' sign). Symptoms and signs of pulmonary embolism (*see* p. 269) may sometimes precede those of the venous thrombosis. Thrombophlebitis is recognized by the presence of a tender palpable cord in one or more segments of the superficial veins with reddening of the adjacent skin.

Venous stasis of long standing leads to secondary changes in the skin. There may be a network of superficial varices, eczema, pigmentation and ulceration. These changes are maximal in the lower part of the leg especially on the medial aspect above the ankle (*see Fig.* 3.43, p. 62). The subcutaneous veins will be tortuous and dilated but this may only be apparent when the patient is standing.

### Disorders of the lymphatics

There are few clinical signs peculiar to disorders of the lymph vessels. Amongst these are the red line around inflamed lymphatics draining an area of infection (*Fig.* 7.86); yellow discoloration of the nails associated with congenital hypoplasia of lymphatics (*Fig.* 6.37); non-pitting lymphoedema due to lymphatic obstruction by malignant disease or radical surgical dissection, and the gross limb swelling of elephantiasis resulting from lymphatic obstruction by filarial parasites (*see Fig.* 12.6). Obstruction of the thoracic duct may lead to a 'chylous' pleural effusion (*see* Chapter 6).

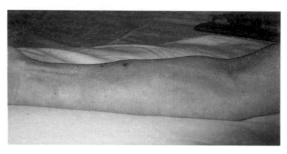

**Fig. 7.86** Lymphangitis secondary to an insect bite on the forearm.

## SPECIAL INVESTIGATIONS

Various radiographic and laboratory procedures are of value in the assessment of peripheral vascular disease. The arteries may be displayed by *retrograde aortography*, for which a catheter is passed into the aorta through the femoral artery. A radio-opaque material is then injected near to or within the origin of the relevant arteries. For *venography*, a radio-opaque material is injected into a vein near the ankle and will be carried upwards to display the veins of the leg and pelvis.

Non-invasive techniques are also available for the investigation of peripheral vascular disease. Doppler ultrasound can be used to assess both arterial and venous blood flow and ultrasound imaging has proved of value in the detection of aortic aneurysm and its differentiation from solid tumour. Plain radiographs of the abdomen or chest may be sufficient to demonstrate an aortic aneurysm, especially one which is calcified, and a radiograph of the thoracic inlet to exclude arterial compression associated with a cervical rib should always be taken in patients with upper limb ischaemia.

Relevant laboratory investigations include measurement of the serum lipoproteins and cholesterol in patients with atheroma; the ESR, tests for auto-antibodies (anti-nuclear and rheumatoid factors, etc.) and muscle or artery biopsy when a vasculitis is suspected; cryoglobulins and cold agglutinins in patients with a Raynaud phenomenon; and a Wassermann reaction to exclude syphilis as a cause of aortic aneurysm or regurgitation.

The investigation of a patient with hypertension consists mainly of excluding renal and endocrine causes (*see* Chapters 5 and 11).

## The haemopoietic system

Under this heading are included the blood and those tissues concerned in its production or destruction, namely, the bone-marrow, the lymph nodes, the spleen and the liver.

### ■ SYMPTOMS AND SIGNS OF HAEMATOLOGICAL DISEASE

The symptoms and signs of haematological disease include:
1. Symptoms and signs of anaemia.
2. Symptoms and signs of haemorrhage.
3. Enlargement of lymph nodes.
4. Enlargement of the spleen and liver.
5. Changes in the fundus oculi.
6. Changes in the mouth.
7. Changes in the skin.

These symptoms and signs are never sufficient for a diagnosis without examination of the blood and often of the bone-marrow. For this reason, this chapter is not restricted to a description of symptoms and physical signs.

### ANAEMIA

This term means a deficiency in the haemoglobin content of the blood and usually a decrease in the number of red cells. The iron-containing pigment haemoglobin, which is responsible for the normal pink coloration of the mucous membranes and skin, carries the necessary oxygen to all the organs and tissues of the body.

*The signs and symptoms, which result from a deficiency of haemoglobin, are—*

#### Pallor of the skin and mucous membranes

Pallor of the skin without a corresponding loss of colour in the lips, tongue, buccal cavity and nailbeds can frequently be disregarded, as many persons normally have a pallid complexion. In true anaemia, pallor occurs both in the skin and in the mucous membranes and varies in grade from a slight loss of colour, only appreciable to the experienced eye, to the extreme pallor of profound haemorrhageic anaemias or the lemon-yellow tint which is present occasionally

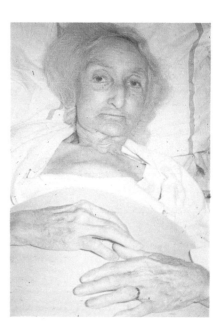

**Fig. 8.1**
Pallor due to pernicious
anaemia.

in pernicious anaemia (*Fig.* 8.1). In anaemias due to malignant disease an earthy pallor is often seen, and in bacterial endocarditis the skin colour has been likened to *café au lait*. The degree of pallor of the mucous membranes is only a rough guide to the severity of the anaemia, which should always be corroborated by a haemoglobin estimation. It is important not to rely solely on the conjunctivae for evidence of anaemia in the mucous membranes, as infection of the former from other causes not uncommonly gives a false redness.

### Symptoms and signs of oxygen deficiency

In the face of the reduced oxygen carrying capacity of the blood, both the respiratory and cardiovascular systems adapt in order to maintain tissue oxygenation. Dyspnoea may be as great as in certain forms of heart or lung disease, but the patient is only breathless at rest in very severe anaemia. With only a moderate anaemia the heart-rate is increased both at rest and on exertion. This compensatory mechanism is more marked in the elderly when both palpitations and angina are common symptoms. Sometimes right-sided heart failure may occur (*see* p. 268). The deficient oxygenation of the blood also affects adversely most of the organs and tissues of the body. Dizziness, throbbing in the head and tinnitus are common and the patient complains of general lassitude and inability for physical or mental work. The function of the gastrointestinal tract may be affected, and loss of appetite, nausea, and constipation or diarrhoea may occur. Slight albuminuria is not unusual, and renal function may be impaired occasionally. A mild or moderate degree of fever is common when the anaemia is severe. It should be pointed out that the severity of the symptoms is not necessarily related to the degree of anaemia.

## HAEMORRHAGE

Haemorrhage, especially in the form of melaena or occult bleeding from the gastrointestinal tract, is an important cause of anaemia (p. 307). Spontaneous bleeding into the skin and from the mucosae—epistaxis, haemoptysis, haematuria, menorrhagia—is characteristic of certain forms of purpura (*Fig.* 8.2 *and see* p. 314). In haemophilia haemorrhage is usually provoked by minor trauma and consists of haemarthroses and excessive bleeding from small breaches of the skin or mucosae.

## ENLARGED LYMPH NODES

The common haematological diseases which present with lymph node enlargement are described on p. 313.

Enlargement of the lymph nodes (*Fig.* 8.3) is so common that a brief description of the characteristics of the nodes is necessary in differential diagnosis. The following points should be noted:

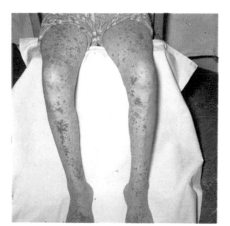

**Fig. 8.2**
Purpura. From a case of leukaemia in its terminal stages.

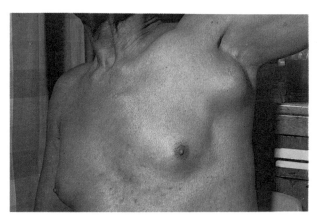

**Fig. 8.3** Enlarged axillary lymph nodes due to lymphoma.

### The group or groups of nodes affected

The student should examine the area which the nodes drain. This is of particular importance when lymph node enlargement is due to local infection or malignant diseases. A more generalized enlargement may be found in infectious mononucleosis (glandular fever), the lymphomas and some blood diseases (p. 312). In some parts of the world syphilis and plague are not uncommon causes of generalized enlargement.

### The consistency

A stony hardness, especially when accompanied by irregularity, suggests carcinoma. Nodes of moderate firmness are found in tuberculosis and other chronic infections and also in the infiltrations of leukaemia and the lymphomas. Sepsis and more rarely tuberculosis may cause abscess formation with characteristic 'fluctuation' on palpation.

### The attachments of the nodes

They tend to remain discrete in the lymphomas and leukaemias. Inflammatory changes often result in adherence of the nodes to the skin and subcutaneous tissues, which can no longer be moved freely over them. Carcinoma has a similar effect but with greater infiltration which anchors the nodes to the deeper structures.

### The presence of tenderness

Tenderness usually accompanies acute inflammatory changes in the nodes, especially those due to coccal infections. In these the superficial lymphatic vessels can frequently be seen as red streaks on the the skin between the inflamed nodes and the original focus of infection (lymphangitis: *see Fig.* 7.86, p. 294).

A palpable lymph node, if soft, is not necessarily abnormal; a few lymph nodes can be felt in most healthy people, especially in the groins and axillae and in the necks of children.

## ENLARGEMENT OF THE SPLEEN AND LIVER

The spleen may attain such huge dimensions that it causes a sense of weight and discomfort in the abdomen, of which the patient complains. More often the enlargement is moderate and only detected upon abdominal examination. Pain due to perisplenitis may also occasionally draw attention to splenic enlargement. It is experienced in the left hypochondrium and over the left lower ribs but is sometimes referred to the left shoulder (*see* Abdominal Pain, p. 75).

If the spleen is grossly enlarged, it may be seen on inspection occupying the left hypochondrium and, in extreme cases, extending across the middle line of the abdomen.

Palpation is the most useful method of determining splenic enlargement (*Fig.* 8.4). The patient should be in a recumbent posture with the head on one pillow and the knees drawn up. Palpation should start well away from the spleen, below and to the right of the umbilicus, and the fingers of the right hand be gradually brought upwards until they encounter the sharp margin of the enlarged organ. At the same time the left hand is placed behind the lowermost ribs which are

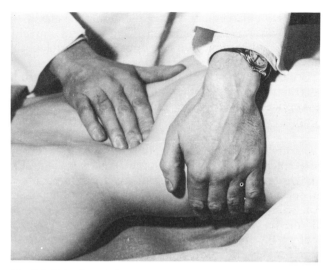

**Fig. 8.4** Palpation of the spleen. The fingers of one hand are pressed gently into the abdomen and the patient is asked to take a deep breath. With the other hand the lowermost ribs are pressed forwards. This helps to bring an enlarged spleen in contact with the examining fingers.

pressed forwards as the patient inspires deeply. A very large spleen can be missed completely if the hand is pressed down on top of it. When the spleen is only slightly enlarged, it may be more easily felt with the patient lying half turned to his right side.

Two of the most distinctive features of an enlarged spleen are that it is sharp-edged and superficial, so that a light touch should be tried before resorting to deeper palpation. The edge should be defined and its medial border followed until the notch can be felt, although this is not always evident. The consistency of the organ should be noted, firmness being the usual characteristic in most haematological diseases. In infections the spleen is frequently soft and sometimes difficult to feel. Small degrees of splenic enlargement may not be detectable, as the organ must be moderately enlarged before it is palpable below the costal margin. When very large it may resemble the kidney in filling the left groin but can generally be distinguished by the sharp edges and the notch, if present. Moreover, it is impossible to get above the spleen on palpation. Rarely, in cases of perisplenitis, a friction rub may be heard.

Percussion may help to outline the borders of the spleen, especially when this is enlarged upwards. Dullness may be found between the ninth and eleventh ribs in the mid-axillary line, and as high as the eighth or seventh rib in cases of great splenic enlargement. Percussion is less satisfactory than palpation in determining enlargement of the spleen except when doubt exists as to the nature of a large tumour in the left hypochondrium which also fills the loin. In these circumstances the percussion note anteriorly is dull with a splenic tumour and resonant with renal enlargement.

The main causes of enlargement of the spleen may be classified as follows:

*Haematological disorders*: Leukaemias, lymphomas, myelofibrosis, poly-cythaemia vera, haemolytic anaemias (except sickle cell anaemia), megaloblastic and iron-deficiency anaemias.

*Vascular*: Portal venous obstruction by cirrhosis of liver or thrombosis; disseminated lupus erythematosus (and other collagen disorders).

*Infections*: Septicaemias (bacterial endocarditis), infectious mononucleosis, brucellosis, enteric infections, miliary tuberculosis, tropical diseases (malaria, kala-azar).

*Infiltrations*: Amyloidosis, sarcoidosis, lipoidoses (e.g. Gaucher's disease).

The degree of splenomegaly can be of some diagnostic value. Extreme enlargement suggests chronic myeloid leukaemia, myelofibrosis, some forms of lymphoma, or, in certain tropical areas, chronic malaria or kala-azar. Conversely in acute infections, acute leukaemias and in the megaloblastic and iron-deficiency anaemias only the tip of the spleen may be felt.

Enlargement of the liver is a common accompaniment of splenomegaly in haematological diseases (*see also* Chapter 4, p.96).

## CHANGES IN THE FUNDUS OCULI

These include retinal haemorrhages in thrombocytopenic purpura, leukaemia and severe anaemia. They may be punctate, splinter and flame-shaped, often with white centres. Flame-shaped haemorrhages around the optic disc are common in severe anaemia from any cause and do not necessarily signify an associated bleeding disorder. After sudden massive haemorrhage, particularly from the gastrointestinal tract, severe changes may occur with gross retinal haemorrhages and exudates, papilloedema and rarely permanent optic atrophy. Vitamin $B_{12}$ deficiency may produce optic atrophy, which has occasionally been observed in the absence of anaemia. Leukaemia can cause retinal exudates and, when there is meningeal involvement, papilloedema also. Venous engorgement may occur in patients with polycythaemia.

## CHANGES IN THE MOUTH

More can be learnt about blood disease by examination of the mouth than of any other part of the body. A smooth depapillated tongue (*see Fig.* 8.9, p. 309) is seen in cases of advanced iron deficiency, while the tongue in anaemia due to vitamin $B_{12}$ or folic acid deficiency tends also to be red and raw. Spontaneous bleeding from the gums is commonly observed in thrombocytopenic purpura and sponginess of the gums associated with pain is characteristic of acute leukaemia; sponginess and hypertrophy also occur in some patients with scurvy (*see Fig.* 8.13, p. 316). It should be remembered, however, that the commonest cause of spongy bleeding gums is chronic infection, i.e. gingivitis. Hypertrophy of the gums (*Fig.* 8.5 and *Fig.* 10.94, p. 454) is sometimes seen in epileptic patients treated with phenytoin sodium (Epanutin) and this drug also can cause folic acid deficiency with megaloblastic anaemia; gum hypertrophy also occurs in myeloid leukaemia (*see Fig.* 8.5) and almost always in the rare acute monocytic leukaemia. Lead poisoning may cause a blue discoloration of the gum margin.

Ulceration of the mouth occurs in a variety of haematological disorders,

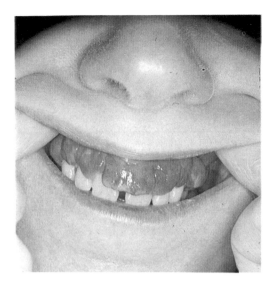

**Fig. 8.5** Hypertrophy of the gums in a child with acute myeloid leukaemia.

especially in acute leukaemia, but also in patients with folic acid or vitamin $B_{12}$ deficiency and agranulocytosis.

Purpura in the mouth is seen in association with thrombocytopenia. The purpuric spots are usually similar to those observed in the skin but sometimes take the form of small blood blisters. Groups of petechiae on the soft palate are not uncommon in acute viral illnesses, particularly glandular fever, even in the absence of thrombocytopenia.

Infection of the mouth and throat, especially moniliasis (or 'thrush'), occurs with leukaemia or aplastic anaemia.

The lymphoid tissue in Waldeyer's ring should be examined in all patients with haematological disorders. It is commonly hypertrophied in patients with lymphosarcoma and chronic lymphatic leukaemia, and in these disorders the tonsils may be so large as to meet in the midline.

### CHANGES IN THE SKIN

The various types of pallor observed in blood disorders have already been noted at the beginning of the chapter. Icterus is commonly found in patients with haemolytic anaemias. Purpura is characterized by haemorrhages into the skin, and the lesions can vary in size from a pin-head ('petechia') to a large bruise ('ecchymosis').

The skin should be carefully examined for areas of infiltration in patients with leukaemia (*Fig.* 8.6) and lymphomas, and for fungal and other infections in those with bone-marrow depression. Ulceration of the skin over the legs may accompany the hereditary haemolytic anaemias.

Polycythaemia vera causes cyanotic suffusion with injection of the superficial blood vessels over the face and upper half of the chest; the extremities tend to be

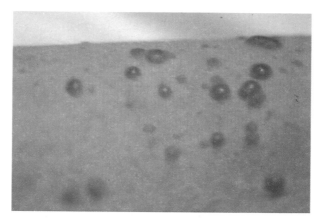

**Fig. 8.6** Chronic myeloid leukaemia: skin infiltration.

warm and red and there are often scratch marks on the skin since pruritus is a common symptom. Pruritus with scratch marks may occur in any of the myeloproliferative disorders and also in Hodgkin's disease. Herpes infections may complicate leukaemia and lymphoma (*see Fig.* 3.22).

A rare connective tissue disorder which may present with abnormal bleeding and bruising is the Ehlers–Danlos syndrome. A characteristic sign of this condition is the abnormal elasticity of the skin (*Fig.* 8.7).

---

## ■ EXAMINATION OF THE BLOOD

Much information can be obtained from examination of the peripheral blood which is readily accessible and should be routinely examined. Venous blood is drawn with minimal stasis into a plastic tube containing the anticoagulant sequestrene.

### Cell counting and electronic counters

Recent years have seen the advent of electronic particle counters so that it is now usual to obtain, accurately and quickly, red cell counts, white cell counts and platelet counts. Hitherto these tests have been performed manually using counting chambers, and the results have been unreliable.

As a result of these technological advances the red cell indices dependent on these have become more valuable. These include the mean cell volume (MCV) and mean cell haemoglobin (MCH).

The most commonly used electronic counter measures red cell count, white cell count, haemoglobin concentration and MCV. With the aid of a small built-in calculator, it then derives the packed cell volume (PCV), mean corpuscular haemoglobin concentration (MCHC) and mean corpuscular haemoglobin (MCH), and prints the results out on a standard card.

**The stained blood film** The films are spread on a glass slide and stained by one of the Romanowsky methods (Leishman, Giemsa). The size, shape and staining

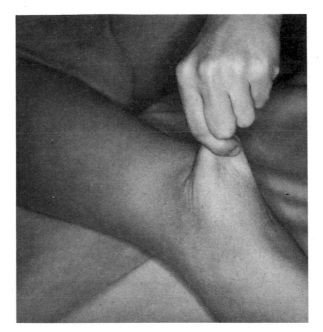

**Fig. 8.7** Abnormal elasticity of the skin in the Ehlers–Danlos syndrome.

characteristics of the cells are observed. Small cells are known as *microcytes* and large cells as *macrocytes*. Microcytosis is produced by iron deficiency, and macrocytosis by an increase in reticulocytes (*see below*), deficiency of vitamin $B_{12}$ and folic acid, excess alcohol intake and cirrhosis of the liver. When there is much variation in size, the phenomenon is known as *anisocytosis*.

Variation in shape is known as *poikilocytosis*, the cells appearing oval, pear-shaped, helmet-shaped or grossly irregular. Poikilocytosis is particularly striking in severe hypochromic and megaloblastic anaemias and in myelofibrosis. The presence of appreciable numbers of cells with spiny projections (burr cells) and red cell fragments (schistocytes) indicates severe damage to the cells and is found frequently in renal failure and sometimes in disseminated carcinomatosis. Spheroidal cells (spherocytes) appear on a stained film as small, round densely staining cells, and they are found in both hereditary spherocytosis and autoimmune haemolytic anaemias.

The pink coloration of the red cells is a criterion of their haemoglobin content. A decrease in haemoglobin is indicated by an exaggeration of their central pallor, and when the anaemia is severe, most of the red cells are colourless discs with a thin pink rim (*hypochromic cells*). Some of these hypochromic corpuscles may have a central stained area (*target cells*). In Britain hypochromic cells are almost always produced by iron deficiency. In many countries, particularly those in the Mediterranean region but also in immigrant areas of Britain, thalassaemia is a common cause.

The recognition of nucleated cells, which are the precursors of mature erythrocytes, is important. These cells are normally only present in the bone-marrow (*see* p. 306). Red cell precursors, which are morphologically normal, are known as *normoblasts*, and those with morphological abnormalities due to deficiency of vitamin $B_{12}$ and folic acid are known as *megaloblasts*. Intermediate in position between mature erythrocytes and these nucleated cells are some large cells without a nucleus. These cells may be stained blue with the methylene blue of Leishman's stain, either uniformly (*polychromasia*) or with a fine blue stippling known as *punctate basophilia*. A *reticulocyte* contains a network or skein of basophilic material, which can only be demonstrated by vital dyes such as brilliant cresyl blue but is seen as a polychromatic cell on the routine smear.

The presence of normoblasts in the peripheral blood may occur after haemorrhage or haemolysis, and may also be produced by various disorders which act as irritants to the bone-marrow (e.g. infiltration of the bone-marrow with leukaemia or metastatic carcinoma). Megaloblasts are sometimes found in the peripheral blood in cases of severe anaemia due to deficiency of vitamin $B_{12}$ and folic acid. Punctate basophilia is a characteristic feature of lead poisoning but occurs in many other types of anaemia. The phenomena of polychromasia and reticulocytosis usually indicate a physiological response by the bone-marrow to some specific stimulus such as haemorrhage, haemolysis or the administration of a specific haematinic (e.g. iron, vitamin $B_{12}$, folic acid) to a subject deficient in this substance.

In certain conditions clumps of red cells form on the blood film. These clumps may appear as agglutinated masses (auto-agglutination) or as intertwining columns (rouleaux). The former occur in severe types of auto-immune haemolytic anaemia, and the latter in diseases in which abnormal globulins are present in the serum, e.g. multiple myeloma.

### The white cells (leucocytes)

**The total leucocyte count** This is carried out by an electronic cell counter (*see* p. 302). The total white cell count is more often of diagnostic value than a red cell count, and fortunately visual counting is less tedious to perform and an error is not so important as in a red cell count. For example, an error of 20 per cent between 8000 and 10 000 cells per $mm^3$ ($8-10 \times 10^9$/l) is not significant.

The normal leucocyte count in adults is from 4000 to 11 000 cells per $mm^3$ ($4-11 \times 10^9$/l). Slight fluctuations in the count occur during the day and also from day to day. In childhood and during pregnancy the count is usually increased by 2000–5000 cells per $mm^3$ ($2-5 \times 10^9$/l), and a more pronounced increase may occur after delivery and with strenuous exercise.

**The stained blood film** The various types of white cell are identified and recorded as a differential count. One hundred white cells are counted and the number of each variety recorded. The cells are of two main types—granular and non-granular.

*Granular cells* These cells, the granulocytes, include the neutrophil, eosinophil and basophil polymorphonuclear leucocytes, which respectively contain fine pink granules, coarse red granules and coarse blue granules. They vary in size from 10 to 15 µm. In severe infections and other toxic conditions vacuoles and basophilic granules are sometimes found in the cytoplasm of the neutrophils. The nuclei of the neutrophil polymorphs normally have two to five lobes, but less than 10 per cent of the nuclei have five lobes. Simplification of the nucleus is known as 'shift to the left', an increase in the number of cells containing multilobed nuclei a 'shift to the right'. An increase in cells with more than four lobes in the nucleus is more probably due to disordered nuclear development than to increased age of the cells and is frequently the result of folic acid and vitamin $B_{12}$ deficiency. A 'shift to the left' occurs in chronic myeloid and acute myeloblastic leukaemia, and in association with the leucocytosis found in various toxic conditions, e.g. burns and pyogenic infections.

*Non-granular cells* These include the large and small lymphocytes (size 7–18 μm) and the monocytes (size 12–20 μm). The small lymphocyte has a darkly staining nucleus with a narrow rim of sky-blue cytoplasm. The large lymphocyte has a broader rim of cytoplasm which often stains less deeply. Usually granules are absent from the cytoplasm, but sometimes several bright red granules are found. Monocytes, often twice the size of a lymphocyte, have a lightly staining reticular and indented nucleus and a variable amount of greyish cytoplasm which is often filled with numerous reddish-blue granules.

The differential count of the white cells is represented by the following average normal figures:

| | |
|---|---|
| Neutrophils | 2·5–7.5 ×10⁹/l |
| Lymphocytes | 1·5–3.5 ×10⁹/l |
| Monocytes | 0·2–0·8 ×10⁹/l |
| Eosinophils | 0·04–0·44×10⁹/l |
| Basophils | 0–0·1 ×10⁹/l |

*Immature white cells* In the examination of a stained blood film the presence of immature white cells, which are normally present only in the bone-marrow, is especially significant, and when these are abundant it generally indicates the presence of a leukaemia. Small numbers of immature white cells (myelocytes and metamyelocytes) may be found in various other disorders, e.g. myelofibrosis, disseminated carcinoma and megaloblastic and post-haemorrhagic anaemias. However, the most primitive form of white cell (blast cell) is usually found only in chronic myeloid (granular) and acute leukaemias.

**Abnormalities of the differential and total white cell counts** An increase in the total number of white cells is termed a *leucocytosis*, and a decrease a *leuco-penia*. Both a leucocytosis and a leucopenia are usually associated with a change in the differential count. For instance, in the leucocytosis which occurs in pneumococcal pneumonia there is an increase in the number of neutrophils, and in the leucopenia which occurs in hypoplastic anaemia there is a decrease in the polymorphonuclear leucocytes (*granulopenia*).

An increase in the number of neutrophils (*neutrophilia*) appears most fre-quently in sepsis (particularly coccal infections) if the body is capable of making a good defensive reaction. The count may rise to between 15 000 and 50 000 per mm³ (15−50×10⁹/l). Neutrophilia of this grade is frequently seen in acute infections such as cellulitis, pneumonia and erysipelas, and where pus has actually been formed, e.g. in empyema, the count attains the higher levels. Neutrophilia may also be found following acute haemorrhage and myocardial infarction and in acute haemolytic anaemias, myelofibrosis, cachectic conditions such as carci-noma, and certain intoxications, e.g. gout, diabetic ketosis, or uraemia. In grave infections leucocytosis is often slight or absent owing to the profound toxaemia, which impairs the function of the bone-marrow. An eosinophilia occurs in parasitic infestations and allergic conditions, e.g. bronchial asthma, in some cases of polyarteritis nodosa, and in Hodgkin's disease. A lymphocytosis occurs in whooping-cough and during the convalescent stage of mumps and rubella. In infectious mononucleosis the blood picture is characterized by a lymphocytosis and monocytosis and by the presence of abnormal mononuclear cells.

The number of neutrophils may be diminished (*neutropenia*) in certain specific diseases, such as typhoid, influenza and measles, and in megaloblastic and hypoplastic anaemias. The syndrome called *agranulocytosis*, in which there is a complete disappearance of granulocytes, is characterized by ulceration of the fauces and often ends fatally. (This usually presents with a sore throat in a patient who is disproportionately ill.) In susceptible persons certain drugs, e.g. sulphonamides and chloramphenicol, among many, may cause agranulocytosis by a direct toxic action on the granulocyte precursors in the bone-marrow. A decrease in the number of both granulocytes and lymphocytes (total leucopenia) occurs only rarely and is found in Felty's syndrome (rheumatoid arthritis, splenomegaly and enlarged lymph nodes) and in disseminated lupus erythrematosus. (*For* Leukaemias, *see* p. 311.)

### The blood platelets (thrombocytes)

The platelets are small spherical, oval or rod-shaped bodies, and on staining they have a light blue cytoplasm packed with azure granules. They are concerned with the production of thrombi and the control of haemorrhage from the capillaries. In health they number 150 000–450 000 per mm$^3$ ($150-450\times10^9$/l). They are increased (*thrombocythaemia*) in polycythaemia vera and sometimes in chronic myeloid leukaemia and after splenectomy or acute haemorrhage. A decrease in the number of platelets is termed *thrombocytopenia*, and the causes of this are discussed on p. 314.

## ■ EXAMINATION OF THE BONE-MARROW

The marrow is obtained by inserting a special needle into the marrow cavity of the upper portion of the sternum, between the second and third ribs, under local anaesthesia. Alternative sites from which marrow may be obtained are the iliac crests, the spinous processes of the vertebrae and the ribs. A small quantity of material (about 0·2 ml) is aspirated into a 10 ml syringe, and stained films are made from it in the same manner as blood films.

In the cytological examination of the bone-marrow particular consideration should be given to the following:

1. The absolute numbers of the myeloid and erythroid series of cells and the ratio between these two groups of cells; this is known as the myeloid : erythroid ratio, and is usually in the region of from 2 : 1 to 6 : 1. These observations will determine whether there is a relative increase in activity of either the myeloid or erythroid series.

2. The morphological appearance of the erythroid series of cells in order to determine whether erythropoiesis is normoblastic or megaloblastic.

3. The morphological appearance of the myeloid series of cells, and in particular whether there is a predominance of primitive 'blast' cells.

4. The presence of cells which are normally either not found in the bone-marrow or are only present in small numbers, such as lymphocytes, myeloma cells or tumour cells. A bone-marrow biopsy rather than an aspirate gives a more reliable guide to marrow infiltration and cellularity.

5. The quantity and morphology of the megakaryocytes, from which the blood platelets are produced.

# ■ THE DIAGNOSIS OF HAEMATOLOGICAL DISEASES

## ANAEMIAS

There are three causes of anaemia: (1) Haemorrhage; (2) Defective erythropoiesis (red cell production); (3) Increased haemolysis (red cell destruction). Of these the commonest is loss of blood.

### Post-haemorrhagic anaemia

The most apparent cause for anaemia is acute haemorrhage, and where it is from obvious sources, e.g. wounds, haematemesis, haemoptysis or epistaxis, it should not escape notice. The loss of blood by profuse haemorrhage causes symptoms of shock, referable to the sudden decrease in blood volume (collapse, low blood pressure, tachycardia, thirst, etc.). These symptoms do not occur when the loss of blood is gradual and should not be confused with those of severe anaemia.

The possibility of concealed haemorrhage must not be overlooked as a cause of rapidly produced anaemia, and when symptoms of haemorrhage occur without obvious cause, such contingencies as melaena, haemorrhage into serous spaces or ruptured ectopic gestation should be considered. The blood picture in acute post-haemorrhagic anaemias shows an equal reduction in red cells and haemoglobin. The red cells are usually normochromic, and there are numerous polychromatic cells which are macrocytic.

### Dyshaemopoietic anaemias (Anaemias due to defective red cell production)

**Iron deficiency** This could have been considered in the previous section on post-haemorrhagic anaemias, as chonic blood loss is the most important cause. However, poor diet, impaired iron absorption and increased iron requirements (childhood, adolescence, pregnancy) are often important contributory factors and may be the chief causes of iron deficiency in the developing countries.

The blood picture is characterized by the low haemoglobin content of the red cells producing hypochromia and microcytosis. The MCH and MCV are reduced.

Iron-deficiency anaemia is most frequently found in women between 20 and 45 years, when the iron requirements are increased by menstrual haemorrhage and repeated pregnancies. When iron deficiency occurs in men, or in women who have passed the menopause, a particularly careful search should be made for sources of occult bleeding, especially from the gastrointestinal tract, e.g. peptic ulcer, hiatus hernia, gastric bleeding induced by aspirin and malignant disease of the stomach or large bowel.

The predominant symptoms are those of oxygen deficiency (p. 296), but stomatitis and glossitis are common. Dysphagia (Plummer–Vinson syndrome) occurs rarely and the spleen may be palpable. Inflammatory and atrophic changes in the gastric mucosa, leading to impaired secretion of hydrochloric acid in the gastric juice, are frequently present. The nails may be spoon-shaped (koilonychia) (*Fig.* 8.8), although this sign is comparatively rare. (*See* Chapter 3, p. 59.)

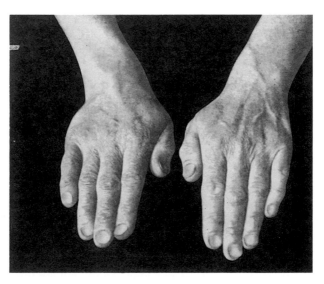

**Fig. 8.8** Koilonychia, From a case of iron-deficiency anaemia. The nails show a spoon-shaped or salt-cellar defect.

**Vitamin B$_{12}$ deficiency** Dietary deficiency of vitamin B$_{12}$ commonly occurs in many developing countries. In this country vitamin B$_{12}$ deficiency is usually caused by impaired absorption, and dietary deficiency only occurs in those people who do not eat any food of animal origin (vegans). The conditions which cause impaired absorption of vitamin B$_{12}$ are:

*a.* Deficiency of gastric intrinsic factor, which occurs in pernicious anaemia and following total gastrectomy and occasionally partial gastrectomy.

*b.* Diseases of the ileum (e.g. Crohn's disease) which is the site of vitamin B$_{12}$ absorption.

*c.* The abnormal growth of bacteria in the small intestine, which assimilate vitamin B$_{12}$ for their own metabolism. This may occur when there are strictures, fistulas and blind loops of bowel.

*d.* Infestation with the fish tape-worm, *Diphyllobothrium latum*. This is confined to Scandinavia.

Vitamin B$_{12}$ deficiency produces a macrocytic anaemia, and, when the anaemia is severe, marked anisocytosis and poikilocytosis. There is usually a decrease in the number of neutrophils and platelets in the blood. The bone-marrow picture is megaloblastic. It is advisable to confirm the presence of vitamin $B_{12}$ deficiency by assaying the level of the vitamin in the serum before committing the patient to life-long treatment. This is usually done by a radio-assay method.

*Pernicious Anaemia* is the most common of the diseases classified above. The disease is rare before the age of 40. Predominant symptoms, in addition to those of Hb deficiency, include sore tongue (*Fig.* 8.9) and loss of appetite and weight. Symptoms due to degenerative changes in the spinal cord and peripheral nerves are now rare (*see* p. 430). Mental symptoms are not uncommon. The tongue is often smooth and red (glossitis), and the spleen may be palpable. Haemolysis results from the defective erythropoiesis and, when severe, gives rise to the characteristic lemon-yellow pallor. Petechiae may also occur. After giving histamine or pentagastrin, there is virtually always an absence of secretion of acid in the gastric juice.

Confirmation of the diagnosis of pernicious anaemia is obtained by demonstrating:

   *a.* A macrocytic anaemia with megaloblastic marrow.

   *b.* A low serum vitamin $B_{12}$ level.

   *c.* Impaired absorption of vitamin $B_{12}$, corrected by intrinsic factor, measured by radioactive isotope techniques.

   *d.* Autoantibody estimation; anti-intrinsic factor and parietal cell.

   *e.* Good response to vitamin $B_{12}$ therapy.

**Folic acid deficiency** The causes of folic acid deficiency are:

   *a. Dietary deficiency*: This is widespread in many of the developing countries. In Western countries it occurs more commonly than was hitherto supposed in persons with impaired appetite, due in particular to psychiatric and gastric disorders.

   *b. Impaired absorption from the jejunum*: Extensive involvement of the jejunal

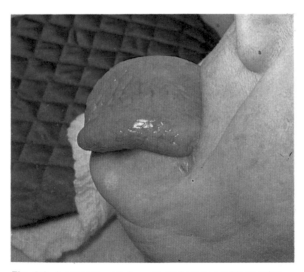

**Fig. 8.9** A smooth, red depapillated tongue with angular cheilosis. These changes may be caused by deficiency of iron, folic acid or vitamin $B_{12}$.

mucosa is required before folic acid absorption is affected, and this occurs in idiopathic steatorrhoea (coeliac disease) and in tropical sprue.

*c. Increased requirements*: Megaloblastic anaemia due to increased folic acid requirements occurs frequently in pregnancy, unless prophylactic folic acid is given, and occasionally in certain other conditions: haemolytic anaemia, repeated haemorrhage, extensive dermatitis and widespread neoplastic disease, e.g. multiple myeloma, myelofibrosis and carcinomatosis.

*d. Impaired utilization*: Certain drugs, notably phenytoin sodium (Epanutin), can antagonize the action of folic acid and thus cause megaloblastic anaemia.

The blood and bone-marrow pictures are indistinguishable from those due to vitamin $B_{12}$ deficiency. Glossitis and icterus may be present, but neurological signs are most unusual. Free acid is frequently present in the gastric juice.

Folic acid deficiency is virtually always the main cause of megaloblastic anaemia of pregnancy. Otherwise it may be necessary to assay the serum levels of vitamin $B_{12}$ and folic acid and to investigate the absorptive function of the gastrointestinal tract in order to distinguish anaemias arising from vitamin $B_{12}$ and folic acid deficiency.

**Other diseases** Other diseases in which red cell production is impaired are:

Lymphomas, *see* p. 313.
Diseases infiltrating the bone-marrow:
  *a.* Leukaemias, *see* p. 311.
  *b.* Myelofibrosis, *see* p. 312.
  *c.* Multiple myeloma (infiltration of bone-marrow; Bence Jones protein in urine; 'M' band in serum globulin on electrophoresis)
Infections, generally subacute or chronic lasting more than a month, e.g. subacute bacterial endocarditis, chronic pyelonephritis
Renal and hepatic failure
Carcinomatosis
Hypoplastic anaemias due to toxic agents, e.g. irradiation, benzine derivatives, cytotoxic drugs, and in sensitive persons chloramphenicol, antithyroid drugs and other therapeutic agents
Endocrine disorders (hypofunction of the thyroid or adrenal cortex may produce a mild anaemia)
Collagen diseases

**Haemolytic anaemias** (Anaemias due to excessive red cell destruction)

These can be classified into two main groups: hereditary and acquired.

**Hereditary** In this group there is an abnormality of the red cells. The main examples are hereditary spherocytosis, thalassaemia (Cooley's anaemia), the haemoglobinopathies, e.g. sickle cell disease, and red cell enzyme deficiencies, e.g. drug-induced haemolysis and favism due to deficiency of glucose-6-phosphate dehydrogenase. The haemoglobinopathies occur mainly in the Negro race. Thalassaemia and glucose-6-phosphate dehydrogenase deficiency have a wide racial distribution in tropical, subtropical and Mediterranean countries, but occur very rarely in Northern Europeans.

**Acquired** In this group the fundamental abnormality is outside the red cells. The main examples are acquired auto-immune haemolytic anaemia and erythroblastosis foetalis, in which there is a specific red cell antibody. Red cell destruction may also be produced by bacterial, metabolic, or chemical toxins and by protozoal parasites, e.g. septicaemia, uraemia, lead poisoning and malaria.

**Clinical description** Haemolytic anaemia may be fulminating and acute or insidious and chronic, and the latter may be punctuated by episodes of more acute haemolysis. By and large the manifestations tend to be more severe in acquired auto-immune haemolytic anaemia than in hereditary spherocytosis, in which the mild cases have been described as 'more yellow than sick'.

During the acute episodes the symptoms often suggest an acute febrile illness with sudden weakness, headache, shivering, vomiting and aching pain in the limbs, back and abdomen. The abdominal pain may occasionally be so severe and be accompanied by such marked muscular rigidity as to simulate an acute surgical condition. Anuria or oliguria may develop, and the urine may be very dark.

Pallor and jaundice of varying degree are found, more pronounced during the phases of acute haemolysis. Jaundice, however, is usually only slight unless the bile duct is obstructed by pigment gallstones. Splenomegaly, except in sickle cell anaemia, is common in acute and chronic haemolytic anaemias. The organ may be just palpable or it may be huge. Moderate enlargement of the liver may also occur. Chronic leg ulcers are common in sickle cell anaemia and may occur in hereditary spherocytosis.

Deformity of the skull with overgrowth of the maxillae occurs in certain congenital haemolytic anaemias. Patients with sickle cell anaemia tend to be tall and thin with long legs and often suffer from oesteoarthrosis of the hip joints.

Haemolytic anaemia is usually associated with an increase in the number of reticulocytes in the peripheral blood and a slight to moderate rise in the levels of serum bilirubin and urine urobilinogen. However, these abnormalities are not only related to the degree of haemolysis but also to the capacity of the bone-marrow response and to liver function. Bile is only found in the urine when the patient develops obstructive jaundice due to the formation of pigment gallstones. When the haemolysis is severe, methaemalbumin can be detected in the plasma by Schumm's test (the spectroscopic detection of a haemochromogen band at 558 µm after the addition of concentrated ammonium sulphide to the serum or plasma), and haemoglobin and haemosiderin may occasionally be present in the urine.

The osmotic fragility of the red cells is always increased in hereditary spherocytosis. It is usually increased in acquired auto-immune haemolytic anaemia depending on the number of the spherocytes present, and it is decreased in thalassaemia. Acquired auto-immune haemolytic anaemia is diagnosed by the detection of an incomplete antibody coating the patient's red cells (direct Coombs test), and quite frequently the incomplete antibody can also be detected in the serum (indirect Coombs test). Occasionally when the evidence for increased haemolysis is equivocal or when splenectomy is being considered in auto-immune haemolytic anaemia, it is of value to determine the red cell survival and the principal sites of red cell destruction by methods using cells tagged with the radioactive isotope [51]Cr. For the laboratory diagnosis of the haemoglobinopathies, thalassaemia and red cell enzyme deficiencies the reader should consult a textbook of haematology.

## LEUKAEMIAS

This is a group of conditions characterized by widespread proliferation of the leucocytes and their precursors in the tissues of the body. They are classified into acute and chronic forms, the distinction resting on the rapidity of the disease and on the stage of maturity of the predominant cells. Both the acute and chronic forms are further subdivided according to the dominant type of cell.

### Acute myeloblastic leukaemia

This occurs particularly in adults and there is a slight predominance among males. The onset is sudden and the course short. Anaemia, fever and prostration rapidly develop. Often there are extensive haemorrhagic manifestations—petechiae, epistaxis, uterine bleeding—and necrotic lesions develop in the mouth and throat. There is usually slight or moderate splenomegaly. Enlargement of the lymph nodes is unusual except in the monocytic form when the cervical nodes may be considerably enlarged. There may be exquisite tenderness over the bones, the sternum and the tibiae especially. Moderate or severe anaemia is usually found, and the number of platelets is often below 100 000 per mm$^3$ ($100 \times 10^9$/l). The total white cell count may be decreased or normal but is usually increased. Myeloblasts may form more than 60 per cent of the circulating white cells. In some cases they are completely absent with a granulopenia, but the bone-marrow is packed with them (*aleukaemic leukaemia*).

### Acute lymphoblastic leukaemia

This variety occurs most frequently in childhood. The symptoms and signs are similar to those of the myeloblastic form but enlargement of the spleen and lymph nodes tends to be more pronounced. The blood and bone-marrow pictures can usually be distinguished from myeloblastic leukaemia by ordinary staining methods but special cytochemical stains and membrane marker studies are available to help.

### Chronic myeloid leukaemia

This disease is rare before the age of 25 and most common between 30 and 65. The sex incidence is equal. The onset is insidious and early diagnosis is often accidental during the routine examination of a blood film. The symptoms may be classified into those resulting from anaemia, those caused by the gross enlargement of the spleen (abdominal discomfort or a visible mass) and those attributable to the increased metabolic rate (loss of weight, cachexia and excessive sweating). Dominant physical signs are the great enlargement of the spleen and to a lesser extent of the liver, and, later, anaemia. A well-marked leucocytosis is the rule with counts ranging from 100 000 to 750 000 per mm$^3$ (100 to $750 \times 10^9$/l). The increase is due to cells of the granulocyte series with neutrophils, metamyelocytes and myelocytes. There is only a small number of myeloblasts. The Philadelphia chromosome and a low leucocyte alkaline phosphatase score are usually present.

### Myelofibrosis

This condition clinically may resemble chronic myeloid leukaemia as there is splenomegaly, leucocytosis and the presence of immature cells of the granular series. Myelofibrosis may be distinguished from myeloid leukaemia by the finding of marrow fibrosis in the former condition and by the presence in the latter of the Philadelphia chromosome (Ph₁) and decreased leucocyte alkaline phosphatase activity.

### Chronic lymphatic leukaemia

In contrast to chronic myeloid leukamia, this occurs mainly in elderly men. Enlargement of the lymph nodes is a salient feature, while splenomegaly is less marked than in myeloid leukamia, and the total leucocyte count tends to be lower, the majority of the cells being mature lymphocytes.

### LYMPHOMAS

This term is used to classify a group of neoplastic diseases that are characterized clinically by enlargement of the lymph nodes and spleen. The principal members of this group are Hodgkin's disease and the non-Hodgkin's lymphomas. In most cases it is impossible to distinguish these disorders from one another, either clinically or from examination of the blood and bone-marrow, and lymph node biopsy is necessary to confirm the diagnosis.

**Hodgkin's disease** This condition may occur at any age but is observed chiefly between the age of 20 and 40 years. Males are affected more often than females. The course of the disease may be variable but the prognosis has improved dramatically with modern treatment. Enlargement of the superficial groups of lymph nodes is usually the presenting symptom, and constitutional symptoms (lassitude, fever, loss of weight), if present, are signs of poor prognosis. The enlarged lymph nodes are usually painless. They remain discrete, have an elastic character on palpation, and do not become adherent to the skin. The fever sometimes exhibits the Pel–Ebstein phenomenon. Palpable enlargement of the spleen and liver and involvement of abdominal and thoracic lymph nodes indicate a later state of the disease.

Anaemia is common and is rarely associated with haemolysis. There may be either a neutrophilia, an eosinophilia or a lymphopenia. The histological appearance of the lymph nodes is characterized by the wide variety of proliferating cells; these include neutrophils, eosinophils, lymphocytes, plasma cells and multi-nucleated giant cells (Reed Sternberg cells).

**Other forms of lymphoma** These non-Hodgkin's lymphomas can be divided into a poor prognosis group with diffuse node involvement (*Fig.* 8.10) and a follicular type in which the course is more benign. The age incidence of these diseases tends to be higher than in Hodgkin's disease and the disease is more often clinically disseminated at diagnosis.

### HAEMORRHAGIC DISEASES

After injury to a vessel, the process of normal haemostasis takes place in three phases: (1) Vessel wall contraction; (2) Platelet aggregation and plugging of the injured area; (3) The formation of an insoluble fibrin clot from soluble fibrinogen due to the activation of the intrinsic and extrinsic blood clotting system; this third step takes a few minutes to get under way. There is, in addition, a fibrinolytic system which actively removes the clot. Thus the haemorrhagic diseases can result from abnormalities of blood vessels, platelets or the intrinsic or extrinsic clotting systems. Diseases affecting the smaller blood vessels or platelets produce the clinical picture of purpura. Disorders of the clotting systems

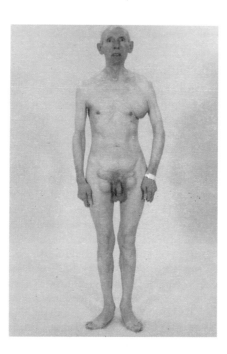

**Fig. 8.10**
Lymphoma: enlargement of axillary and inguinal lymph nodes.

may be congenital (e.g. haemophilia) or acquired (deficiency of prothrombin or fibrinogen).

### Purpura

This is characterized by extravasation of blood into the skin, causing purple spots varying in size from a pinhead (petechiae) to large bruises (ecchymoses). Sometimes haemorrhage also occurs from the mucosae, for example, in the nose, gastrointestinal tract and uterus. Purpura is due to increased capillary permeability and this may result from a deficiency in the number (*thrombocytopenia*) or function (*thrombasthenia*) of platelets, or from damage to the capillary walls by antibodies (*allergic purpura*), vitamin C deficiency (*Fig.* 8.11), drugs and bacterial and metabolic toxins, e.g. bacterial endocarditis and uraemia.

In elderly persons purpura frequently occurs on the back of the forearms and hands. This is called *senile purpura* and results from rupture of small vessels due to increased mobility of the inelastic skin. Similar lesions are caused by prolonged corticosteroid therapy (*Fig.* 8.12).

Thrombocytopenic purpura may be primary (*idiopathic thrombocytopenic purpura*) due to the development of platelet antibodies, or secondary due to suppression of the bone-marrow as in hypoplastic anaemia, pernicious anaemia, acute and chronic leukaemias (*see Fig.* 8.2, p. 297), secondary carcinoma and certain forms of drug therapy. The spleen is rarely enlarged in idiopathic thrombocytopenic purpura, and then it is only just palpable.

One type of allergic purpura is referred to as the Henoch–Schönlein syndrome and is characterized by haemorrhage from the gastrointestinal tract and kidneys,

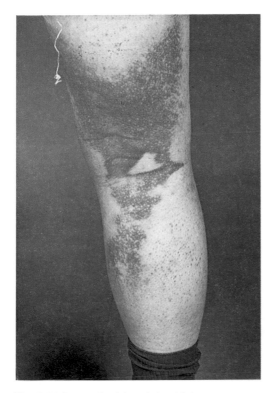

**Fig. 8.11** Scurvy: bruising of the thigh.

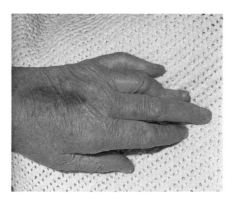

**Fig. 8.12**
Purpura on the back of the hand of a patient receiving corticosteroid therapy for rheumatoid arthritis. Note the deformities of the interphalangeal joints.

serous effusions into the joints and purpuric and urticarial skin rashes. It is frequently related to infection with the haemolytic streptococcus.

The closure of capillaries which occurs after injury depends on normal platelet numbers and function, and therefore the bleeding time is prolonged in cases of thrombocytopenic purpura. In other types of purpura the bleeding time may be prolonged, but sometimes it is normal. The measurement of bleeding time has been made more accurate by modifying the Ivy technique by the use of a template device which allows a standardized incision to be made on the skin of the forearm. The bleeding time using a template is normally between 2½ and 8 minutes.

### Scurvy

Scurvy, both in adult and infantile forms, is due to a deficiency of vitamin C in the diet. There may be extensive ecchymoses on the legs (*Fig.* 8.11), and petechiae occur characteristically around the hair follicles. Haemorrhages from any mucous membrane may take place but are most commonly seen in the mouth (*Fig.* 8.13), where the spongy bleeding gums (if the patient has teeth) are always a suggestive feature in a patient who has been undernourished or incorrectly fed.

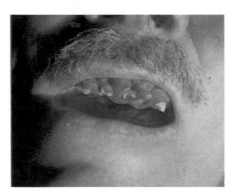

**Fig. 8.13**
Scurvy showing the condition of the gums.

### Congenital clotting disorders (haemophilia)

This is a sex-linked hereditary deficiency of clotting factor (Factor VIII) which is transmitted by females and occurs predominantly in males. A male haemophiliac transmits the carrier state to all his daughters, and they in turn transmit the haemophilic state to 50 per cent of their sons. A careful family history must therefore be taken in bleeding disorders.

The diagnosis of haemophilia should be considered when profuse haemorrhage occurs from such minor causes as cuts and tooth extraction, and when there are episodes of spontaneous haemorrhage into the muscles and joints, peritoneal cavity and the renal and gastrointestinal tracts. Recurrent haemarthroses may lead to ankylosis of the affected joints, especially the knees, with disuse atrophy of adjacent muscles. The initial bleeding time is normal as this depends on capillary contractility and not on the coagulability of the blood. There is a tendency, however, for the bleeding to recommence after an interval of several minutes. The clotting time of the blood is prolonged, but to confirm the diagnosis it is necessary to demonstrate a low or absent anti-haemophiliac globulin.

### Acquired clotting disorders

Haemorrhage due to *vitamin K dependent coagulation factor deficiency* may occur in severe liver disease (*see* Chapter 4) or as a result of anticoagulant therapy.

*Hypofibrinogenaemia* can also result from destruction of the liver but is more commonly produced by release from the tissues into the circulation of thromboplastin, which consumes fibrinogen by bringing about intravascular clotting and secondary activation fibrinolysis. The condition usually occurs as a result of (1) obstetrical complications—abruptio placentae and intra-uterine retention of a dead fetus—; (2) extensive physical trauma; (3) pulmonary surgery. It is termed 'disseminated intravascular coagulation'.

The clinical picture may present with the sudden appearance of severe bleeding from mucous membranes and extensive ecchymoses, or in some cases the bleeding may be only slight. The clotting time of the blood is greatly prolonged. The failure of the blood to clot rapidly after the addition of thrombin distinguishes hypofibrinogenaemia from other disorders of coagulation.

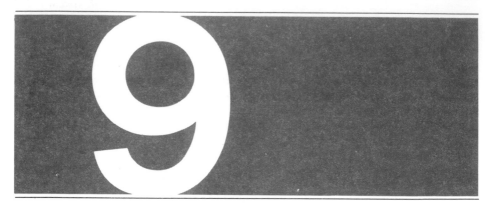

## The skeletal system

The skeletal system provides not only the strength to support the body and to protect vital organs, but also the flexibility to permit a wide range of movement at the joints of the axial skeleton and the limbs. The following description of the symptoms and signs arising in the skeleton especially refers to those generalized disorders affecting bones and joints. The student must be aware, however, of the orthopaedic and traumatic lesions of this system.

### ■ SYMPTOMS

The chief symptoms arising in the skeletal system are pain, deformity, impaired movement and cracking and creaking.

#### Pain

Pain may originate from bone and periosteum, the capsule and synovia of joints, the ligaments, tendons and muscles. Bone pain is usually continuous, aching and disturbs sleep whilst that arising in the joints and their adnexae is more often sharp, related to posture or to movement and accompanied by a feeling of stiffness. Pain in the limb joints is usually well localized with the exception of the hip, when discomfort may be referred to the adjacent knee. In the vertebral column, however, degenerative osteoarthrosis in the cervical or lumbar spine often produces referred as well as local pain. The former is produced by pressure on nerve roots and may indicate the segmental level of the lesion giving rise to brachial neuritis and sciatica (*see* p. 420). Sneezing, coughing and straining at stool may aggravate the discomfort by raising the intraspinal pressure.

#### Deformity

The patient or relatives may notice painless alteration in the appearance of the skull and face (Paget's disease, *Fig.* 9.1, or acromegaly), hands (Heberden's nodes), legs (Paget's disease or rickets), joints (Charcot's neuropathy), or the gradual loss of height and spinal curvature in osteoporosis of the vertebrae.

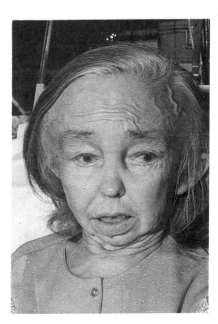

**Fig. 9.1**
Paget's disease: enlargement of the head.

### Impaired movement

When movement is limited by pain and stiffness the skeletal system is usually at fault but diminished movement without these symptoms suggests a neurological lesion. In rheumatoid arthritis stiffness is noted especially on first awakening in the morning and symptoms may improve as the day progresses. However, in osteoarthritis, movement is restricted after using the joints at the end of the day or on first using the joints after a period of immobility.

### Cracking and creaking

Minor clicks in the finger joints produced by passive hyperextension are of no significance nor are clicks arising in the shoulder joint or scapula, sometimes heard during auscultation of the chest. Snowball crunching in the knee during active or passive movement is heard when the articular cartilage is badly damaged as a result of osteoarthritis.

### Constitutional symptoms

Fever and sweating with joint involvement accompany septic arthritis and rheumatic fever, and the latter may be associated with a skin eruption – erythema marginatum. Rashes can be diagnostic in psoriatic arthropathy, Reiter's disease and systemic lupus erythematosus. Breathlessness and pleuritic chest pain may precede or accompany the arthritis in rheumatoid disease and other connective tissue disorders. Eye symptoms such as conjunctivitis in Reiter's disease, dry eyes in Sjögren's syndrome, or a painful iritis in ankylosing spondylitis may give useful clues. Blue sclerae may be noted in children with multiple fractures due to osteogenesis imperfecta (*Fig.* 9.2). Raynaud's phenomenon (*Fig.* 9.3) may herald rheumatoid arthritis, systemic sclerosis or systemic lupus erythem-

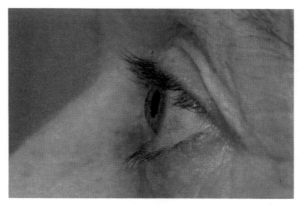

**Fig. 9.2** Blue sclerae in osteogenesis imperfecta.

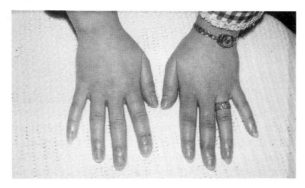

**Fig. 9.3** Cyanosis of the fingers—Raynaud's phenomenon, *see Fig.* 9.4.

atosus (*Fig.* 9.4) and genital symptoms such as urethritis in Reiter's disease or penile and vaginal ulceration in Behçet's syndrome should merit specific inquiry. Alteration in bowel habit may accompany ankylosing spondylitis, Reiter's disease or systemic sclerosis and bulky stools indicating malabsorption may be associated with osteomalacia. Painful recurrent mouth ulcers suggest Behçet's syndrome and in Paget's disease blindness and deafness may be disabling complications.

## ■    SIGNS

Physical examination should first consist of a general inspection of the patient with special attention to stance, gait, posture, height, skeletal proportion and the performance of simple tasks such as dressing, bending or rising from a chair.

The observer should note the appearance of the face and then examine the

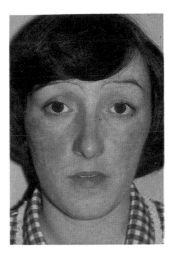

**Fig. 9.4**
Butterfly rash in systemic
lupus erythematosus. Same
patient as *Fig.* 9.3.

skull, jaw, rib cage, spinal column and pelvis, and each limb in turn, comparing one side with the other and noting any abnormality in structure or function of the joints and adjacent tissues: the bones, cartilage, synoviae, bursae, ligaments, tendons, fascia, muscles, subcutaneous tissue and overlying skin.

### Inspection

Inspection will reveal any gross deformity, displacement or enlargement of bone such as occurs in tumours (primary or secondary), Paget's disease (*Fig.* 9.1) and osteomalacia.

On inspection of the joints, the examiner will look for swelling, discoloration and deformities, including ulnar deviation of the fingers, spinal scoliosis (*Fig.* 9.5), flexion of the knee and clawing of the toes. He will then observe the range of active movement and the patient's ability to use the joints for everyday purposes such as gripping, putting on shoes, eating and combing the hair. Nodular lesions, swelling of tendon sheaths and muscle wasting around the joint (*see Fig.* 9.15) are also noted, remembering that muscle wasting can give a false impression of joint enlargement. Particular attention is paid to the distribution of joint changes throughout the body since this may be of prime importance in the differential diagnosis of arthritis (*Table* 9.1).

### Palpation

Palpation must be gentle and sudden sharp movements avoided. The patient's face should be watched for signs of distress when the joints are moved or tender parts are explored. Palpation is used to detect a raised temperature over a bone or joint. For this purpose the back of the fingers may be more sensitive than the palmar surface. An increased temperature indicates a high blood flow (e.g. Paget's disease) or inflammation (e.g. septic arthritis, rheumatoid arthritis or rheumatic fever). Palpation is also used to elicit tenderness over bones or ligaments; to determine the anatomical origin and consistency of any swellings (fluid, synovial, bony, cartilaginous, tendinous, sub-cutaneous); to measure the

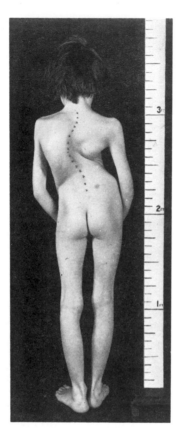

**Fig. 9.5**
Thoracic scoliosis: idiopathic
or adolescent type.

| Table 9.1 | **Arthritis: distribution of joint changes** |
|---|---|
| *Disease* | *Joints most commonly affected* |
| Rheumatic fever | Large ('flitting') |
| Rheumatoid arthritis | Small peripheral (MP and proximal IP) |
| Ankylosing spondylitis | Central (sacro-iliac, spine, hip) |
| Infective arthritis | Large (usually one only) |
| Osteo-arthritis | Weight bearing. Terminal IP (Heberden's nodes) |
| Gout | Small peripheral (1st metatarsophalangeal especially) |

MP, Metacarpophalangeal/metatarsophalangeal; IP, interphalangeal.

range and power of movement at each joint and, at the same time, to note crepitus or abnormal mobility. Examples of unusual mobility are observed in Charcot's knee joints and the Ehlers–Danlos syndrome in which lax ligaments permit hyperextensibility (*Fig.* 9.6). Fluid accumulations within the joint or adjacent bursae can be recognized by the presence of fluctuation. This is most easily detected in a knee joint, when a brisk depression of the patella causes displacement of the fluid and a slight knock of the patella against the underlying bone (patella tap).

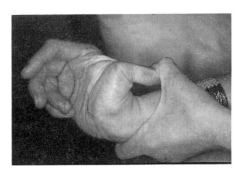

**Fig. 9.6**
Hyperextensibility of the right thumb joint in Ehlers–Danlos syndrome.

### Movement

To assess the range and power of a joint is an important part of the clinical examination. Active movements test the function not only of the joint under consideration but also the tendons, muscles and nerves, whereas passive movements test the state of the joint itself and are therefore more useful. When movement is limited by pain or fixation an attempt should be made to determine the cause. If the bone, cartilage or synovial membrane is diseased, movement is limited in all directions and tenderness is generalized. If the capsule or ligament is damaged, movement towards the affected structure relieves the pain. Tenderness will be detected locally and an effusion may be present. If an intra-articular structure is present, such as a detached semilunar cartilage in the knee, movement is restricted by pain when the joint is compressed towards the detached fragment and relieved by movement away from it.

Complete lack of joint movement because of pain is due to recent trauma or acute inflammation, but if painless, is due to ankylosis or arthrodesis.

The direction and degree of passive movements to be found in the joints of a healthy subject are shown in *Table* 9.2 and these should be recorded in all patients presenting with an arthropathy. Joint movement is measured by the goniometer, a protractor with long hinged arms, preferably transparent (*Fig.* 9.7). Movement is recorded by the neutral zero method whereby all joints are considered to be neutral when the subject is standing upright to attention with the hands flat against the thighs.

A rough measure of temporomandibular movement is given by the distance between the incisor teeth when the mouth is fully opened. Shoulder movements may be scapulo-thoracic in origin; mobility of the gleno-humeral joint itself can only be measured after fixation of the scapula. For examination of forearm pronation and supination, the arm is adducted at the shoulder and the elbow held in

| Table 9.2 | Joint movements: system of examination |
| --- | --- |
| *Joint* | *Movements* |
| Jaw | Open and shut<br>Protrusion and retraction<br>Side to side |
| Spine (cervical and thoracolumbar) | Flexion and extension<br>Lateral flexion (R & L)<br>Rotation (R & L) |
| Shoulder | Flexion (180) and extension (60)<br>Abduction (180) and adduction (45)<br>Internal (80) and external (60) rotation |
| Elbow | Flexion (150) |
| Wrist (and forearm) | Flexion and extension (70)<br>Ulnar (30) and radial (20) deviation<br>Pronation (80) and supination (80) |
| Fingers: MP joints<br>IP joints | Flexion (90) and extension (45)<br>Flexion (90) |
| Hip | Flexion (120) and extension (30)<br>Abduction (45) and adduction (30)<br>Internal (80) and external (60) rotation |
| Knee | Flexion (135) |
| Ankle and foot | Plantar (50) and dorsal (20) flexion<br>Eversion (5) and inversion (5) |
| Toes: MP joints<br>IP joints | Flexion (40) and extension (40)<br>Eversion (15) and inversion (5)<br>Flexion (90) |

The figures in parentheses indicate range of movement in degrees.
MP, metacarpophalangeal/metatarsophalangeal; IP, interphalangeal.

the flexed position. An index of the range of lumbar spine flexion can be obtained by making a mark at the lumbosacral junction and a second mark 10 cm higher with the spine extended. On full flexion of the spine, the distance between these two points should increase by 4–6 cm in the healthy adult (*Fig.* 9.8). The sacro-iliac joints are virtually immobile but can be examined by local palpation and by lateral compression or 'springing' of the pelvis. These manoeuvres may induce pain or discomfort, a useful early sign of ankylosing spondylitis. Examination of the knee joint should include an assessment of the stability of the joint with particular reference to any undue 'play' in the lateral or anteroposterior plane. The range of knee joint movement is illustrated in *Fig.* 9.9.

Active movements are used to measure the power of joint action which may be impaired not only if the bones or joints are deformed but if tendons are disrupted or muscles wasted, as in rheumatoid arthritis. Power should be recorded

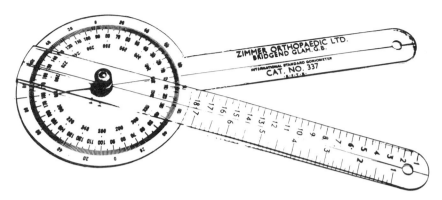

**Fig. 9.7** The goniometer.

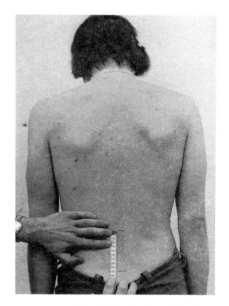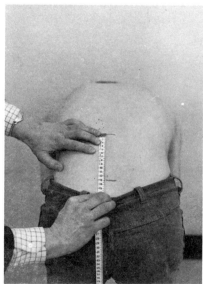

**Fig. 9.8** Evaluation of lumbar spine mobility. With the patient standing upright 10 cm is measured upwards from the lumbo-sacral junction. The patient is then asked to bend forwards and the 10 cm should extend to 15 cm in an individual of average build. This affords a reproducible and readily repeated test of the lumbar spine mobility.

on a simple scale, such as one recommended by the British Medical Research Council:

0 No movement
1 Flicker of movement
2 Movement with gravity eliminated
3 Movement possible against gravity
4 Movement possible against gravity and resistance
5 Normal power

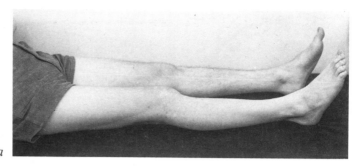

*a*

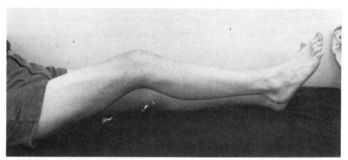

*b*

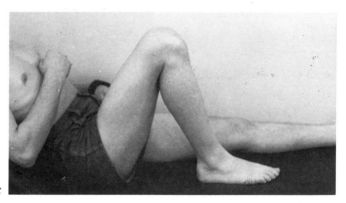

*c*

**Fig. 9.9** Examination of the knee. This is conventionally recorded as three figures, e.g. 0—30—130. *a*, 0 in this instance shows that, when extended, the knee is straight. *b*, 30 indicates a 30° extension lag on straight-leg raising and reflects impairment of quadriceps function. *c*, 130 demonstrates that flexion is possible to 130°.

■　　　ILLUSTRATIVE DISEASES

### DISEASES OF BONE

#### Osteomalacia

Osteomalacia or softening of the bones, results most commonly from deficiency of vitamin D, a vitamin concerned with the absorption and metabolism of calcium and phosphate and with the normal mineralization of osteoid tissue. The plasma levels of calcium and phosphate are usually reduced and the alkaline phosphatase raised. At one time, the commonest form of osteomalacia was rickets, a condition due to deficient dietary intake of vitamin D from the small intestine (see Malabsorption Syndrome, p. 112). The chief manifestation of osteomalacia is bone pain, which is usually generalized and persistent but may become acute and localized when 'pseudo-fractures' (*Fig.* 9.10) occur. Muscle weakness, skeletal deformities and tetany due to hypocalcaemia are features of severe cases. Other signs of malabsorption may also be found (*see* p. 113). The clinical features of childhood rickets are similar to those of adult osteomalacia with the addition of tender swellings at the ends of long bones due to increased epiphyseal activity (*Fig.* 9.11) and characteristic deformities of the skull, chest and legs.

#### Osteoporosis

Osteoporosis is a condition in which there is a decrease of bone mass due to loss of the glycoprotein matrix. Plasma levels of calcium, phosphate and alkaline phosphatase are usually normal. Osteoporosis occurs most commonly in elderly women (senile or postmenopausal osteoporosis), but bone resorption may also result from prolonged inactivity, deficient intake or absorption of cal-

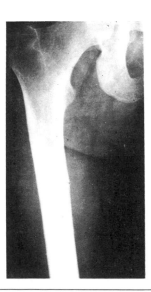

**Fig. 9.10**
Osteomalacia. Pseudo-fractures are seen in the cortex of the femoral shaft and in the pubic ramus.

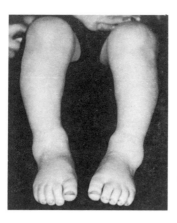

**Fig. 9.11**
Epiphysial enlargement.
Marked enlargement of the
epiphyses of the ankles in a
case of rickets. Note also
bow-legs.

cium and from certain endocrine disorders, e.g. hyperthyroidism, Cushing's syndrome and corticosteroid therapy.

Episodic backache is a characteristic symptom of osteoporosis, the principal signs of which are attributable to compression and collapse of the vertebrae resulting in kyphosis and loss of height. In severe cases the lower ribs may override the pelvis and characteristic horizontal skin folds then appear over the lower chest and abdomen. In the senile group especially there is an increased susceptibility to fracture of the femoral neck and the lower end of the radius.

### Paget's disease (Osteitis deformans)

This is a chronic progressive bone disease of unknown cause, the incidence of which increases with age. It is characterized by rapid bone formation and resorption which at first is localized but later may extend to involve much of the skeleton. The skull and the weight-bearing bones of the spine, pelvis and leg are most commonly affected.

The clinical features include enlargement of the skull (*see Fig.* 9.1), kyphosis and thickening and bowing of the long bones of the leg (*Fig.* 9.12). The disease may be symptomless but bone pains are common, and there is an increased skin temperature over areas of active disease due to the high blood flow through the bone; this increased blood flow may lead to dyspnoea from high output cardiac failure. The excessive bone growth can encroach upon neural structures adjacent to skull or spine and cause such symptoms as nerve deafness and paraplegia. Osteogenic sarcoma is a rare complication. The plasma level of alkaline phosphatase is raised and the urinary excretion of hydroxyproline increased.

### Disseminated neoplasia of bone

Perhaps the most common serious disorder of bone in medical practice is metastatic carcinoma secondary to a primary lesion in the breast, prostate, lung, kidney or thyroid. Bone metastases usually present with pain, a 'pathological' fracture or a bony swelling at the site of a malignant deposit. The plasma alkaline phosphatase (and, in the case of prostatic carcinoma, the acid phosphatase also) is raised with osteosclerotic metastases (e.g. breast and prostate). There may be evidence of primary or secondary tumours in other organs.

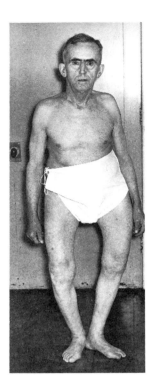

**Fig. 9.12**
Paget's disease. Note the
large head and the bowing of
the legs.

Diffuse neoplastic bone disease can also be secondary to malignant change
within the bone-marrow itself, as in the case of certain lymphomas (e.g. Hodgkin's
disease) and leukaemias (*see* p. 311). A special example of this is multiple myeloma, a neoplasm of the plasma cells in which there is widespread destruction of
the skeleton associated with anaemia, hypercalcaemia, impaired renal function
and an increased susceptibility to infections.

### Hyperparathyroidism

(*see* p. 468).

### DISEASES OF JOINTS: INFLAMMATORY

### Rheumatic fever

This disease is the result of a reaction to infection with β-haemolytic
streptococci and therefore generally appears 2–3 weeks after a sore throat. It now
occurs mainly in those areas where overcrowding and poor economic conditions
still prevail. The relative rarity of rheumatic fever today is also due to the effective
antibiotic treatment of streptococcal infections.

Rheumatic fever usually presents in the school-age child or sometimes during
pregnancy. The onset is generally sudden with high fever and profuse sweating.
The large joints are most often attacked, but the active signs of inflammation
usually manifest themselves in one joint at a time and remain 24 hours on average,
before they appear in another joint. The arthritis, however, does not pass away

completely from the joint first affected but remains in a subacute form. Thus it is common for one joint to show acute inflammation signs while several others are affected to a lesser extent. Each affected joint is hot, swollen and exquisitely tender. The skin over it may be reddened.

The illness may be accompanied by other rheumatic manifestations, including skin rashes (e.g. erythema marginatum), subcutaneous nodules, choreiform movements and evidence of cardiac involvement, such as a pericardial rub, systolic murmur or tachycardia disproportionate to fever. Chronic disease of the mitral and aortic valves are important complications (*see* Chapter 7, p. 255) which may present in adults whose original rheumatic illness was too slight to be recalled.

### Rheumatoid disease

Rheumatoid disease is an inflammatory condition in which immunological mechanisms play an important role. Arthritis is its principal manifestation, but the disease can affect the lungs (fibrosing alveolitis), eyes (episcleritis and kerato-conjunctivitis (*Fig.* 9.13)), pericardium and peripheral nerves. Splenomegaly and lymphadenopathy also occur. Rheumatoid nodules may be found in the subcutaneous tissues, especially over the elbow, forearm and hand, but also in the lungs and other organs (*Fig.* 9.14). Anaemia is common and amyloidosis a rare complication. A rheumatoid form of polyarthritis may accompany systemic disorders such as systemic lupus erythematosus and polyarteritis nodosa.

Rheumatoid arthritis is more common in women than in men and most often presents in the fourth or fifth decades. The onset may be acute or insidious and the course remittent or progressive. Although the disease process may eventually become inactive, some degree of permanent dysfunction and deformity is the rule, and in many cases disability is severe and lasting.

Although any joint in the body may be involved, the inflammation typically affects the small joints of the hands and feet in a symmetrical manner, notably the proximal interphalangeal and the second and third metacarpophalangeal joints (*Fig.* 9.15). The terminal interphalangeal joints are usually spared (in contrast

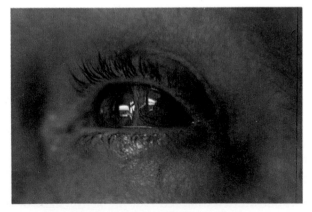

**Fig. 9.13** Rheumatoid disease: recurrent scleritis has led to gross scleral thinning and secondary glaucoma.

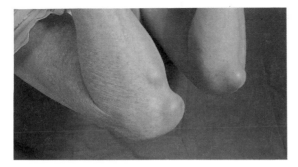

**Fig. 9.14** Rheumatoid nodules over the elbows and forearms.

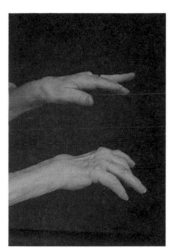

**Fig. 9.15**
Rhematoid arthritis showing muscle wasting, nodules, flexion deformities and joint swelling.

with gout and the psoriatic form of arthritis). Other joints commonly involved include the wrists, elbows, knees, ankles, joints of the feet, cervical spine and, occasionally, the temporomandibular joints.

The chief symptom of rheumatoid arthritis is painful joint stiffness, especially on first wakening in the morning, but constitutional symptoms such as fatigue, anorexia and weight loss also occur. In acute disease the affected joints are swollen and warm, tender to touch and painful on motion. In advanced cases there will be diminished range of joint movement, disuse atrophy of muscles, and characteristic deformities, including spindle-shaped swelling of the proximal interphalangeal joints (with compensatory hyper-extension or even subluxation of the distal joints), ulnar deviation at the metacarpophalangeal joints and flexion deformities of the wrists, fingers and knees (*Fig.* 9.16).

## Ankylosing spondylitis

Like rheumatoid arthritis, ankylosing spondylitis is an inflammatory condition of uncertain cause which may be associated with systemic lesions, notably iritis, aortic regurgitation and apical pulmonary fibrosis. Ankylosing spon-

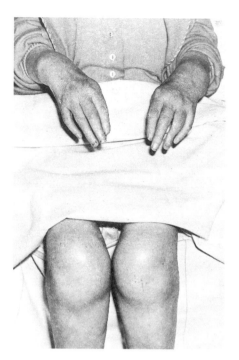

**Fig. 9.16**
Rheumatoid arthritis, showing
deformity of the wrists,
metacarpophalangeal joints
and knees.

dylitis differs from rheumatoid arthritis in that it occurs most often in young men and chiefly involves the proximal or 'central' joints of the body: the sacro-iliac, intervertebral, costovertebral, hip and, occasionally, the shoulder joints.

The patient complains of back pain especially in the early stages when there may be tenderness over the sacro-iliac joints. Later, examination will show abnormal rigidity of the spine, reduced chest expansion and fixation of the hip joints. In untreated cases, a flexion deformity of the spine may develop with forward displacement of the head (*Figs.* 9.17, 9.18).

### Reiter's syndrome

This disorder is largely confined to young men and is characterized by conjunctivitis, non-bacterial urethritis or enterocolitis, various mucosal and skin lesions and a polyarthritis. It is usually venereal but not gonococcal in origin. The arthritis particularly affects the lower limb and consists of an acute inflammatory reaction which can be followed by permanent joint damage.

### Infective arthritis

Bacterial infection, which usually involves only one or two of the larger joints, has become infrequent as a cause of arthritis since the development of effective antibiotics. Gonorrhoea, tuberculosis, typhoid, dysentery and pneumococcal and staphylococcal infection are among the commoner causes. Pyogenic infection may also occur in a rheumatoid joint, especially after intra-articular corticosteroid injections.

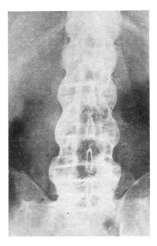

**Fig. 9.17**
Ankylosing spondylitis:
radiograph of the lumbo-sacral
spine showing bony bridging
between the vertebral bodies.
Note also obliteration of the
sacro-iliac joints.

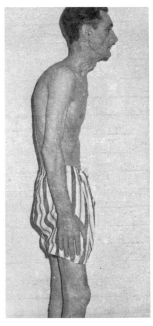

**Fig. 9.18**
Characteristic posture in
ankylosing spondylitis. Due to
the dorsal kyphosis, the neck
is hyperextended to maintain
horizontal gaze.

## Other forms of arthritis

Varying patterns of inflammatory joint disease occur in association with psoriasis, ulcerative colitis, Crohn's disease, brucellosis, erythema nodosum and many other conditions. Some of these may resemble rheumatoid arthritis. In psoriatic arthritis the terminal interphalangeal joints are typically involved, whereas in rheumatoid arthritis they are often spared (*Fig.* 9.19). Psoriatic nails show thimble pitting, thickening, crumbling and discoloration of the nail plate indistinguishable from fungal changes and separation of the nail from the nail plate produces onycholysis (*Fig.* 9.20).

## DISEASES OF JOINTS: DEGENERATIVE

### Osteo-arthritis

This degenerative non-inflammatory condition of the joints increases in frequency with age. It is by far the commonest cause of arthropathy in the elderly but may come on at an earlier age as a result of repeated trauma from postural and mechanical defects, occupational stresses or obesity. It follows that the weight-bearing joints—the spine, hip and knee especially—are chiefly involved. In contrast to rheumatoid arthritis, the distal interphalangeal joints are

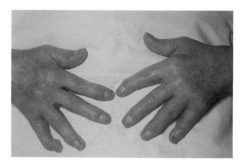

**Fig. 9.19**
Psoriatic arthritis involving the
terminal interphalangeal joints
and nails.

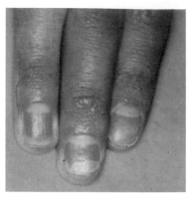

**Fig. 9.20**
Psoriatic nails showing
thimble pitting and
onycholysis (separation of nail
from nail plate).

commonly affected to produce the characteristic Heberden nodes, especially in women (*Fig.* 9.21). Joints with a large range of mobility such as the neck, shoulders and base of the thumb are also specially prone to osteo-arthritis.

The patient most often complains of aching pain and stiffness on using the joints especially after a period of immobility. Those patients having vertebral arthritis may also suffer from root pains due to neural compression from osteophytes or disc protrusions. Examination may show enlargement of the affected joint due to bony hypertrophy, and there may be transient effusions, particularly in the knee. Passive motion of the joint may be accompanied by pain and palpable crepitus but, except in the hip, the range of movement is often unrestricted.

**Fig. 9.21**
Heberden's nodes.

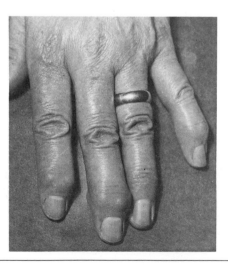

### Neuropathic joint disease

In certain neurological disorders, loss of pain and proprioceptive sensations deprive the joint of its normal protective reactions. The resulting impairment of joint posture and stability leads to degenerative changes resembling those of osteoarthritis. The final state is a grossly enlarged and disorganized joint with an excessive range of painless mobility ('Charcot joint') (*Fig.* 9.22). The hip and knee are most commonly affected in tabes, the foot in diabetic neuropathy and the shoulder and elbow in syringomyelia.

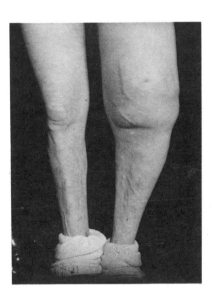

**Fig. 9.22**
Charcot's joint. The left knee joint is disorganized but painless.

## ■ METABOLIC DISORDERS

### Gout

This is a syndrome characterized by an excess of uric acid in the blood. Often there is an inherited factor, with either increased synthesis of uric acid or its decreased excretion by the kidney, or both. Gout may also be secondary to increased cellular breakdown (as in polycythaemia and chronic myeloid leukaemia) or to the use of certain drugs (e.g. thiazide diuretics) which impair the renal excretion of urates. Sodium urate is deposited in the joints, cartilage (e.g. of the ear) and kidneys to produce the three principal features of the disease: arthritis, tophi and renal failure.

Gout usually presents in middle life and is uncommon in women. A family history can often be obtained. The classic attack consists of a rapidly developing painful swelling of one joint, usually the first metatarsophalangeal, which is extremely tender with shiny hot redness of the overlying skin and oedema of the surrounding parts. The temperature may be raised and the illness can be mistaken for a bacterial infection such as cellulitis. The attack usually subsides within a week and may be followed by a complete remission. However, in some cases, the deposition of urates in the joints and periarticular tissues may gradually cause a crippling form of polyarthritis with gross deformity. The feet, ankles, knees, fingers, hands, wrists and elbows are the joints most frequently affected.

When gout is suspected as a cause of arthritis, the clinical examination should include a careful search for tophi and for evidence of renal damage (albuminuria, hypertension etc.). Tophi may be seen under the skin, especially in the helix of the ear (*see Fig. 9.23b*) and around the joints (*Fig. 9.23a*); they consist of pale yellow deposits of sodium urate, sometimes forming large masses that ulcerate and discharge a pasty material through the skin. However, tophi are found in only a small proportion of cases, and the clinical diagnosis is usually made from the history alone.

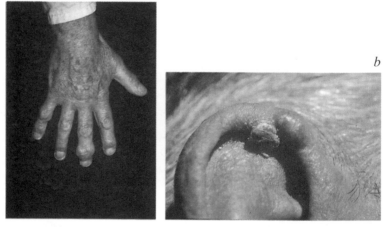

**Fig. 9.23** Gouty tophi. *a*, Around interphalangeal joints. *b*, In the ear (one has ulcerated).

## ■  SPECIAL INVESTIGATIONS

*Radiology* plays an important part in the investigation of bone and joint disease. Radiographs of bone reveal fractures and pseudo-fractures, deformity and areas of resorbtion or thickening. CAT scans show bone structure in greater detail and radioactive bone scanning reveals increased activity in Paget's disease and bony metastases not visualized on conventional radiographs.

In disease of the limb joints it is advisable to compare one side with the other. It should be noted that radiology is usually unhelpful in diagnosing early gout since punched out areas in the bone do not appear until there are clinical tophi. In osteoarthritis, the involved bone margins show sclerotic thickening with loss of joint space and outgrowth of bony spurs—osteophytes. In the early stages of rheumatoid arthritis, soft tissue swelling over the affected joint may be visualized

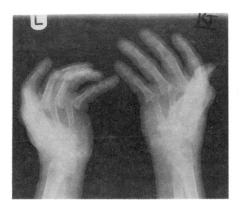

**Fig. 9.24** Advanced rheumatoid arthritis: radiograph showing subluxation of MP joints, ulnar deviation, erosions and cystic changes in metacarpals and phalanges.

but later typical erosions appear at the margin of the articular surfaces which eventually are destroyed and subluxation can occur (*Fig.* 9.24). The sacro-iliac joints in ankylosing spondylitis show subtle marginal sclerosis in the early stages but later there may be fusion of vertebral bodies and calcification of ligaments spreading upwards from the sacrum producing the characteristic bamboo spine (*see Fig.* 9.17).

Investigations of value in the differential diagnosis of bone disorders include the plasma and urinary levels of *calcium* and *phosphorus*, the plasma alkaline and acid phosphatases and the urinary total hydroxyproline excretion.

The erythrocyte sedimentation rate (ESR) is raised in the presence of inflammation and may thus help to differentiate active inflammatory from degenerative forms of arthropathy. The finding of a raised antistreptolysin titre (evidence of recent streptococcal infection) would support a diagnosis of rheumatic fever while the presence of rheumatoid factor (positive Latex flocculation test) suggests rheumatoid arthritis. Detection of LE cells or anti-nuclear antibodies in the blood may indicate systemic lupus erythematosus and ankylosing spondylitis occurs almost exclusively in those who have the HLA B27 antigen. In septic arthritis, the causative organism may be recovered from cultures of the synovial fluid, and a positive complement fixation test may be found in those cases due to gonorrhoea. In gout, the serum uric acid is raised, monosodium urate crystals are present in the synovial fluid of the affected joints and tests of renal function may be abnormal. Tabes can be identified as the cause of a neuropathic arthrosis by the Wasserman reaction and fluorescent treponema antibody test, and diabetes by the finding of impaired glucose tolerance.

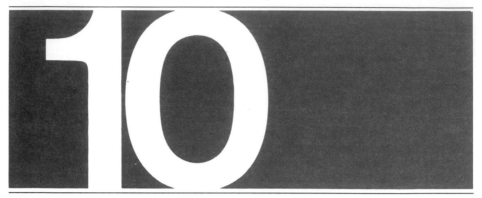

## The nervous system

The diagnosis of nervous diseases offers an excellent example of the importance of grouping symptoms and signs together so as to present a picture of the underlying pathological processes. This should be the physician's aim and should not be obscured by mere names such as 'syringomyelia' and 'Parkinsonism', unless these names are qualified by full details of the cause and extent of the disease. For example, in the case of Parkinsonism, it is essential to know the origin of this—ischaemic, drug-induced (e.g. phenothiazines), post-encephalitic and so forth.

In arriving at a full diagnosis, careful history-taking is of great importance as in other systems; age, sex incidence and time relationships play a great part in deciding the pathological nature of the lesion. The anatomical diagnosis, as will be explained, depends upon careful assessment of changes in motor power and sensation, alteration in reflexes and disturbances of the special functions of the brain, cranial nerves and spinal cord. Some of the signs are due to paralysis of function in the damaged areas and are likely to be lasting, as are the various 'release' phenomena due to loss of control of one part of the nervous system over another. Others are more transient, e.g. irritative fits or abolition of function due to shock to the brain or spinal cord, but they are none the less valuable evidence of the anatomical site of the lesion.

## ■ CEREBRATION AND CONSCIOUSNESS

The brain is concerned in the higher functions of cerebration and consciousness apart from its work in connection with motor power, sensory reception and the control of vital functions, such as respiration and cardiac action.

The examination of these higher functions of the brain is chiefly based upon systematic questioning and upon observation of the patient's behaviour, habits and mode of life. Physical examination plays a smaller part in the diagnosis of cerebral disease than accurate history-taking, though associated lesions of the motor or sensory cortex and of the cranial nerves frequently form an integral part of the clinical picture, which must be considered as a whole.

### Cerebration

The general *intelligence* of different individuals varies enormously, but the patient's relatives are often able to assist in determining whether his mental activity has changed of late. *Memory* and *orientation* in space and time should be tested by asking the patient to state the names of his nearest relatives, the address of his home, the date of his birth, the place where he is at the present time and the day of the week. His ability to obey simple commands should also be noted.

Loss of memory for recent events is more common than loss of long-term memory. It can be tested by asking the patient to recall something he has just read or to repeat something he has just been told. Episodes of unconsciousness due, for example, to trauma or epilepsy may be followed by a period of memory loss which can precede the onset of the coma (*retrograde amnesia*). In Korsakov's pyschosis an attempt is made to disguise the memory defect by the elaborate invention of recent happenings (*confabulation*).

Many mental symptoms such as hallucinations, delusions and abnormalities of conduct may result from organic brain disease an in cerebral arteriosclerosis and neoplasm. These are briefly discussed on p. 457.

### Disturbances of consciousness

Mental function naturally depends upon full consciousness. This may be lost partially, *stupor*, or completely, *coma*, apart from the physiological cyclical loss of consciousness which we know as sleep. The partial unconsciousness which is accompanied by restlessness of the body and mind is called *delirium*. All phases of this state are seen, from tossing and turning in bed with periodic chattering, to the wilder types in which the patient throws himself about and struggles violently, frequently shouting at the top of his voice. These changes in consciousness are often found in severe cerebral lesions such as trauma, vascular insults and tumours but may be caused by fever and toxaemias, which exert an indirect effect upon the brain.

**Coma** The differential diagnosis of this deep state of unconsciousness is discussed on p. 12 as it causes include many that are not primarily neurological. (*See also Fig.* 1.3, p. 14.)

---

■ **SPEECH DEFECTS**

---

Speech is one of the highest functions of the human brain. It is not surprising, therefore, that it is disordered in many gross diseases of the brain which affect other mental functions. For speech to be carried out normally not only must the higher centres be intact, but the motor mechanism which controls the muscles of articulation must be perfect. Disorders of speech can thus be divided at once into two groups: (1) Those affecting the higher centres in the brain—*dysphasia* or *aphasia*, a disturbance of speech as an intellectual function; (2) Those interfering with the motor execution of speech—*dysarthria* or *anarthria* (*see* The 12th Cranial Nerve, p. 368, and Bulbar Paralysis, p. 406).

## Aphasia

The older view that two principal types of aphasia, sensory and motor, exist still has much to commend it from the point of view of simplicity, providing the student does not draw too sharp a distinction in his mind between the two but allows for mixtures of both types, which occur in many cases. The conception of sensory and motor aphasia arises from a consideration of the way in which language is built up in the child's mind. Sight and hearing take the first part. The repetition of the same sound evokes in the child's mind a particular mental impression. Similarly a visual impression repeated in association with a word causes that word to be identified with the object seen. The two types of sensory impression, auditory and visual, are usually received at the same time. We point to a book and say 'book' to the child, and, with repetition, the word 'book' eventually produces the mental image of that article. Similarly the sight of a book recalls to the mind the sound of the word.

Other sensations besides hearing and sight take part in the formation of speech, notably the appreciation of the form and size of objects (stereognosis).

In time the child learns to speak, that is, to call into action those parts of the brain which control the mechanism for understanding and emitting words. The use of a word conjures up in the mind an auditory, visual or other sensory image. With mental development, not only in the child but in the adult, this process of speech becomes more intricate, but the later acquired faculties of speech, for example, foreign languages, do not take such deep root as those upon which the foundations were laid. Further, speech has an emotional as well as an intellectual character and the former is more primitive and less disturbed by lesions of the speech centre. For example, the patient may be able to sing an old familiar song using words which he cannot speak.

The symptom aphasia implies above all a loss of speech comprehension. It is possible, and indeed not uncommon, for an aphasic person to speak words which he does not understand. On the other hand, speech may be impossible owing to paralysis of the articulatory mechanism (anarthria) without aphasia being present.

**Sensory aphasia** In sensory aphasia impressions upon which speech is based become meaningless. The patient may hear words which convey nothing to him (*word-deafness*), or may see written words which have lost all meaning (*word-blindness*). These types of aphasia may be recognized by asking the patient to perform some simple command. A spoken command—'Put out your tongue'— will not be executed if the patient does not grasp the meaning of the words. The same command in writing will test whether he appreciates the meaning of written words. In sensory types of aphasia the patient often misnames objects shown to him.

In testing for different types of aphasia certain pitfalls must obviously be avoided, e.g. deafness or the possibility of paralysis of the muscles of articulation or of the right hand when the patient is asked to write. Sensory aphasia arises from lesions in the (left) superior temporal gyrus (area 42) (*see Figs*. 10.36, 10.37, p. 372) and is valuable in the recognition of the site of a cortical lesion. Care must be taken to distinguish it from mental disorders affecting speech.

**Motor aphasia** Motor aphasia may be surmised if the sensory appreciation of words appears normal and the articulatory apparatus is unharmed, yet the patient is unable to speak words which have a meaning both to him and to the listener.

This type of aphasia may be obvious if the patient is quite unable to speak at all or if he utters unintelligible sounds. Often the earliest change is the loss of names (*nominal aphasia*), so that the patient circumvents the use of the name by a phrase, as one does with a limited knowledge of a foreign language. It may be specifically tested by asking him to name common objects after first ascertaining that no gross sensory aphasia is present. In motor aphasia the faculty of writing is usually lost (*agraphia*), but in testing for its loss the possibility of paresis of the right arm or hand must first be excluded. Motor aphasia is commonly associated with a right hemiplegia from left middle cerebral artery thrombosis which also affects the area of the (left) inferior frontal gyrus known as Broca's centre (area 44) (*see Figs.* 10.36, 10.37, p. 372; *also Fig.* 10.1).

Although aphasia is often accompanied by impairment of intellect, many patients retain some understanding of the spoken word, and this must be borne in mind when discussions are held at the bedside.

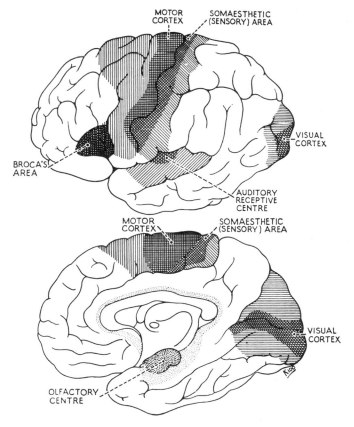

**Fig. 10.1** Lateral and medial aspects of the brain showing motor and sensory areas (dark shading) and respective association areas (lighter shading). These figures should be compared with *Figs.* 10.36, 10.37, p. 372.

**Localizing value of aphasia** If the patient is right-handed, the presence of aphasia establishes the lesion in the left side of the brain (and vice versa) with very few exceptions. Motor aphasia is usually caused by lesions in front of the central sulcus, while lesions behind it may cause sensory aphasia. The whole area which may be involved in aphasia is considerable, and extends from the posterior end of the inferior frontal gyrus to the upper temporal area and the lower part of the parietal region. The zone includes the insula.

The vascular lesions, especially thrombosis and embolism, which cause aphasia can usually be localized with greater certainty by the extent of concomitant paralysis, but aphasia may sometimes have a topographical diagnostic value in cerebral tumours.

### Dysarthria

Speech is often altered in character without being lost. Some types of abnormal speech may be recognized spontaneously, but others are made apparent when the patient attempts to repeat certain difficult phrases. In lesions of the basal ganglia speech is unusually slow and monotonous; in cerebellar ataxia (e.g. disseminated sclerosis) it has an interrupted character described as *staccato* or *scanning* (sometimes with an explosive element). The speech in cases of palatal paralysis has a nasal quality as air escapes through the nose. Lesions of the recurrent laryngeal nerve cause whispered speech due to paralysis of the vocal cord (aphonia) and this is usually accompanied by a bovine cough. In bulbar paralysis, whether of nuclear or supranuclear origin, all stages between difficult speech and complete absence (*anarthria*) may be present, and the patient frequently mumbles indistinguishable sounds although fully aware of what he wishes to say.

■       ## THE CRANIAL NERVES

A systematic examination of the cranial nerves is essential in every neurological case. Not only may primary lesions of the nerves, their nuclei or their cerebral controlling centres be found, but the secondary involvement of these by diseases of the brain or its meninges frequently gives most important localizing data.

If there are signs of paralysis of muscles supplied by a cranial nerve, it is necessary to consider whether the lesion is situated in the upper or lower motor neuron, just as in the case of paralysis of the limbs. The cranial nerve lesion may then be described as either *supranuclear* or *infranuclear*.

When the lesion has been localized, its pathology must be determined. The common pathological processes responsible for cranial nerve paralysis are similar to those mentioned for the nervous system as a whole (p. 434).

### The 1st or olfactory nerve

The olfactory nerves are not of great clinical importance. Their anatomical position renders them liable to damage by tumours, especially subfrontal meningioma, or by head injuries, especially when a fracture involves the anterior fossa. The result will be loss of the sense of smell, *anosmia*, which is particularly significant if unilateral. The patient often confuses this with loss of the sense of taste, as flavours depend upon the sense of smell, not the sense of taste. In total olfactory lesions, only the primary sensations of taste (sweet, bitter, sour and salt) remain.

The perception of smell appears to be situated in the uncus and pyriform cortex, lesions of which may be associated with perversions of smell. Similar perversion may occur as an aura in epilepsy, and in mental disorders.

**Examination** The olfactory nerves must be tested by substances which do not stimulate the sensory endings of the 5th nerve. Ammonia and acetic acid, therefore, must not be used. Peppermint, turpentine and oil of cloves are suitable and should be applied to each nostril in turn.

### The 2nd or optic nerve

This is the most important of the cranial nerves. Not only does it serve the most highly organized special sense, that of sight, but it spreads out into the retina, the examination of which so often reveals signs of disease in other parts of the body.

A few important anatomical facts must be recalled. The impressions of light from the whole of each retina are taken in the optic nerve to the optic chiasma. Here the fibres from the left half of each retina pass into the left optic tract, those from the right half to the right optic tract. Most of the fibres of each optic tract pass on to the lateral geniculate body; some to the pretectal area which presides over the reflex action of the pupils and movements of the orbital muscles. From these lower visual centres the fibres make their way, via the optic radiation on each side, to the occipital cortex. Through the medial part of each optic tract communication is established between this optical system and the oculomotor nuclei. The pupillary reflexes are also controlled through special fibres in the optic nerve which leave the optic tract to reach the pretectal area, which in its turn communicates with the 3rd nerve nucleus.

The various parts of these optical paths may now be considered in relationship to surrounding structures. The nerve itself may be involved as it enters the orbit, or by lesions in the anterior fossa of the skull or of the frontal lobes. The chiasma lies in close contact with the pituitary gland and the internal carotid arteries and may be damaged by lesions of these structures such as pituitary tumour or carotid aneurysm; also by meningeal changes such as arachnoiditis following skull injury. Each optic tract, as it diverges from its fellow in front of the interpeduncular space, winds round the corresponding crus in close association with the posterior cerebral artery which supplies it. The tract may be affected by disease, either of the artery or of the crus. Finally, each optic radiation passes through the posterior limb of the internal capsule and sweeps round the posterior horn of the lateral ventricle to the visual cortex (area 17), the lower fibres having first descended through the temporal lobe.

The effects of lesions in the different parts of these visual pathways will be seen in *Fig.* 10.2.

### Examination of the optic nerve and its connections

The patient must first be asked whether he has noted any visual changes. His visual acuity may then be tested, and an ophthalmoscopic examination of the retina and optic discs made. Finally the visual fields may be tested.

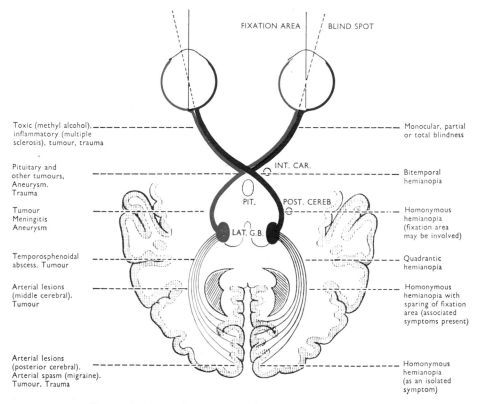

FIXATION AREA    BLIND SPOT

Toxic (methyl alcohol), inflammatory (multiple sclerosis), tumour, trauma ——— Monocular, partial or total blindness

Pituitary and other tumours, Aneurysm. Trauma ——— Bitemporal hemianopia

INT. CAR.

PIT.

POST. CEREB.

Tumour Meningitis Aneurysm ——— Homonymous hemianopia (fixation area may be involved)

LAT. G.B.

Temporosphenoidal abscess. Tumour ——— Quadrantic hemianopia

Arterial lesions (middle cerebral). Tumour ——— Homonymous hemianopia with sparing of fixation area (associated symptoms present)

Arterial lesions (posterior cerebral). Arterial spasm (migraine). Tumour. Trauma ——— Homonymous hemianopia (as an isolated symptom)

**Fig. 10.2** Course of visual fibres. On the left side are shown the common lesions in the various parts of the course of the fibres, on the right the results of the lesion. INT. CAR., Internal carotid artery; PIT., Pituitary gland; POST. CEREB., Posterior cerebral artery; LAT. G. B., Lateral geniculate bodies. (*Diagram constructed by Mr A. McKie Reid.*)

## Visual acuity

Acuity of vision is tested by means of special charts (Snellen types) with lines of print varying in size (*Fig.* 10.3). Each eye is tested separately. Central visual acuity is conventionally recorded as a fraction. For example, if the patient standing at 6 metres' distance can read only the largest type, which he should be able to read at 60 m, his visual acuity is said to be 6/60. Similarly, if he can read no further down the type than that line which should be read at 18 m, his visual acuity is stated to be 6/18, and ability to read the penultimate line (line 7 in the diagram) is expressed as 6/6, i.e. normal vision.

## Ophthalmoscopic examination

The retinae and optic discs (*Fig.* 10.4) can be examined with an ophthalmoscope (*Fig.* 10.5) even by the inexperienced, and it cannot be overemphasized that the student should use every opportunity of becoming familiar with

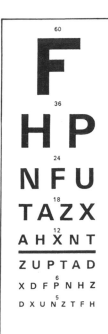

**Fig. 10.3**
Snellen's test types. Reduced
in size from standard chart
seen at 6 m. (*By courtesy of
Messrs Hamblin.*)

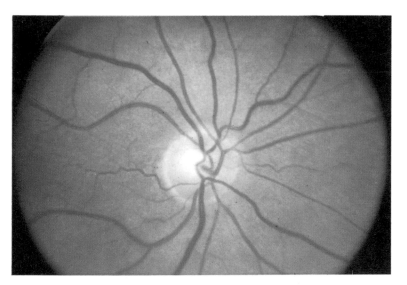

**Fig. 10.4** Normal retina and optic disc. Note the well-defined
margin and paler shade of the disc. The vessels radiate from
the centre of the disc, the veins being broader and deeper in
colour than the arteries.

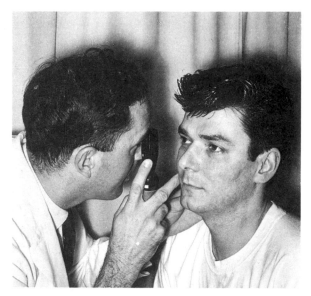

**Fig. 10.5** Method of using the ophthalmoscope.

the physiological variations in the fundus and the commoner types of pathological changes. These include changes in the optic disc, such as pallor, swelling (papilloedema and optic neuritis), cupping and atrophy; and various forms of retinitis and retinopathy, either primary or associated with systemic disease, such as hypertension, blood dyscrasias, renal disease and diabetes.

**The optic disc** The optic disc is as individually characteristic as a fingerprint. Its pattern is probably only repeated in identical twins.

Inspection of the disc calls for a definite plan. Colour—pink or paler; margin—clear-cut, blurred or absent; contour—elevated, flat or cupped; crescents—at the temporal margin as in myopia; the distribution of the vessels; lamina cribrosa—the floor of the disc—whether abnormally obvious as in glaucoma or not visible as in oedema; and finally, abnormalities such as neuroglia, pigment deposition, haemorrhages and opaque nerve fibres.

**Papilloedema** Papilloedema or choked disc (*Fig.* 10.6) is a non-inflammatory swelling of the optic disc or nerve head usually associated with increased intracranial pressure such as results from space-occupying lesions in the cranium, malignant hypertension and chronic carbon-dioxide retention. Papilloedema may also arise from occlusion of the retinal veins or cavernous sinus by thrombosis or other causes. Unilateral papilloedema with contralateral optic atrophy (Foster Kennedy sign) occurs when a tumour presses upon the optic nerve and blocks the posterior opening of the optic canal, while increased intracranial pressure causes papilloedema in the other eye.

**Pathogenesis of papilloedema** (*Fig.* 10.7) The subarachnoid space of the optic nerve sheath is in direct communication with the cerebral subarachnoid space. The retinal artery, vein, and lymphatics run in the nerve, and cross the subarach-

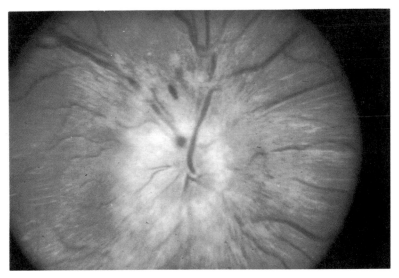

**Fig. 10.6** Papilloedema due to cerebral tumour. Note blurring of the disc margin and of the lamina cribrosa. Most of the vessels disappear near to the margin of the disc (cf normal retina, *Fig.* 10.4). Note also the exudates radiating from the disc and two small haemorrhages immediately above the disc.

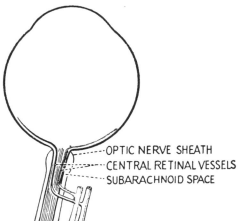

**Fig. 10.7**
Pathogenesis of papilloedema. (*Diagram by Mr A. McKie Reid.*)

OPTIC NERVE SHEATH
CENTRAL RETINAL VESSELS
SUBARACHNOID SPACE

noid space of the nerve sheath about 1 cm behind the eyeball. Increased pressure in the cerebral subarachnoid space is transmitted into the nerve sheath. The relatively thin walls of the vein and lymphatics, with the low pressure of their fluid contents, permit them to be compressed more than the artery. The inflow of blood to the retina is practically unchecked, while the outflow of venous blood and lymph is obstructed. This results in increased transudation of lymph into and oedema of the optic disc.

The swelling may be measured by the ophthalmoscope. Both eyes of the examiner should be kept open and unaccommodated as if looking at a distance. A vessel near the centre of the disc is brought into focus with the highest possible plus lens. The same vessel is followed until it leaves the disc and is focused again. The difference, e.g. between +6·0 and +3·0 dioptres, is the measure of the swelling. In this case it would be 3 dioptres (3 dioptres = 1 mm of swelling).

Other features to be noted are the engorgement of the veins, blurring of the disc margin, and apparent disappearance of the blood vessels as they 'mount' the elevated disc.

**Optic neuritis** Inflammation or demyelination may affect the optic nerve at any point. When the anterior part of the nerve, the optic disc, is involved the disc is oedematous, but the swelling is not as great as in papilloedema; the disc colour is usually more red, and the disc appears cloudy due to inflammatory exudates not only in the disc but in the overlying vitreous. The differential diagnosis between papilloedema and optic neuritis is, however, not always easy. In neurological practice disseminated sclerosis is the only common cause.

Retrobulbar neuritis is the condition in which the nerve lesion lies behind the lamina cribrosa. There is little if any disturbance of the disc, but there is often a central scotoma.

This state of affairs has been described as one in which 'neither the ophthalmologist nor the patient sees anything'. The most common cause of retrobulbar neuritis is disseminated sclerosis. Other causes are meningitis and avitaminosis. Optic atrophy may follow.

**Optic atrophy** (*Fig.* 10.8) The common feature of all varieties of optic atrophy, whatever their aetiology or pathogenesis, is pallor of the optic disc and loss of visual acuity. Optic atrophy may be classified in the following manner:

1. *Primary*, which is observed in tabes and other diseases of the central nervous system, after injury, compression to or ischaemia of the optic nerve, or in consequence of certain exogenous toxins such as methyl alcohol, lead and quinine. The disc is bluish-white and the margins are sharply defined. Cupping or depression of the disc is observed and the calibre of the vessels, both veins and arteries, is narrowed.

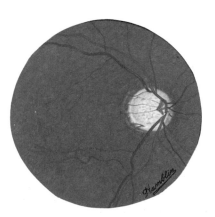

**Fig. 10.8**
Primary optic atrophy. The disc is pale and stands out vividly against the red fundus; the margin is sharply defined. The vessels are attenuated. (*By kind permission of the Oxford University Press. Drawing by Messrs Hamblin*).

2. *Secondary*, in which optic atrophy occurs when the ganglion cell layer of the retina has been damaged by observable pathological processes such as choroido-retinitis or pigmentary degeneration (retinitis pigmentosa). The general picture of the retina shows the cause of which the atrophy is the secondary effect.

3. *Consecutive* optic atrophy in which the atrophy follows papilloedema as a continuous process. Exudate in the disc undergoes organization, the margins of the disc are blurred, the lamina cribrosa is hidden, the vessels are ensheathed in neuroglia, and the disc appears shaggy.

4. *Glaucomatous*. The disc is white or pale grey and is deeply cupped. The lamina cribrosa, with its perforations, is clearly displayed, and the vessels emerging from the disc are pushed right up to the margin. This condition is caused by the long-continued increase of intra-ocular tension which occurs in glaucoma.

**The retinopathies** The most important retinopathies are (1) hypertensive and (2) diabetic.

*Hypertensive* vascular changes in the retina have been classified into four stages according to the appearances and life prognosis (*Fig.* 10.9).

Grade I: narrowing of the vessels. Grade II: marked variation in the calibre of the vessels with pressure by the artery on the vein at arteriovenous crossings, so that the vein is kinked and its peripheral calibre is engorged while the part central to the crossing is attenuated. Grade III: the addition of flame-shaped or round retinal haemorrhages and cottonwool patches of exudate. Grade IV: the addition of papilloedema and increased haemorrhages and exudates.

**Diabetic retinopathy** (*Fig.* 10.10) The retina is spattered sparsely or thickly with minute red dots which are micro-aneurysms. Larger blot and dot haemorrhages appear next; then waxy-looking exudates with harder edges than the cotton-wool patches in hypertensive retinopathy. Larger haemorrhages appear wiht irregular veins, and, later, new-formed vascular plexuses, venous loops and coils which may protrude into the vitreous. Vitreous haemorrhages and detachment of the retina may follow with blindness as a result.

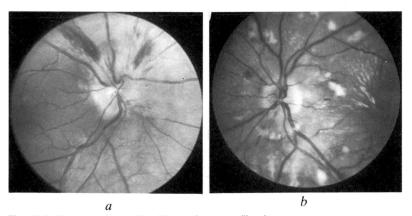

*a*          *b*

**Fig. 10.9** Hypertensive retinopathy. *a* shows papilloedema, flame-shaped haemorrhages, and arterial narrowing. Contrast with *b*, which shows a few haemorrhages and many exudates, some of which appear as a star-shaped figure near the macula.

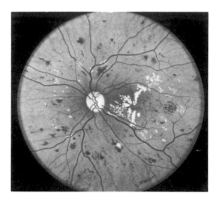

**Fig. 10.10**
Diabetic retinopathy, showing microaneurysms, 'blot and dot' haemorrhages, and waxy-looking exudates.

The diabetic changes are sometimes associated with hypertensive changes in the retina as already described.

### Fields of vision

Whenever the visual field is found to be abnormal by rough tests, accurate charts should be prepared by perimetry. As a rough test, the examiner may compare the patient's visual fields with his own. The examiner and the patient sit facing each other, with opposite eyes closed and each fixes his gaze upon the other's nose. The examiner then holds out his arm to its full extent and asks the patient to say when he sees any movement of the examiner's finger. If no movement is detected, the hand is brought in, kept still and the finger moved again. The examiner compares his own first sighting of the movement with the patient's. When a perimeter is used, a record must be made of the visual field for each colour separately (white, red, green and blue). The colour fields are the first to be restricted in most cases. Lastly, it is essential not to overlook central scotomas, i.e. patches of impairment in the central area of the field of vision.

Blindness in the whole of the visual field occurs from lesions of the retina or optic nerve, less commonly from occipital lobe lesions. Blindness in one-half of each visual field is known as *hemianopia*. If it affects the same—that is, right or left—half of each field, it is called right or left *homonymous hemianopia* (*Fig.* 10.11). This occurs, for example, in lesions of the optic tract and also of the optic radiation. If the right side of one field and the left side of the other are affected, the condition is known as *crossed* or *heteronymous hemianopia*. There are two types of this, *bitemporal hemianopia* (*Fig.* 10.12) when the outer half of each visual field is affected, and *binasal hemianopia* when the inner halves are involved. Bitemporal hemianopia not infrequently results from tumours of, or adjacent to, the pituitary gland and binasal hemianopia may be caused by calcification and expansion of both internal carotid arteries. A field defect affecting one eye only indicates a lesion anterior to the chiasma, either of the optic nerve or of the retina itself.

*Quadrantic defects* ('quadrantic hemianopia') (*Fig.* 10.13) occur from lesions involving the optic radiations or, less commonly, the occipital lobe. The restriction of the visual field is less than one-half, usually about one-quarter. It is to be

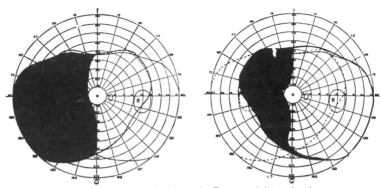

**Fig. 10.11** Left homonymous hemianopia. Tumour right parietal lobe; male, aged 50. Visual acuity; right and left eyes 6/6. Fixation area spared. Perimetry with white object 5 mm in diameter—daylight. (*Constructed by Mr A. McKie Reid.*)

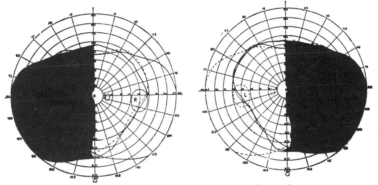

**Fig. 10.12** Bitemporal hemianopia. Pituitary tumour, 6 years' history. Visual acuity: right eye 6/9, left eye 6/24. Sparing of fixation area. Perimetry with 5-mm white object—daylight. (*Constructed by Mr A. McKie Reid,*)

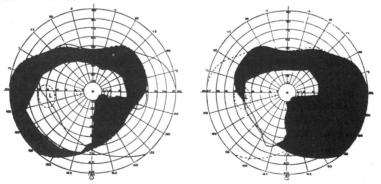

**Fig. 10.13** Quadrantic hemianopia. Subcortical haemorrhage left parietal lobe; male, aged 58. Accompanied by weakness of right arm and leg and blurring of speech. Visual acuity: right eye 6/12, left eye 6/9. Perimetry 4 months after onset with 2-mm white object—daylight. (*Constructed by Mr A. McKie Reid.*)

observed that most forms of hemianopia are irregular, and in their early stages both homonymous and crossed hemianopia may appear quadrantic. This is particularly so when the temporal loop of the optic radiation is affected.

## Oculomotor and pupillary innervation (the 3rd, 4th, 6th and sympathetic nerves) (see Figs. 10.19, 10.20, p. 356)

**Anatomical considerations** The muscles which move the eyeball and those which are responsible for the pupillary reactions are all innervated by the 3rd, 4th, 6th and sympathetic nerves, and these nerves are tested together. The 3rd and 4th nerves have their nuclei in the midbrain and the 6th nerve nucleus is in the floor of the fourth vertricle in the pons.

*The 3rd nerve* emerges at the upper border of the pons, passes through the cavernous sinus and superior orbital fissure and supplies all the orbital muscles except the superior oblique and lateral (external) rectus. It also sends fibres to the levator palpebrae superioris, and, through the ciliary ganglion, controls the muscles of accommodation (the sphincter of the pupil and ciliary muscle).

*The 4th nerve* and its fellow decussate before emerging lateral to the frenulum veli and each winds round the crus and enters the orbit through the superior orbital fissure to supply the superior oblique.

*The 6th nerve* appears between the pons and medulla and also passes through the cavernous sinus and superior orbital fissure to enter the orbit. It supplies the lateral (external) rectus.

The *sympathetic* fibres concerned with the oculomotor mechanism arise in medullary centres and run in the spinal medulla to the 1st and 2nd thoracic nerves, through which they emerge to pass upwards in the cervical sympathetic trunk to the superior cervical ganglion where they synapse. Postganglionic fibres pass upwards from the ganglion in company with the internal carotid artery to be distributed by way of the nasociliary branch of the ophthalmic division of the trigeminal nerve and the long ciliary nerves to the dilator pupillae, and by way of the upper branch of the oculomotor nerve to the involuntary fibres in the levator palpebrae superioris.

The oculomotor muscles work in unison so as to secure conjugate movements of the eyes in a vertical or lateral plane, during which the visual axes remain parallel and in convergence. This simultaneous action of the oculomotor muscles is obtained by special centres in the brainstem, in close association with the nuclei of the 3rd, 4th and 6th nerves. These centres probably control the reflex movements of the eyes, while similar conjugate movements of voluntary origin are under control of the higher cortical centres.

**Examination** The patient should be asked if he sees double (*diplopia*), and note should be taken of squint (*strabismus*), drooping of the eyelid (*ptosis*) or oscillation of the eyeballs (*nystagmus*).

The condition of the *pupils* should be observed, whether they are equal in size and regular in outline, whether abnormally dilated or contracted, and whether they react normally to light and accommodation.

In testing the reaction to light the patient should focus on a distant point and the light should not be too bright. A strong light is then shone into each eye in turn, ensuring that the light does not fall on the other eye and the pupil contracts.

Sometimes the pupil size slowly waxes and wanes as the light source remains constant. This is known as hippus and implies an intact 3rd nerve nucleus.

A *consensual* reflex may be obtained by shining a light into one eye and noting the contraction of the pupil in the other. The value of this reflex is in the recognition of retrobulbar neuritis, one of the earliest signs of disseminated sclerosis. If the afferent path of the reflex arc for pupillary reactions is interrupted by retrobulbar neuritis, the direct response to light will be lost. But the efferent limbs of the reflex arc (from the 3rd-nerve nuclei) are intact, so when a light is shone into the normal eye, the other pupil will contract, though it may show no response to direct light.

In testing the reaction to accommodation the patient is told to look at the far wall of the room. The observer's finger is then suddenly held vertically about 15 cm in front of the patient's nose, and the patient is told to look at it. The pupils should contract equally as he accommodates for the finger, and dilate as the finger is moved away.

To test the *ocular movements* (*Fig.* 10.14) the patient's head must be fixed, and he must be asked to move the eyes in turn to the right, to the left, upwards and downwards as far as possible in each direction. Any limitation of movement is noted (*see Figs.* 10.14–10.17).

**Common lesions** These are usually lower motor neuron lesions, i.e. affecting the nuclei or nerves. The causes include trauma, meningeal infection or haemorrhage, disseminated sclerosis, peripheral neuropathy and local lesions within or behind the orbit (e.g. tumour, aneurysm). Upper motor neuron lesions, e.g. cerebral haemorrhage, or thrombosis affecting the cortical or midbrain centres, are often transient and produce paralysis of conjugate movements rather than of individual nerves or muscles (*see* p. 369). In myasthenia gravis, ocular pareses, especially ptosis, tend to be bilateral, to vary from time to time and to increase with fatigue.

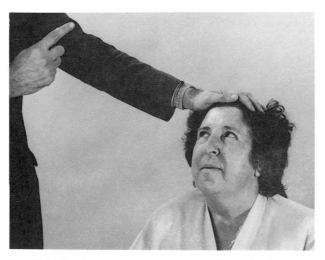

**Fig. 10.14** Testing the ocular movements. The patient's head must be fixed by the examiner's hand.

*Third-nerve paralysis* If this is complete, the eye is immobile except in the direction it is moved by the lateral (external) rectus (*Figs.* 10.15–10.17). It cannot be moved upwards, downwards or inwards. There is usually external strabismus owing to the unopposed action of the 6th nerve. Diplopia results in most cases, the type varying with the muscles principally involved, but it may be masked by ptosis. Ptosis gives a narrow palpebral fissure (*Figs.* 10.15, 10.18, 10.23), owing to paresis of the levator palpebrae superioris, and there is compensatory wrinkling of the forehead on the same side. This wrinkling, due to overaction of the frontalis muscle, may raise the eyelid and mask the narrowing of the palpebral fissure, especially if the ptosis is slight. If the fingers are pressed firmly on the eyebrow against the bone, however, so as to prevent the eyelid from being raised by the frontalis, the ptosis at once becomes apparent. The pupil is fixed and dilated owing to unopposed action of the sympathetic on the dilator pupillae. In 3rd and 6th nerve paralyses secondary deviation may also be observed, i.e. the non-paralysed muscles force the eye farther to the lateral angle than normal and this in its turn results in erroneous projection, so that the patient points farther to one side than the object really is.

Sometimes only portions of the nucleus of the 3rd nerve are affected, and the result is paresis of individual orbital muscles such as the superior or inferior rectus or the inferior oblique. This happens especially with central lesions involving the 3rd nucleus, while peripheral lesions of the nerve give complete paralysis. Paral-

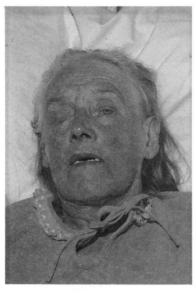
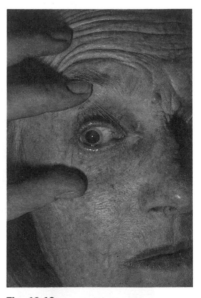

**Fig. 10.15**
Right 3rd-nerve paralysis. Complete ptosis obscures the other physical signs.

**Fig. 10.16**
Same patient as *Fig.* 10.15. Note the large pupil and that the eye looks downwards and outwards due to the unopposed action of the 4th and 6th cranial nerves.

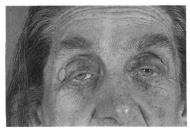

**Fig. 10.18**
Bilateral partial ptosis due to
carcinomatous neuromyopathy.

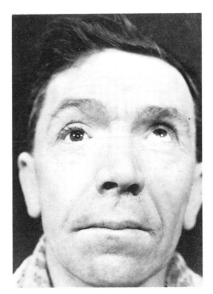

**Fig. 10.17**
Another case with residual
3rd-nerve paralysis of the
right side following meningitis.
Shows failure of the superior
rectus when the patient
attempts to look upwards.

ysis of the superior rectus becomes apparent in abduction or in attempting to look upwards, which also reveals the paralysis of the inferior oblique. Adduction shows up the paralysis of the medial (internal) rectus. A lesion affecting the anterior part of the third nerve, as in some forms of neuropathy, will spare the fibres to the pupil.

*Fourth-nerve paralysis* Superior oblique paralysis is difficult to determine objectively, but on looking downwards the patient complains of diplopia, particularly when the eye is adducted, i.e. turned towards the nose. Isolated lesions of the 4th nerve are extremely rare.

*Sixth-nerve paralysis* The patient is unable to move the eyeball outwards (*Fig.* 10.14). Unopposed contraction of the medial rectus eventually leads to internal strabismus with corresponding diplopia.

If the 6th nucleus is paralysed abduction is limited, i.e. the patient is unable to look towards the side of the lesion with the affected eye, but the unaffected eye moves normally.

Some of these points are illustrated by *Figs*. 10.19 and 10.20.

*Diplopia* Double vision has been referred to under paralysis of the oculomotor muscles. The patient may complain spontaneously or only after questioning that he sees double. The diplopia may be present in all positions of the eye but increases when an attempt is made to move the eye in that direction towards which the paralysed muscle would normally move it.

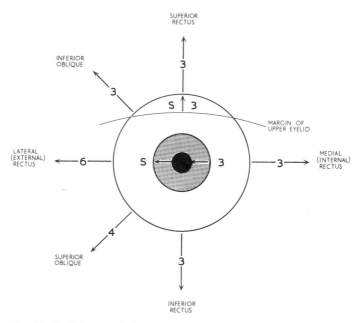

**Fig. 10.19** Right eye. Action and nerve-supply of the ocular muscles. (S=sympathetic.) (*See also Fig.* 10.20 *for action of oblique muscles.*)

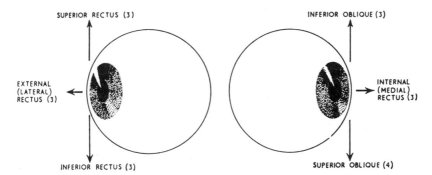

**Fig. 10.20** Movements of the right eye and paralysis of individual muscles. *Left*, The right eye is abducted, that is looking towards the temple, by the external (lateral) rectus (6th nerve). In this position the eye is elevated or moved upwards by the superior rectus (3rd nerve) and downwards by the inferior rectus (3rd nerve). *Right*. The right eye is adducted, that is pulled towards the nose, by the internal (medial) rectus (3rd nerve), and in this position it is *elevated* by the *inferior* oblique (3rd nerve) and *depressed* by the *superior* oblique (4th nerve).

The symptom results from strabismus because the images from the two eyes do not fall on corresponding parts of the retina and two images are seen instead of the one, which is the normal result of binocular vision (*Fig.* 10.21). The visual axis is a line drawn from the point of fixation through the nodal point of the eye so as to reach the retina at the macular lutea. If an image falls on the retina to the temporal side of the macula, it is projected to the nasal side of space (in front of the observer), and vice versa. In paralysis of the internal rectus it may be impossible to direct the eye so that the image of the fixation point falls on the macula. The image falls on the retina to the temporal side of the macula, and the object is falsely projected to the nasal side of the fixation spot. True fixation and projection take place in the unaffected eye, and hence crossed diplopia occurs. When the squint is of long standing the patient may learn to disregard the false image, and diplopia no longer occurs.

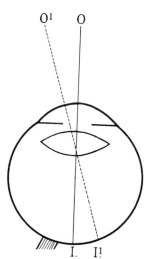

**Fig. 10.21**
Diplopia and false projection
(*see text*). O, Fixation spot;
O¹, Fixation spot or object
falsely projected to nasal side
of space; I, Image at macula;
I¹, Image on temporal side of
macula. (*Diagram by Mr A.
McKie Reid.*)

The position of the images as seen by the patient is often useful in determining the nature of the ocular paresis. The false (more peripheral) image is the one seen by the paralysed eye, the true one by the normal eye.

**Strabismus (squint)** This sign has been mentioned as occurring in oculomotor paralysis (*Fig.* 10.22). Concomitant strabismus is due to an imbalance in the action of opposing muscles. Many cases of squint are non-paralytic and are called 'concomitant'. The main differences between paralytic and concomitant squint may be summarized as follows:

*Paralytic Strabismus*

1 Known cause and sudden onset
2 Diplopia present
3 Limitation in ocular movements
4 Deviation of visual axis varies as the gaze is turned in different directions
5 No amblyopia (blindness)
6 False projection
7 Vertigo may occur

*Concomitant Strabismus*

1 Gradual onset in early childhood
2 No diplopia
3 No limitation of movement
4 Deviation of visual axis does not vary
5 Eye may be amblyopic
6 No false projection
7 No vertigo

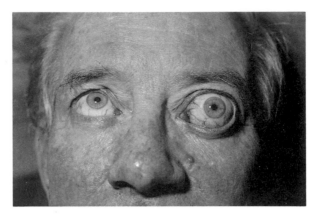

**Fig. 10.22** Left exophthalmic ophthalmoplegia.

The descriptions which have been given of an oculomotor paralysis apply only to lower motor neuron lesions. If the lesion is supranuclear, individual orbital muscles are not affected, therefore squint and diplopia do not occur. Instead, muscles controlling a particular movement are paralysed. In most cases this results in *conjugate deviation*, in which the eyes are persistently turned towards the side of the lesion, as the centres enabling the patient to gaze to the side opposite from the lesion are paralysed. In irritative processes there may be conjugate deviation towards the side opposite the lesion due to overaction of the affected muscles.

*Cervical sympathetic paralysis* (*Fig.* 10.23) The sympathetic may be involved by diseases in the cervical cord such as syringomyelia, or by lesions in the neck, such as trauma, surgical resection (*Fig.* 10.23) or malignant lymph nodes (*Fig.* 10.24). The pupil is contracted owing to unopposed action of the 3rd nerve. Slight ptosis occurs from paresis of the involuntary muscle fibres in the upper eyelid giving the impression of recession of the eyeball (enophthalmos), and sweating may be absent on the affected side of the head and neck. This combination of myosis, ptosis, and anhidrosis is known as Horner's syndrome.

*Pupillary abnormalities* Make sure first that no mydriatics have been used recently.

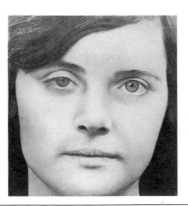

**Fig. 10.23**
Sympathetic nerve paralysis. The right sympathetic nerve was resected at operation (Mr J. B. Oldham). The corresponding eye shows ptosis, causing narrowing of the palpebral fissure, and myosis from unopposed action of the 3rd nerve.

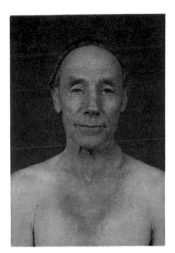

**Fig. 10.24**
Right Horner's syndrome due
to malignant lymph nodes in
the neck seen on both sides,
especially the left.

The pupils may be abnormally dilated (*mydriasis*) in conditions of sympathetic overactivity, e.g. hyperthyroidism and anxiety, or from the adhesions of iritis. They are contracted (*myosis*) in cerebrospinal syphilis, especially tabes, and in morphine poisoning.

*Inequality* in the size of the pupils in lesions of the 3rd nerve or sympathetic affecting one side only, and in diseases such as syphilis or iritis which may produce more advanced changes on one side.

*Irregularity* may result from the synechiae of iritis, but syphilis and encephalitis are sometimes responsible.

*Argyll Robertson pupil*: Argyll Robertson described the pupil in neurosyphilis as small, constant in size and unaltered by light or shade; contracts fully on convergence and dilates when effort to converge is relaxed. The pupils are also unequal, irregular in outline and eccentric, and the central part of the iris may be depigmented. The site of the lesion causing these changes in the pupil is probably in the pre-tectum of the midbrain behind the optic tract and 3rd-nerve nucleus. Diabetes is now a more common cause than tabes for pupillary changes of this kind ('diabetic pseudotabes').

*The myotonic pupil* is a rather rare condition which may erroneously suggest tabes, especially as the knee jerks or ankle jerks are sometimes absent. The abnormality is, however, usually unilateral, and the affected pupil is of normal size or dilated. The reaction to light is lost and that to accommodation sluggish. The condition is generally found in young women and is unexplained, but it is not associated with clinical or spinal-fluid signs of syphilis. It is also known as the Adie–Holmes syndrome.

*The pupil in cerebral injury*: Changes in the pupils provide important diagnostic and prognostic information after head injuries or cardiac arrest. Inequality of the pupils may indicate rising intracranial pressure due, for example, to an expanding haematoma. Dilated pupils unreactive to light for several minutes suggest that brain damage is irreversible and that further attempts to resuscitate the patient are unlikely to succeed.

## The 5th or trigeminal nerve

**Anatomical considerations** This nerve has motor and sensory roots. Both have their nuclei in the medulla oblongata. The sensory nucleus also makes connections with the medulla and spinal cord through the substantia gelatinosa. The motor and sensory roots emerge from different parts of the brain but come closer together as they approach the trigeminal ganglion on the petrous portion of the temporal bone. Into this ganglion the sensory root enters, but the motor portion lies beneath the ganglion and later joins the mandibular division of the 5th nerve.

From the trigeminal ganglion the three divisions of the 5th nerve emerge: (1) Ophthalmic; (2) Maxillary; (3) Mandibular. These divisions are responsible for reception of sensation from the greater part of the face, forehead, parietal and temporal regions, nasal and buccal mucosae and conjunctivae.

The mandibular division makes connections through the lingual and facial nerves with the chorda tympani, which is responsible for the sensation of taste in the anterior two-thirds of the tongue. Motor fibres innervate the muscles of mastication, of which the most important are the temporals, masseters and pterygoids.

**Examination** The sensory and motor functions of the nerve must be tested.

*Sensation* Sensation may be tested as elsewhere in the body by the use of cotton-wool and a pin over each area of the face and buccal mucosa supplied by the three divisions of the 5th nerve. A light wisp of cottonwool touching the cornea normally produces closure of the eye, but if there is anaesthesia of the cornea the reflex will be abolished. Loss of the corneal reflex may precede other signs of a trigeminal nerve lesion. If the 5th nerve has been paralysed for some time, serious effects may appear, especially ulceration of the cornea and dryness of the nasal and buccal mucous membrane, with anosmia and difficulty in chewing.

*Motor power* The position of the teeth should be noted to see if there is any deviation of the jaw. The temporal and masseter muscles should then be palpated while the patient clenches his teeth; any difference in the strength of contraction on the two sides is noted. The side-to-side movements (pterygoids) may be tested by asking the patient to move the jaws in a ruminating manner against the resistance of the observer's fingers. If the lesion is in the upper neuron the paresis is rarely marked owing to bilateral cortical innervation. The jaw jerk, scarcely detectable in health, is brisk when there is a bilateral upper neuron lesion above the level of the trigeminal motor nucleus. Wasting of the muscles of mastication will be present in lower neuron lesions of considerable standing, giving the face and temple on the affected side a hollowed-out appearance.

**Lesions** Pontine lesions (vascular and neoplastic) which involve the 5th nucleus produce pyramidal tract and other characteristic signs. Outside the pons the nerve may be involved by tumours at the base of the brain, especially in the cerebello-pontine angle, and more rarely the trigeminal ganglion or individual branches may be affected by tumours or neuropathies. Lesions of the upper cervical cord, such as syringomyelia, may involve the spinal prolongation of the trigeminal sensory nucleus to cause loss of facial sensation, especially over the forehead.

**Trigeminal neuralgia** This affection of the 5th nerve needs special consideration in view of its frequency. It is commoner in old age, especially in women. Any or all of the three sensory branches may be involved, and the patient complains of sudden severe lancinating pain over the distribution of the affected divisions. The attacks are often provoked by touch, cold or the movements of the face in eating or talking. The second and third divisions are usually primarily affected, but the first may follow. Localized tenderness is usually present over the same area, but there is never any sensory loss. Trigeminal neuralgia comes in attacks, at first short, but later of long duration. Long periods of freedom are common. The cause is unknown. It must be distinguished from other types of facial pain, e.g. those associated with dental and sinus disease, in which the classic paroxysms do not occur. A good history is imperative.

**Ophthalmic herpes** (*Fig.* 10.25) Herpes zoster commonly affects the first division of the trigeminal nerve and may result in severe and intractable pain, especially in older patients. Sensory loss and corneal ulceration may occur.

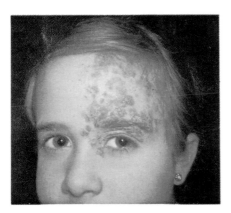

**Fig. 10.25**
Left ophthalmic herpes.

### The 7th or facial nerve

**Anatomical considerations** The facial nerve arises from its nucleus in the pons, where its fibres course around the nucleus of the 6th nerve. The nerve emerges in the cerebello-pontine angle in company with the 8th nerve. Both enter the internal (auditory) acoustic meatus, but later the 7th nerve leaves the 8th and runs in the facial canal to its point of exit at the stylomastoid foramen. Thereafter the nerve is distributed to the facial muscles, all of which it supplies except the levator palpebrae superioris (3rd nerve). In its course through the aqueduct the facial nerve gives off two branches which have localizing value: (1) the nerve to the stapedius; (2) the chorda tympani.

In cases of facial paralysis it is often possible, if these anatomical data are borne in mind, to determine fairly accurately the part of its course in which the nerve has been damaged. Simultaneous involvement of the 6th nerve is suggestive of a pontine lesion; concurrent affection of the 7th and 8th nerves is common in lesions at the cerebello-pontine angle; excessive response to sounds in one ear ('hyperacusis') indicates that the lesion has also affected the nerve to the stapedius in the aqueduct; and loss of taste over the anterior two-thirds of the tongue implies that the 7th nerve has been damaged in the aqueduct before the origin of the chorda tympani. In the commonest type of facial lesion, Bell's palsy, these collateral signs are not commonly present, as the nerve is affected either at or after it has left the stylomastoid foramen, or sometimes in its course through the temporal bone.

**Examination** The examination of the facial nerve is primarily designed to test the movements of the facial muscles. The patient should be asked in turn to show the teeth, puff out the cheeks, wrinkle the forehead by looking upwards and close the eyes (*see Fig.* 10.27).

Taste on each half of the anterior two-thirds of the tongue should be tested as described on p. 367, but the loss of taste is often more easily determined by questioning. Finally, note should be taken of any abnormal acuity of hearing on the affected side.

**Lesions** Facial paralysis results quite commonly from both upper and lower neuron lesions.

*Upper neuron paralysis* This only affects the muscles of the lower part of the face, as the occipito-frontalis and orbicularis oculi muscles are bilaterally innervated from the cortex (*Fig.* 10.26). Vascular lesions of the brain are commonly responsible, the paralysis occurring on the opposite side to the lesion (*see also* p. 402). The angle of the mouth droops, the paralysed cheek is puffed out loosely with each expiration. On the other hand, the forehead can be wrinkled normally and the eye closed (cf. lower neuron lesions).

*Lower neuron paralysis (Bell's palsy)* If the paralysis is complete the whole side of the face is smooth and free from wrinkles (*Figs.* 10.27, 10.28). The lower eyelid droops and the angle of the mouth sags. Saliva may dribble away from the mouth and tears flow over the lower lid. In attempting to look upwards or frown, the wrinkling on the normal side contrasts with the smoothness of the affected side. The patient is unable to close the eye, and also rolls it upwards in the attempt,

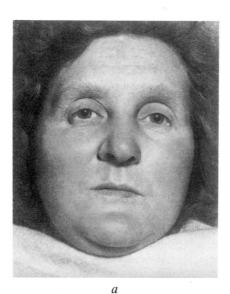 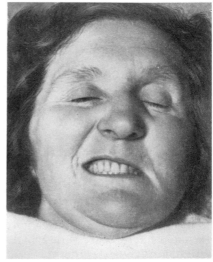

|       |       |
|-------|-------|
| *a*   | *b*   |

**Fig. 10.26** Upper neuron facial paralysis (left), *a*, Face at rest. *b*, Showing the teeth; note normal eye closure.

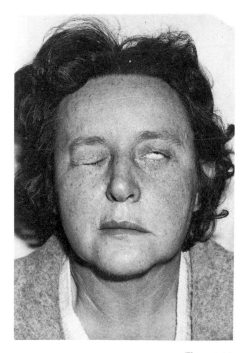

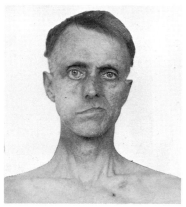

**Fig. 10.27**
Lower motor neuron facial paralysis (Bell's palsy) showing inability to close the left eyelids with upward rolling of the eye. Note also the drooping of the left angle of the mouth and loss of the nasolabial fold.

**Fig. 10.28**
Long-standing lower motor neuron lesion. Right facial paralysis with contractures.

due to the mechanical effect of the fibres of the levator palpebrae superioris, supplied from the 3rd nerve, which are partially inserted into the eyeball (*see Fig.* 10.27). The mouth cannot be moved so as to expose the teeth, and when the cheeks are puffed out the paralysed side balloons more than normal. Attention should be paid to complaint of alterations in taste or hearing in view of the anatomical connections of the 7th nerve.

If the paralysis does not improve quickly, conjunctival infections may result from inability to close the eye.

Although in Bell's palsy the cause is often unknown, it is usually associated with inflammation and compression of the nerve within the facial canal. Other causes include tumours of the pons or cerebello-pontine angle (*Fig.* 10.29), osteomyelitis of the petrous temporal bone due to chronic middle ear infection, parotid tumours and herpes zoster affecting the geniculate ganglion. This last condition may be associated with a herpetic eruption on the pinna of the ear (Ramsay–Hunt syndrome, *Fig.* 10.30).

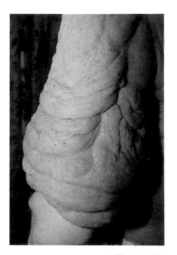

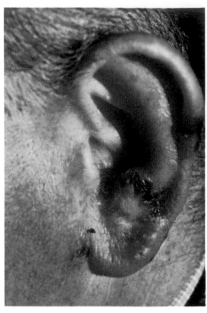

**Fig. 10.29**
Plexiform neurofibroma of the upper arm. This patient also has a cerebellopontine neurofibroma of the 8th cranial nerve.

**Fig. 10.30**
The Ramsay–Hunt syndrome. Geniculate herpes.

## The 8th or vestibulo-cochlear nerve

It is convenient under this heading to consider the functions and disturbances of the inner ear which contains three different organs: (1) The cochlea, the true organ of hearing; (2) The three semicircular canals, constituting the organ of dynamic equilibrium; (3) The two otolith organs, utricle and saccule, constituting the organ of static equilibrium.

*The cochlear nerve* carries impulses from the spiral ganglion in the modiolus of the cochlea via cochlear nuclei in the medulla and thence, via the lateral lemniscus and medial geniculate body, to the superior temporal gyrus of the opposite cerebral hemisphere.

*The vestibular nerve* conveys impulses from the organs of equilibrium and terminates in nuclei within the medulla which then communicate with the cerebellum and midbrain and, by the way of the vestibulo-spinal tract, with the spinal cord.

The two nerves run as a common trunk in close association with the 5th and 7th in the cerebello-pontine angle and are usually involved in pathological conditions affecting the region, e.g. cysts, acoustic neuromas and cerebellar abscesses.

**Disturbances of the cochlear system** These manifest themselves essentially with deafness and tinnitus.

**Deafness** The existence of significant hearing loss can easily be established by testing the patient's ability to hear a watch or a soft whisper. Each ear is tested separately, the other being firmly occluded by the finger. The tests should be carried out in a room free of distracting noise, and the examiner should know beforehand the distance at which a normal ear can hear his watch or his voice. A soft whisper whould normally be audible at about three feet.

**Tinnitus** This symptom is variously described by the patient as 'ringing', 'buzzing', 'hissing', 'singing' or other form of noise in the ear. It may precede deafness as a symptom of 8th-nerve disease. It is also common in ischaemia of the auditory apparatus due to anaemia, atheroma or postural hypotension and after high dosage of salicylates and quinine. It is most commonly present when the inner ear is actively deteriorating but can also occur in the course of middle ear disease. In some cases, fortunately rare, distressing tinnitus can be caused by disease in the central nervous system, and cases have been recorded in which even section of the 8th nerve has failed to suppress the sensation.

*Tuning-fork tests*: Tuning-forks emit pure tones and enable more accurate information to be obtained by comparison of AC (air-conditioned) hearing with BC (bone-conducted) hearing.

*Principles of tuning-fork tests*: In AC hearing the sound traverses the outer and middle ears to reach the cochlea where it stimulates the organ of Corti. In BC hearing the sound traverses the skull bones to reach the organ of Corti.

Thus pathological conditions in the outer and middle ear will reduce AC hearing but will have no effect on BC hearing, i.e. conductive deafness. Pathological conditions in the inner ear or central pathways will reduce both AC and BC hearing, i.e. perceptive deafness.

In other words, if BC is normal, the inner ear must be normal, but if BC is reduced, the inner ear or central pathways are at fault.

*Schwabach's* test is the simplest of all. The examiner, assumed for simplicity to have normal hearing, strikes the fork and places it on the subject's mastoid asking him to indicate when the sound becomes inaudible. The examiner then places the fork on his own mastoid. If he can still hear it, the patient's BC is reduced and the diagnosis is perceptive deafness.

*Rinne's* test compares the patient's AC hearing with his BC hearing. In the normal ear AC hearing is better than BC hearing (written AC>BC or Rinne positive). If a tuning-fork held on the mastoid until it is inaudible is then transferred to the external auditory meatus, it will be audible once more for a number of seconds. Let us assume for example that it is heard for 40 s on the mastoid and a further 10 s at the meatus. Now test a case of conductive deafness.

> BC remains normal at 40 s but
> AC will be reduced, say, to 30 s
> i.e. AC<BC=Rinne negative.

In such a case the fork obviously will be held at the meatus till inaudible and then placed on the mastoid when it will become audible once more. Lastly in perceptive deafness the hearing will be impaired by both routes since the devitalized neural mechanism is less responsive to sound by either route. If, for example, its efficiency is reduced by 50 per cent.

> AC becomes 25 s
> BC becomes 20 s
> i.e. AC>BC=Rinne positive (compare normal ear).

*Weber's test*: If a tuning-fork is placed in the midline of the skull, the sound reaches both inner ears by bone conduction (i.e. not by the normal route through the middle ears). Thus so long as the inner ear is normal (as in middle ear deafness) the sensation aroused by such a fork is unaffected. If, however, the inner ear is impaired the sensation evoked is also impaired. Now consider a patient with unilateral deafness. If the lesion is in the inner ear, the sensation is quieter on that side than on the normal side, i.e. the patient lateralizes to the healthy ear. But in unilateral conductive deafness the sensation from the deaf ear is just as great as from the normal ear and therefore the sound does not lateralize. Indeed, the sound may actually lateralize to the deaf ear because the conduction defect has excluded background noise. The student should test this observation for himself by occluding one external meatus and applying the tuning fork to the centre of his forehead. The sound will be louder on the side of the occlusion.

*Limitation of tuning-fork test*: The above tests often give valuable qualitative information but are unable to give quantitative estimates of auditory acuity. For the latter purpose the otologist now depends on the audiometer. A more serious weakness of tuning-fork tests is that bone-conducted vibrations reach all parts of the skull irrespective of where the fork is placed. Thus the examiner ostensibly testing BC on the right ear may obtain misleading answers because the patient will also be hearing with his left ear. In audiometry this error is obviated by masking the opposite ear, i.e. temporarily obtunding it with a special noise which blocks out the testing tone. For a full account of audiometry the student is referred to specialist textbooks on otology.

**Disturbances of the vestibular system** These include vertigo and nystagmus.

*Vertigo* Many conditions, including some of psychological origin, are associated with vague sensations of dizziness or light-headedness. True labyrinthine vertigo involves a sense of movement, usually rotation, in relation to the environment. In its most severe form, vertigo is accompanied by vomiting, pallor, sweating and an inability to remain upright. The spinning sensation is made worse by movement, and the patient usually lies motionless with the eyes tightly closed.

*Positional vertigo* is a transient feeling of dizziness when the head is placed in certain positions, especially dorsiflexion. This can be due to disorder of the otolith mechanism, but similar symptoms can result from vertebral artery compression (*see* p. 435).)

*Ménière's syndrome* is caused by pathological changes within the inner ear. Usually all three end-organs are affected to a greater or lesser degree. Thus: (*a*) The semicircular canals set up sensations of movement of varying severity as described above; (*b*) the cochlea disturbance reveals itself with tinnitus and deafness; (*c*) The otolith organs can produce vague sensations of muscle weakness (*see below*).

In a typical attack the patient complains of intense rotational dizziness, sweats, nausea and vomiting and may show nystagmus. The episode lasts for some hours and slowly subsides although some unsteadiness, deafness and tinnitus may persist for weeks and, in severe cases, may become permanent. Remissions last for months if not years.

*Nystagmus* Nystagmus, i.e. uncontrollable pendular movement of the eyes, can arise from: (1) Disturbance of visual function; (2) Disturbance of labyrinthine function; (3) Disturbance of the central nervous system.

In congenital blindness the eyes, lacking a focal point, oscillate aimlessly. Miner's nystagmus is not fully explained, but may have some connection with poor illumination. Optokinetic nystagmus is characteristically seen in railway passengers gazing at the passing scenery. The eyes fix on a certain point (e.g. a telegraph pole) and follow it until further fixation becomes impossible. They then rapidly jerk back to a new focal point and so the process continues.

Labyrinthine nystagmus is due to disturbance of the semicircular canals. As there are three sets of canals, in three planes in space, nystagmus can occur in three directions, i.e. horizontal, vertical and rotary. Characteristically, there is a slow component and a quick component.

Nystagmus of central origin occurs in lesions which involve the cerebellum and vestibular apparatus, or the pathways in the pons and medulla between these. The commoner neurological disorders include disseminated sclerosis, tumours and other lesions of the cerebellum, and more rarely tumours and syringomyelia affecting the pons or medulla, and Friedreich's ataxia.

Irrigation of the ear, either with hot water or with cold water, sets up convection currents in the endolymph of the semicircular canals and so produces nystagmus. A similar effect can be produced by rotating the patient in a special rotating chair. By evaluating the nystagmus under such controlled conditions of stimulation, useful information can be obtained, not only about the labyrinth but also about the vestibular tract in general. The absence of nystagmus when the ear is irrigated with cold water is one of the criteria used for the diagnosis of brain death.

For details of caloric and rotary tests otological textbooks should be consulted.

## The 9th or glossopharyngeal and 10th or vagus nerves

**Anatomical considerations** The glossopharyngeal and vagus nerves are usually considered and examined together owing to their close association. They arise in medullary nuclei and leave the base of the skull through the jugular foramina, where they are rarely damaged. Brainstem affections also tend to involve the vagal nuclei.

The 9th nerve carries taste fibres from the posterior third of the tongue and innervates certain of the muscles concerned in swallowing, but in its motor function the nerve overlaps with the vagus.

The 10th nerve has a wide distribution and constitutes an important part of the autonomic nervous system, carrying parasympathetic fibres to the heart, lungs and gastrointestinal tract. Special physiological tests are needed to examine the visceral functions of the vagus nerve, although some of its autonomic effects may be evident in such signs as bradycardia (vagal over-action) or diarrhoea (vagal suppression). Direct clinical examination of the vagus depends chiefly upon testing the function of the branches to the voluntary muscles of the pharynx, soft palate and larynx.

**Examination**   1. The sensation of taste is tested in suspected lesions of the 7th and 9th nerves. The anterior two-thirds of the tongue may show loss of taste sensation in 7th-nerve lesions, and the posterior third when the glossopharyngeal nerve is affected.

Substances that are sweet, salt, sour and bitter (sugar, salt, vinegar and quinine) should be used in turn by placing a little on one-half of the anterior two-thirds of the tongue. The patient should not speak, but write down what he tastes. A weak galvanic current is recognized as a metallic taste and is particularly useful in testing the posterior third (glossopharyngeal nerve).

2. Test the pharyngeal reflex by tickling each side of the pharynx with a wooden spatula. Unilateral abolition of the reflex only results from organic lesions. In these cases the pharynx will move like a curtain towards the normal side. Bilateral abolition of the palatal reflex is sometimes found in hysterical subjects.

3. Ask the patient to say 'Ah'. Normally the uvula moves backwards in the median plane, but in vagal paralysis it is deflected to the normal side.

4. Note any difficulty in deglutition or speaking. In vagal paralysis regurgitation of food through the nose and a nasal voice sometimes occur.

5. Hoarseness or aphonia calls for a laryngoscopic examination. The left recurrent laryngeal branch of the vagus may be damaged by mediastinal tumours, causing abductor paralysis.

The effects of a supranuclear lesion of the vagus are discussed under Pseudo-bulbar Paralysis (p. 405).

### The 11th or spinal accessory nerve

The spinal accessory nerve supplies the sternomastoid and trapezius muscles. It emerges from the skull through the jugular foramen, and has relations centrally with the 9th and 10th nerves.

**Examination** The patient should be asked to shrug his shoulders, when the trapezii come into action, and then to rotate the head against resistance, in which the sternomastoid of the opposite side is employed (*Figs.* 10.31–10.33). Sometimes in 11th-nerve paralysis the vertebral border of the scapula stands out, rather like the 'winged scapula' of serratus anterior paralysis.

### The 12th or hypoglossal nerve

The hypoglossal nucleus is in the medulla and in intimate contact

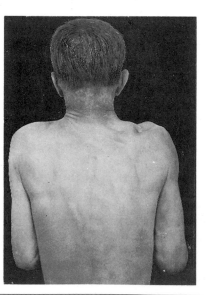

**Fig. 10.31**
Paresis of the right trapezius in 11th-nerve paralysis. The patient is shrugging the shoulders: the left moves upwards normally, but not the right: there is also wasting of other muscles of the shoulder-girdle.

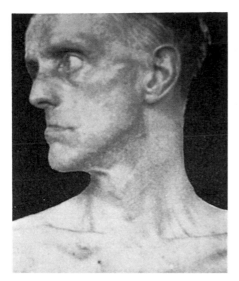 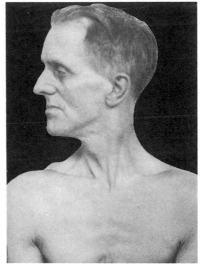

**Fig. 10.32**
Paresis of left sternomastoid due to 11th-nerve paralysis. The patient is turning his head to the right but the sternomastoid does not stand out as it should. (Cf *Fig. 10.34.*)

**Fig. 10.33**
Control. No paresis of the left sternomastoid, the belly of which stands out well on movement of the head to the right.

with the nuclei of the 7th nerve which control the orbicularis oris. Paralysis of the tongue and of the lips are therefore often found together in medullary lesions, e.g. progressive bulbar paralysis. The 12th nerve leaves the skull by the hypoglossal canal foramen and is subject to injury in its subsequent course in the neck.
**Examination** The patient should be asked to protrude the tongue. In lower neuron paralysis the affected side is wasted, wrinkled and may display fasciculation (*Fig.* 10.34). The tongue deviates to the affected side as in cases of facial paralysis, but in the latter the deviation can be rectified by straightening the corner of the mouth with the fingers. Dysarthria is often present. More commonly, as in motor neuron disease, there is bilateral involvement of the tongue. Abnormality can then be detected by noting crenation of the edges of the tongue and generalized fasciculation; the latter should be looked for when the tongue is at rest within the mouth. In supranuclear lesions of the 12th nerve the tongue may be small and immobile, resulting in dysphagia and dysarthria (*see also* p. 407).

■　　**THE MOTOR SYSTEM**

### ANATOMICAL AND PHYSIOLOGICAL CONSIDERATIONS

The neurons responsible for voluntary motor action run in two relays. The first extends from the cortical cells in the motor area, which is found

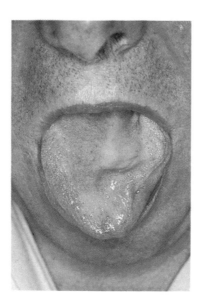

**Fig. 10.34**
Left hypoglossal palsy
showing atrophy of the
tongue and its deviation to
the left.

in the precentral gyrus, and is distributed to cranial nerve nuclei and to different parts of the spinal cord, there to terminate with internuncial neurons in the grey matter of the ventral horns. These in turn synapse with the anterior horn cells which give rise to the roots of the nerves supplying voluntary muscles. To the first relay the name *upper motor neuron* is given; to the second *lower motor neuron* (*Fig.* 10.35).

All forms of organic paralysis, except those due to uncommon primary muscular disorders and mechanical fixation from bone, joint or muscle disease, are due to an interruption in one of these neurons. The clinical signs are similar in every upper neuron lesion and again in every lesion of the lower neuron, but the contrast between the physical signs of upper and lower motor neuron affections is so pronounced that the examiner is at once able to localize the lesion to one or the other. The differences in these signs are indicated in *Table* 10.1 on p. 372.

### The upper motor neuron

The upper motor neuron starts in the precentral gyrus (area 4) in groups of cells which control movements rather than individual muscles. These cells are arranged in a fashion which has been proved experimentally and is shown on the accompaning diagram (*Fig.* 10.36). It will be observed that the motor area covers a considerable region of the cortex, and it follows that a small lesion may pick out only a small part of the motor area, e.g. that governing movements of the hand, and lead to a strictly limited paralysis.

From these cortical cells, projection fibres known as the *corticospinal (pyramidal) tract* pass through the substance of the brain in the *corona radiata*, converging towards the *internal capsule*, where they are densely packed. The result of quite a small lesion in this region will be an extensive paralysis—usually the face, arm and leg on the contralateral side. The position of the fibres in the anterior two-

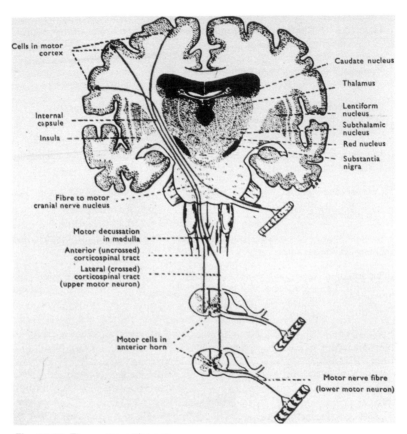

**Fig. 10.35** The motor pathways.

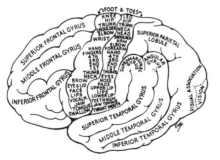

**Fig. 10.36**
Surface of cerebrum showing localization of function. (*See also Fig.* 10.37.)

thirds of the posterior limb and in the genu of the internal capsule is shown in *Fig.* 10.38. The relative position of the motor fibres for different parts of the body is not the same as in the motor cortex. (Cf. *Figs.* 10.36, 10.37.)

Sensory fibres and visual paths in the capsule may be involved simultaneously with the motor fibres but lie more posteriorly.

Table 10.1    **Clinical distinction between upper and lower motor neuron lesions**

| Upper neuron | Lower neuron |
| --- | --- |
| Paralysis affects movements rather than muscles | Individual muscles or groups of muscles affected |
| Wasting only from disuse, therefore slight. Occasionally marked in chronic severe lesions | Wasting pronounced |
| Spasticity of 'clasp-knife' type. Muscles hypertonic | Flaccidity. Muscles hypotonic |
| Cyanosis and oedema may result from disuse; no gross trophic changes (except in infantile hemiplegia) | Skin often cold, blue and shiny. Ulceration may result |
| Tendon reflexes increased (see pp. 388–400). Clonus often present | Tendon reflexes diminished or absent |
| Superficial reflexes diminished or modified (see p. 396). Note especially absent abdominal reflexes, Babinski and Hoffmann signs, and increased jaw jerk | Superficial reflexes often unaltered unless sensation is also lost or when appropriate LMN is interrupted |
| Associated movements sometimes present (see p. 382) | No associated movements. Fasciculations and myotatic irritability often present |

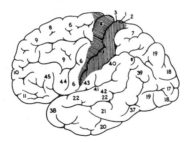 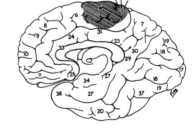

**Fig. 10.37** Brodman's areas.

From the internal capsule the fibres pass through the *crus* and *pons* to the *medulla (oblongata)*, where the bulk of them decussate and travel down the lateral columns of the *spinal cord* as the crossed corticospinal tract. The few fibres which do not decussate, but form the uncrossed corticopinal tract, have little clinical importance.

In the brainstem some of the fibres terminate in relationship with the neclei of the cranial nerves. They form the upper neurons of these nerves, the lower neurons starting from each cranial nerve nucleus.

As in the internal capsule, the dense aggregation of corticospinal tract fibres in the crus, pons and medulla renders a lesion in these parts unusually disastrous in

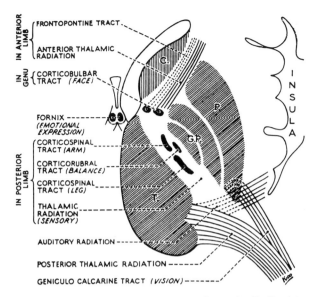

FRONTOPONTINE TRACT

IN ANTERIOR LIMB

ANTERIOR THALAMIC RADIATION

IN GENU

CORTICOBULBAR TRACT *(FACE)*

FORNIX *(EMOTIONAL EXPRESSION)*

CORTICOSPINAL TRACT *(ARM)*

IN POSTERIOR LIMB

CORTICORUBRAL TRACT *(BALANCE)*

CORTICOSPINAL TRACT *(LEG)*

THALAMIC RADIATION *(SENSORY)*

AUDITORY RADIATION

POSTERIOR THALAMIC RADIATION

GENICULO CALCARINE TRACT *(VISION)*

I N S U L A

**Fig. 10.38** Horizontal section of internal capsule. C., Caudate nucleus; T., Thalamus; P., Putamen; G.P., Globus pallidus of lentiform nucleus.

its results. Paralysis is often extensive and bilateral, and other brainstem structures (sensory fibres, cranial nerve nuclei, etc.) may be damaged.

The fibres of the corticospinal tracts pass along the spinal cord for a varying distance, some ending in the upper and some in the lower segments of the cord in close proximity to the anterior horn cells. Between the terminations of the corticospinal fibres and the anterior horn cells there appear to be short internuncial neurons.

The results of corticospinal tract destruction will vary with the level at which the tract is interrupted: for example, if in the cervical regions, both arms and legs will be paralysed; if in the lower thoracic regions, only the legs. Certain movements, notably of the upper part of the face, the jaw and the larynx, are bilaterally represented in the cortex and are therefore little affected by unilateral lesions of the corticospinal system. Bilateral lesions may cause dysarthria and dysphagia (*see* p. 71). In the parietal lobes centres also exist which exercise the highest control over motor power, namely, the will to movement. Sometimes movements are performed without the patient realizing it, which indicates that the pyramidal system is intact, yet if the patient consciously wishes to make the same movements he is unable to do so. For example, a patient without paralysis of the hand may be unable to take a match from a box and strike it. This is known as *motor apraxia*.

### The lower motor neuron

From the anterior horn cells, fibres pass out as the anterior nerve roots to become eventually the peripheral nerves, in many of which sensory fibres are present. The motor fibres end in the voluntary muscles. This lower neuron may be interrupted by lesions in the anterior horns, in the nerve roots, in the peripheral nerves, or at the termination in the muscle (motor end-plate). The results will differ in the distribution of the paralysis, and the effects of a lesion of the anterior horn cells or nerve roots will be entirely motor; in peripheral nerve damage sensory changes often occur as well.

The lower motor neuron is influenced by the upper neuron and also by the extrapyramidal system, and modifications of muscle tone and reflexes result when the correct balance between these neurons is lost (*see* Distinctions between Upper and Lower Neuron Lesions, *below*). The trophic changes often found in diseases chiefly affecting the lower neuron are due mainly to associated damage to the sensory and autonomic systems.

### The extrapyramidal system

Much obscurity still exists concerning the exact connections and functions of this system. It includes the striospinal fibres from the striatum and subthalamic nuclei, the vestibulospinal tract descending from the vestibular nucleus, the rubrospinal tract from the red nucleus, the tectospinal tract from the midbrain and the reticulospinal tract from the reticular formation of the brain-stem. These tracts bring the anterior horn cells of the spinal cord under the influence of the cerebellum and subcortical nuclei.

Lesions involving the extrapyramidal system do not result in paralysis comparable with those of the corticospinal tracts, but some degree of weakness is common. More important is the interference with that delicate precision which characterizes perfect movement. Such interference is manifested in abnormal muscle tone or posture, inco-ordination and tremors (*see* p. 412).

Both the extrapyramidal and cerebellar systems exert considerable influence on posture by the part they play in regulating muscle tone.

### The cerebellum

This part of the brain lies closely packed below the tentorium in intimate contact with the pons and medulla and the cranial nerves which take origin in the neighbourhood. It is not surprising, therefore, that lesions of the cerebellum are frequently accompanied by signs of involvement of these neighbouring structures.

The cerebellum has elaborate connections with other parts of the nervous system, notably with the vestibular nerve, the cerebral cortex and pons, and the spinal cord. These connections make the explanation of cerebellar symptoms complex, but, in general, muscular co-ordination depends upon the connections of the cerebellum with the higher parts of brain, while tone and equilibrium are more particularly associated with its connections with the lower parts. Modern work tends to assign disturbances of equilibrium to the flocculo-nodular lobe, while hypotonia and disorders of movement appear to be related to the neo-cerebellum.

## SYMPTOMS OF DISEASE OF THE MOTOR SYSTEM

The chief symptoms of motor system disease are weakness, stiffness, unsteadiness and tremor.

### Weakness

The patient may complain merely of weakness in a limb or other part of the body. To this the name *paresis* is given. When the part is immovable or nearly so the term *paralysis* is applied. A paralysis affecting one side of the body is known as *hemiplegia*; if it is confined to one limb, *monoplegia*; if it affects both legs, *paraplegia*; or both arms and both legs, either *tetraplegia* or *quadriplegia*. Paralysis is as obvious to the patient as to the doctor; paresis may only be discovered on examination.

In upper neuron lesions paralysis is, to some extent, selective. The limbs are affected more than the trunk, and smaller and more precise movements of the hands are usually interfered with more than the grosser movements, e.g. of the shoulders (*Fig.* 10.39). In the lower limb dorsiflexion of the toes and feet is usually affected and also flexion at the knee and elbow, while extension at the knee and hip is little affected.

Paralysis arising from the lower neuron lesions affects individual muscles or groups of muscles controlled by particular segments of the cord. Knowledge of the segmental control is of localizing value, e.g. in spinal cord compression, and the table indicates the motor distribution of the main spinal segments. (*Table* 10.2.)

| Table 10.2 | **Principal segmental representation of muscles** |
|---|---|
| C4<br>Scaleni, trapezius, levator scapulae, diaphragm | Th5 to 11<br>Abdominal muscles |
| C5<br>Levator scapulae, scaleni, supraspinatus, rhomboids, infraspinatus, teres minor, biceps, brachioradialis, deltoid, supinator longus, serratus anterior, pectoralis major (clavicular part) | L1<br>Quadratus lumborum<br><br>L3<br>Sartorius, adductors of hip, iliopsoas |
| C6<br>Subscapularis, pronators, teres major, latissimus dorsi, serratus anterior, pectoralis major | L4<br>Quadriceps femoris, abductors of hip<br><br>L5<br>Flexors of knee |
| C7<br>Triceps, extensors and flexors of wrist and digits | S1<br>Calf muscles<br><br>S2<br>Small foot muscles |
| C8<br>Small hand muscles | S3, 4<br>Pelvic muscles |
| Th1<br>Interossei and small hand muscles | |
| Th1 to 10<br>Intercostals | |

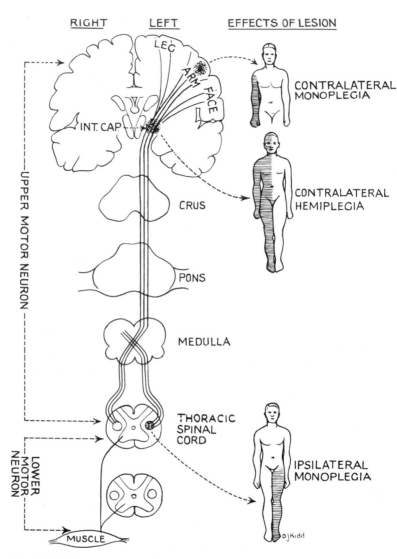

**Fig. 10.39** Diagram to show the extent of the upper and lower motor neurons and the effects of a lesion in different parts of the motor system. Only the common positions for a lesion have been illustrated.

## Stiffness

Stiffness in one or more limbs may be due to spasticity from interruption of the corticospinal tract. The rigidity of extrapyramidal disease is more generalized and may lead to a painful stiffness of the neck and trunk muscles as well as the limbs. Dysphagia and dysarthria may also occur in extrapyramidal or bilateral pyramidal lesions.

### Unsteadiness

Patients with cerebellar dysfunction will complain of loss of balance with a tendency to fall towards the side of the lesion. They may feel unable to control the movements of their hands for everyday purposes such as writing, shaving and eating. They may also notice inco-ordination of speech.

### Tremor (*see also* p. 381)

A persistent rhythmic tremor can be one of the most disabling symptoms of extrapyramidal disease; the patient may find that the tremor is influenced by emotion. The action or intention tremor of cerebellar origin occurs mainly when a movement is attempted so that the patient's purpose is frustrated. The clonic tremor of pyramidal disease usually affects the lower limb and tends to occur when the foot is held in certain positions.

## PHYSICAL SIGNS OF DISEASE OF THE MOTOR SYSTEM

The prime function of the motor system is to permit precise and well-ordered voluntary movements of the muscles. The examinaton of the motor system is firstly concerned, therefore, with testing this movement. Many incidental observations are made, however, which have a direct or indirect bearing on the integrity of the motor neurons. Briefly these fall under the following headings: trophic changes, atrophy or hypertrophy of muscles; fasciculations and myotatic irritability; contractions and contractures; involuntary movements; abnormal postures and gaits. Inspection is the chief method by which these physical signs are elicited, and they are often noted before muscular power and tone are tested. In the interpretation of these abnormal signs, the integrity of the sensory system and reflex arcs must be taken into account (*see below*), but the signs are more conveniently described in the present section.

### Trophic changes

The colour, temperature and texture of the skin should be recorded and any oedema or ulceration noted.

Such changes may result from neurological disease which causes sensory loss, e.g. peripheral neuropathy and syringomyelia, from disturbances of the autonomic nervous system and sometimes from disuse.

### Atrophy and hypertrophy

The contour and size of the muscles should be noted.

*Atrophy* is a characteristic of lower motor neuron lesions (*Figs.* 10.40–10.42), but also occurs in the myopathies (p. 410) and to a lesser extent from disuse, especially in rheumatoid arthritis. The limb loses its normal rounded contour.

For accuracy the circumference should be measured and compared with the normal side. Each limb must be measured at the same level. In the case of the legs, for example, the measurement may be made 15 cm below the lower border of the patella with the limbs extended. The distribution of the atrophy helps in diagnosis, tending to be distal in neuron disease and proximal in certain myopathies.

*Hypertrophy* is more difficult to recognize. Slight grades may result from

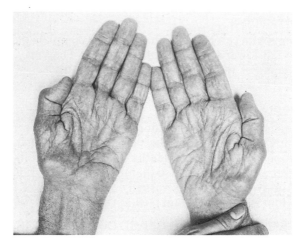

**Fig. 10.40** Wasting of the small muscles of the hand. From a case of progressive muscular atrophy. Note especially the flattened thenar eminences.

**Fig. 10.42** Muscular dystrophy. Shows atrophy of thigh muscles and apparent hypertrophy of calf muscles.

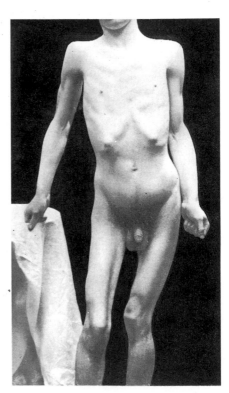

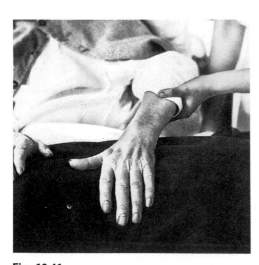

**Fig. 10.41** Wasting of interosseous muscles. Case of progressive muscular atrophy.

increased occupational use of certain groups of muscles, or occasionally as a developmental defect. Without such cause, the presence of apparent muscular hypertrophy usually suggests muscular dystrophies. In the pseudohypertrophic form of muscular paralysis the relatively great calves and buttocks stand out in marked contrast with the atrophic flexor muscles of the thighs.

### Fasciculations and muscular irritability

Fasciculations are not uncommonly seen in chronic degenerative lesions of the anterior horn cells, particularly progressive muscular atrophy and amyotrophic lateral sclerosis and other lesions of the lower neurons. They may be provoked by tapping. The muscle fibres produce a quivering of the skin by their slow irregular contractions. The muscles affected are usually those which are seriously wasted, but fasciculation can be an important early sign of motor neuron disease. Fasciculations may occur even in health and should not be regarded as pathological unless the patient is warm and relaxed, for shivering from any cause may give rise to similar movements. Nor should they be confused with *myokymia*, a familiar and harmless phenomenon in which there is twitching of the orbicularis oculi or less commonly other muscles ('live flesh'). Wasting muscles as in lower neuron lesions are often irritable and contractions can be produced easily by a light tap.

### Contractions and contractures

When a group of muscles is paralysed the action of unopposed groups causes the limb to assume an abnormal position. This happens by virtue of *muscular contraction*. In time fibrotic changes take place in the paralysed muscles and their tendons, resulting in true contractures (*Fig.* 10.43), which are of a permanent and progressive nature. The effects of contraction (*see* Muscle Tone—Rigidity, p. 388) can be overcome by passive movement, but this is not possible with contractures unless considerable force is used.

In upper neuron lesions affecting the corticospinal tracts alone, e.g. cerebral hemiplegia and spinal paraplegia, the limbs are in an extended position; but if

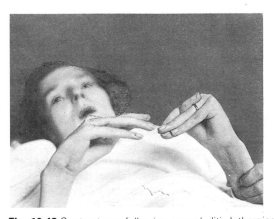

**Fig. 10.43** Contractures following encephalitis lethargica.

the lesion also involves the extrapyramidal tracts below the vestibular nucleus, an attitude of flexion in the limbs results. *Paraplegia in flexion* is thus indicative of a more severe lesion of the spinal cord than *paraplegia in extension*.

The attitude resulting from these types of paralysis may become permanent if contractures are allowed to ensue.

## Involuntary movements

If movements of the limbs, face or trunk are observed, their exact distribution and type must be recorded. Factors aggravating or diminishing the movements should also be noted, especially the effect of voluntary movement, sleep and emotion.

**Choreiform movements** Choreiform movements are irregular and spontaneous. They are quick and apparently purposeless and may occur anywhere in the body. Emotion and voluntary effort usually increase them, but during sleep they disappear.

They are seen in *rheumatic chorea* (Sydenham's chorea), popularly but incorrectly called 'St Vitus's dance', a disease which has now become uncommon. Children are most frequently affected, and the involuntary movements cause the child to drop things and to 'pull faces'. Chorea frequently affects one side of the body more than the other, hemichorea. Weakness of the affected side is common, and may be so extreme as to be called 'paralytic chorea'. Particular signs such as the jack-in-the-box tongue, a rapid protrusion and withdrawal of the tongue, depend upon the inability to perform sustained voluntary movements. The syndrome of chorea is in all probability attributable to lesions in the extrapyramidal system though possibly cortical.

In *Huntington's chorea* similar involuntary movements are seen, but as this disease is familial and occurs in the fourth and fifth decades and is associated with progressive dementia, no difficulty is found in distinguishing it from rheumatic chorea. Moreover the movements are slower. Unlike the movements of rheumatic chorea they are probably a release symptom due to a lesion of the basal ganglia.

**Athetosis** In cases of hemiplegia of long duration, especially infantile hemiplegia, peculiar slow 'snake-charming' movements may be seen, known as 'athetosis'. They chiefly affect the hands and consist of alternate flexion and extension at the wrists and fingers, with spreading of the latter.

Athetosis is only seen when some degree of voluntary movement is retained by the paralysed limb. Occasionally the movements occur in the feet (hyperextension of the big toe), and great facial contortion may result if the affection is bilateral. The phenomenon is thought to arise from a lesion in the extrapyramidal system and its cortical connections and is sometimes found without upper neuron signs. It is in the nature of a release symptom.

**Habit-spasms and tics** Some difficulty may be experienced by the junior student in distinguishing choreiform movements from the more purposive movements seen in habit-spasms and tics. These are of many different types. Some are very simple, such as shrugging the shoulders or blinking the eyes; others are highly complex, affecting many groups of muscles and perhaps associated with verbal abnormalities such as the frequent uncontrollable repetition of the same word or sentence. A more common and special form is a stammer.

The most important point of distinction from chorea is the repetition of the same movements, though a new movement may replace an old one. The movements may go on for much longer than chorea, e.g. months, without much variation in intensity. Habit-spasms and tics have a psychogenic origin. The patient often has an unstable personality, but some physical cause may originally sow the seed of a habit. Disease of the eyelids may, for example, cause blepharospasm, which normally passes away when the local cause is cured, but may persist in the psychoneurotic patient.

**Tremors** Tremors are shaking movements, fine or coarse, which are usually most evident in the hands but may affect the head ('titubation') or other parts of the body.

Tremors of *metabolic* origin may be fine, as in hyperthyroidism (*see* Chapter 11), or irregularly coarse or flapping as in hepatic, renal and respiratory failure (*see* Chapters 4, 5 and 6). Fine or coarse tremors may also be seen in certain *toxic* states such as alcoholism. If the patient is asked to extend the arms, the tremor can be felt by touching the fingers lightly or seen by using the technique shown in *Fig.* 10.44. Flapping tremors are brought out by full extension of the wrists when the arms are outstretched.

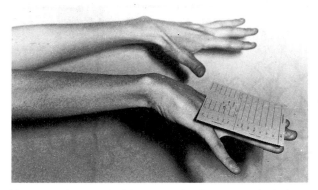

**Fig. 10.44** A method of demonstrating fine tremors by laying a thin piece of cardboard on the outstretched hand.

Tremors of *neurological* origin are of three kinds: essential, static and action. *Essential* tremors are common in adults and, although possibly congenital, they tend to increase with age and are aggravated by emotional tension. The tremors are fine, mainly affecting the hands and head. *Static* tremors are those which are relatively independent of movement or posture. The classic example is the rhythmic 3–5 per second coarse tremor of Parkinsonism which often first affects the index finger and thumb of one hand ('pill-rolling') but may later spread to involve the whole body. *Action* tremors are usually evident only on voluntary movement and are characteristic of cerebellar dysfunction (intention tremor). The usual way of eliciting this tremor is to ask the patient to touch the tip of the nose accurately with the tip of the index finger when the excursion of the involuntary movement will increase as the finger approaches the nose (*see Fig.* 10.64, p. 401). Another form of action tremor is the clonic tremor of a pyramidal tract lesion. Although this may occur spontaneously, it is usually provoked by dorsiflexion of the foot when the patient puts his toes on the ground.

**Associated movements** These are sometimes noticed in upper motor neuron lesions with severe spasticity, though they may occur in intact persons. They are reflexes, similar to those observed in decerebrate animals, and are really changes in posture rather than movements. For example, when an attempt is made to raise one leg while the patient is recumbent, the other leg is firmly pressed against the bed. This can be noted by the observer placing his hand between the heel and the bed. In hemiplegia of organic origin the pressure against the hand increases, but in functional paralysis it is not so great as normally.

**Convulsive movements** These are described on p. 439.

A rarer type is *myoclonus* (sudden shock-like contractions) see in many neurological disorders, e.g. encephalopathies, epilepsy and in toxaemias such as uraemia. A physiological example is hiccup.

## Abnormal postures

The posture of the patient, both erect and recumbent, must be observed when possible. Abnormal postures may be observed when the proper control of muscular tone and movement is affected. Lesions of the motor neurons—upper, lower and extrapyramidal—and of those tracts such as the posterior columns and cerebellar tracts which convey proprioceptive sensations may each result in altered posture.

**Upper neuron lesions** In hemiplegia the paralysed arm is adducted, the fingers and wrist flexed, and the forearm pronated. The hip also is adducted, the knee extended and the foot often inverted and plantar flexed. (*See Fig.* 10.66.)

Mention has already been made of the two types of paraplegia—in extension and in flexion—according as to whether the corticospinal tracts are affected alone or with the extrapyramidal tracts.

**Lower neuron lesions** These include lesions of the anterior horn cells, nerve roots and peripheral nerves. They cause different types of posture dependent upon the groups of muscles paralysed. The posture will result at first chiefly from unopposed action of antagonistic groups of muscles, but later the contractures in the paralysed muscles may overcome this and cause a more permanent abnormal attitude of the limb.

Thus a lesion which picks out the extensor muscles of the wrist will result in the familiar 'wrist drop', seen in certain cases of peripheral neuropathy or lesions of the radial nerve. (*See also* Erb–Duchenne paralysis, p. 408.) Other examples include the posture of the hand in ulnar and median nerve paralysis and in progressive muscular atrophy (*Fig.* 10.45) and the result of paralysis of the long thoracic nerve (winged scapula, *Fig.* 10.46).

**Extrapyramidal system** Lesions may result in Parkinsonism and cause an increase of tone in the flexor muscles in particular, and the result is an attitude of flexion (*Fig.* 10.47). The patient stands with the knees slightly bent, the shoulders drooping and the chin sunk into the chest. The arms are partially flexed at the elbows and the hands at the metacarpophalangeal joints; but extension occurs at the wrists and interphalangeal joints. The rigidity of the facial muscles is responsible for the vacant expression (*Fig.* 10.76).

**Lesions of sensory and cerebellar systems** An example of the former is *tabes dorsalis* (affecting the posterior columns, *see* p. 427) which leads to loss of tone in the muscles and sometimes modifies the posture. In tabes the hypotonus may

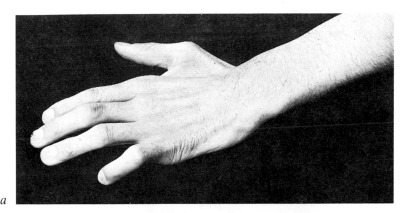

*a*

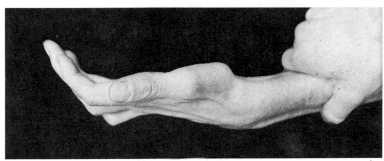

*b*

**Fig. 10.45** *a*, Claw hand (*main-en-griffe*) from a case of
progressive muscular atrophy. Showing the wasting of the
interosseous muscles.
*b*, Another view of the same hand.

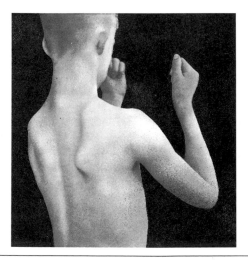

**Fig. 10.46**
Winged scapula from serratus
anterior paralysis.

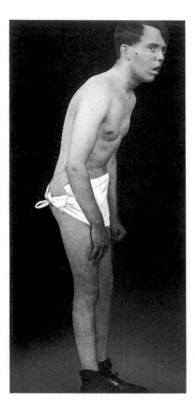

**Fig. 10.47**
Postencephalitic state
(Parkinsonism). The attitude is
one of flexion, especially
marked in this case at the
hips.

result in abnormal extension at the knee joints—genu recurvatum. To preserve balance the patient stands with the feet well apart. Cerebellar lesions have a similar effect.

**Abnormal postures at rest** Even when the patient is confined to bed, suggestive postures may be discovered. The retraction of the head and arching of the back (opisthotonos) are valuable signs of meningeal irritation; deviation of the head and eyes to one side is often seen in cerebral haemorrhage.

All forms of bizarre postures may be assumed in *hysteria*; they have the distinguishing characteristic that they cannot be explained on an anatomical or physiological basis.

### Gaits (*Table* 10.3)

The study of the gait is complementary to that of the posture in a neurological case.

The patient should be asked to walk across the floor with the legs uncovered and unhampered by clothes.

*Spastic* gaits are probably the commonest abnormal type. They result from upper motor neuron lesions such as hemiplegia and paraplegia.

In *hemiplegia* the affected limb is stiff and extended with the foot plantar-flexed. To avoid catching the toe against the ground at each step, the limb is sometimes circumducted in the arc of a circle (*Fig.* 10.48).

| Table 10.3 | **Abnormal gaits** | |
|---|---|---|
| *Descriptive Term* | *Explanation* | *Site of Lesion* |
| Spastic (arm still) | Increased tone Circumduction | Upper motor neurone |
| Scissors | Bilateral adduction and contractures | Bilateral upper motor neurone |
| Wide based ataxia | Hypotonia | Post columns |
| Drunken ataxia | Hypotonia and inco-ordination | Cerebellum and connections |
| Festinating (arm still) | Hypertonicity Bradykinesia | Extrapyramidal |
| High stepping | Foot drop | Peripheral neuropathy Poliomyelitis Progressive muscular atrophy |
| Waddling | Hip muscle weakness | Muscular dystrophy Hip damage |
| Limping | Short or painful leg | Leg or foot |
| Astasia-abasia | Cannot stand or walk | Hysteria |

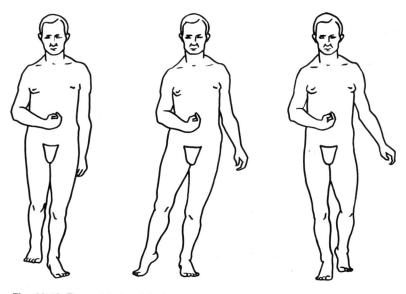

**Fig. 10.48** The gait in hemiplegia.

The 'scissors' gait of *diplegia* results from contractures in the adductors of the thighs and is rarely seen save in the cerebral diplegia of children (Little's disease). The legs cross in the act of walking (*Fig.* 10.49).

Various types of *paraplegia* resulting from spinal cord compression, disseminated sclerosis, etc. cause bilateral stiffness of the legs and plantar flexion of the feet so that the patient walks on the toes.

Lesions involving the posterior columns and cerebellum cause *ataxia*, i.e. an unsteady, uncontrolled gait.

In *tabes* the hypotonia necessitates 'taking in the slack' in the muscles before these can be used effectively. The patient in walking, therefore, picks his feet well off the ground and then slams them down unnecessarily hard.

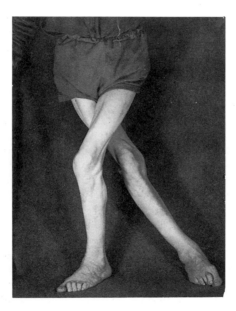

**Fig. 10.49**
Congenital cerebral diplegia. Cross-legged progression. 'Scissors' gait.

A somewhat similar gait results from other posterior column lesions, as in subacute combined degeneration and occasionally disseminated sclerosis, though in these two diseases the spasticity resulting from corticospinal tract involvement may mask the ataxia. In Friedreich's ataxia the disorder of gait is due to involvement of the cerebellar tracts and posterior columns.

The ataxia of *cerebellar disease* (tumours, vascular lesions, etc.) is shown by a characteristic reeling or 'drunken man's' gait with a special tendency to fall to one side, usually to the side of the lesion owing to the loss of muscle tone on that side. Sometimes the affected arm does not swing as the patient walks, and in some cases there is a lack of co-ordination between the trunk and limbs.

The gait in *extrapyramidal lesions* (Parkinsonism) is stiff, and the short steps taken by the patient give a quick shuffling appearance, a phenomenon known as *festination*. In classic cases, if pushed gently forwards, the patient appears 'to hurry after his centre of gravity' (*propulsion*). If pushed backwards he continues in the same direction until he falls or is stopped (*retropulsion*). Lateropulsion is a similar movement sideways, more rarely seen. As in cerebellar disease, the arms do not swing freely.

Another characteristic of the gait in Parkinsonism is that, on being asked to walk away and then turn round, the patient carries out a 'military' turn in three or four steps instead of swinging around on the ball of the foot.

*Peripheral neuropathy* commonly leads to foot-drop as a result of peroneal muscle weakness. The patient adopts a characteristic *high steppage* gait to avoid dragging the toes along the ground.

When pain is produced by weight-bearing the patient puts the foot down carefully and takes a short step to remove the weight off the painful limb as soon as possible. A *limping gait* may also be associated with a short leg or a deformed foot.

Other special types of gait, less frequently observed, are the *waddling gait* of muscular dystrophies caused by weakness of the glutei, also seen in congenital dislocation of the hips, and the contorted gait of Huntington's chorea.

Hysteria may also produce many peculiarities of gait. One special, though uncommon form, generally seen in children, is known as *astasia-abasia*, an inability to stand or walk.

Lastly it is necessary in suspected *myopathies* to watch the way in which the patient rises from the recumbent to the erect posture. In the Duchenne type of muscular dystrophy this is highly characteristic. The patient rolls over, gets on to his hands and knees and takes the weight of the body with the hands while he extends the knees. He then levels the trunk upright with the hands placed on the thighs. Occasionally paralysis of the extensor muscles of the thighs – e.g. from anterior poliomyelitis – has a similar result.

### Motor power

When the preliminary observations have been made the examiner proceeds to test the muscular strength of the limbs and trunk. If there is obvious paralysis it is merely necessary to determine the distribution and degree of this. When slight weakness of a limb is the complaint, and also when other neurological symptoms are present without subjective weakness, the examination of motor function must be systematic.

At each important joint the action of the extensors and flexors, abductors and adductors, pronators and supinators, etc. must be tested without any load and then against the resistance of the physician's hand and compared with the same muscles in the opposite limb. Movements of head and trunk (flexion, extension and rotation) must be similarly tested. The hand grip is important but allowance must be made for the normal variation in power according to handedness. Attention must also be given to the patient's ability to perform more complex but everyday movements such as buttoning a coat or combing the hair. Loss of skilled movements may be an important early sign of an upper motor neuron lesion. *Bradykinesia*, a slowness in initiating and maintaining movement, is seen especially in Parkinsonism.

The importance of the distribution of muscular weakness has already received attention in the discussion of the anatomy of the motor system. To recapitulate: in cerebral lesions the paralysis is usually of one or more limbs, or of large groups of muscles such as those controlling the movements of the hands. In spinal disease affecting the tracts, groups of muscles are put out of action corresponding with the level of the lesion. In lower neuron lesions muscular paralysis may also be extensive, as in anterior poliomyelitis; but more commonly the paralysis is localized to smaller groups of muscles according to the segment of the cord, nerve roots or nerves affected. The distribution of the paralysis has considerable localizing value but must be considered in conjunction with sensory changes and those signs which distinguish upper from lower neuron lesions (*see* table on p. 372).

### Muscle tone

The muscle spindles probably act as stretch receptors and help to maintain basic tone in the muscles which can be diminished by destruction of any part of the reflex arc or increased by interference with the descending extrapyramidal pathways which exert an inhibitory effect on the lower motor neurons (a release phenomenon). These extrapyramidal fibres derive from cortical areas 6 and 8 (*see also Fig.* 10.37, p. 372), but tone may also be influenced by the anterior cerebellum independently of the muscle spindle mechanism.

Tendon reflexes and clonus are also related to tone, the former evoked by a single stimulus to the stretch reflex, the latter by repeated stimuli.

For the testing of muscle tone, it is essential that the patient should be warm and relaxed. The limb is then held on either side of the joint to be tested and passively moved through the full range of the joint. Muscle tone at the wrist can also be tested by shaking the forearm and observing the movements of the hand which, in hypotonia, may be flail-like.

**Hypertonia** Hypertonia occurs in lesions of the upper motor neuron and extrapyramidal system.

*Spasticity* ('clasp-knife' effect) is typical of an upper motor neuron lesion. When the limb is moved the maximum resistance is noticed almost at once, but it gives way suddenly after some effort on the part of the examiner and allows the limb to be moved with comparative ease. Spasticity is usually maximal in the flexors of the arms and the extensors of the legs.

*Rigidity* is a feature of Parkinsonism and may be of two kinds: 'cog-wheel' rigidity, in which the resistance to movement diminishes in jerky steps; this is probably due to a combination of tremor and rigidity. In cases without tremor, rigidity is of the 'lead pipe' variety. Extrapyramidal rigidity is often greater in the head, neck and trunk than in the limbs. This may be demonstrated when the patient lies flat in bed and, whilst distracting him, the examiner suddenly flicks the occiput forward. In Parkinsonism the head returns to the pillow slowly instead of dropping back at once.

**Hypotonia** Hypotonia occurs in lower motor neuron and cerebellar lesions. Passive movement is unduly free, often through a greater range than normal.

---

■ **REFLEXES**

---

Reflex action is an immediate motor or secretory response to an afferent sensory impulse. For clinical purposes such reflex action is spoken of as a 'reflex', of which several types are differentiated:
1. Deep or tendon reflexes.
2. Superficial or skin reflexes.

---

3. Organic or visceral reflexes.

In health these should be present, and, in the case of deep and superficial reflexes, equal on the two sides of the body. It must be recognized, however, that past disease, or some present disability not necessarily of neurological significance, may modify them. Thus the abdominal reflexes may be absent owing to laxity of the abdominal wall after repeated pregnancies.

The clinical importance of reflexes depends partly on their localizing value (*Table* 10.4), and partly on the information they give as to the integrity of the neurons, sensory and motor, which form the reflex arc. If the tendon reflexes of the arm are altered, this will place the lesion higher than if those of the legs only are modified. Again, exaggeration of the deep reflexes is an important sign of an upper motor neuron lesion, while their loss is commonly found in lesions of the lower motor neuron or afferent sensory path.

| Table 10.4 | **Segmental levels of some of the commoner reflexes*** |
|---|---|
| *Deep reflexes* | *Superficial reflexes* |
| Ankle jerk S1, 2 | Plantar reflex S1, 2 |
| Knee jerk L3, 4 | Abdominal reflexes T7–11 |
| Biceps jerk C5, 6 | Cremasteric reflex L1 |
| Triceps jerk C7, 8 | |
| Radial jerk C6 | |
| Jaw jerk pons | |

*Variations of these levels are given by different authors.

## DEEP OR TENDON REFLEXES

These reflexes are elicited by striking a tendon and so stretching it. This forms the sensory impulse which passes up afferent nerve fibres to the spinal cord. Internuncial fibres convey the impulse to the anterior horn cells, which discharge a motor impulse to the muscles supplied from that segment (*Fig.* 10.50).

*Diminution or absence* will result if the reflex arc is interrupted by injury or disease. It may be interrupted in the motor limb, in the sensory limb or in the spinal cord itself. Peripheral neuropathy and root lesions are the commonest causes for absent tendon reflexes. Tendon reflexes are also abolished by spinal cord shock, e.g. severe injury to the cord. Lesions of the muscles themselves (dystrophies, involvement in scar tissue) will, of course, prevent the muscular contraction which is the visible evidence of the reflex. Loss of tendon reflexes is bilateral in states of coma. Lastly it must be borne in mind that in some persons the deep reflexes are sluggish and occasionally absent without pathological cause, especially the ankle jerks in the elderly. Abolition of a reflex by a segmental lesion of the cord is particularly valuable in localization (*see Table* 10.4 *above*).

*Exaggeration* of the deep reflexes is an important sign of an upper motor neuron

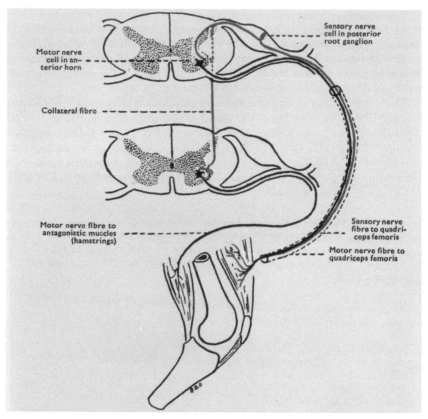

**Fig. 10.50** Diagram of knee jerk.

lesion, especially if unilateral or accompanied by other signs. The reason for this exaggeration (a 'release phenomenon') is not fully understood, but it appears that the higher centres in the pyramidal (corticospinal) and extrapyramidal systems restrain the overactivity of the stretch reflexes, and when the restraint is lost these reflexes are more easily excited.

Moderate exaggeration of the tendon reflexes without other signs may occur in nervous persons and in conditions of hyperexcitability of the nervous system, e.g. tetanus.

The more important deep reflexes follow, and the methods by which they are elicited.

### Knee jerk

If the patient is able to sit, he should cross one leg over the other and allow the upper leg to hang loosely. A more mobile patient should be asked to sit with both legs hanging loosely over the edge of the couch or bed (*see* *Fig*. 10.52). This position permits a more rapid comparison of the two knee jerks. The tendon hammer is held lightly between index finger and thumb, raised by extension of the wrist and then allowed to fall and strike the tendon by virtue of its own weight (*Figs.* 10.51, 10.52). A sharp tap on the patellar tendon then produces a contraction of the quadriceps extensor of the knee, which can be felt if the observer's hand is placed over the lower part of the front of the thigh. The leg is momentarily shot forward if the contraction is sufficiently great, owing to the extension of the knee joint.

Alternatively the patient may be recumbent, and his legs should be supported behind the knee with one hand and the patellar tendon tapped (*Fig.* 10.51).

When the knee jerks are apparently absent they may be reinforced. The patient is asked to lock his hands and try to pull them apart while the physician strikes the patellar tendon (*Fig.* 10.52). This is one method of producing a slight general increase of tone.

Apart from diminution or exaggeration of the knee jerks, certain special responses may be observed occasionally. In chorea they may be sustained, that is, after the contraction of the quadriceps has occurred, the leg seems to hover momentarily before falling to the resting position. Somewhat similar is the pendular knee jerk of acute cerebellar disease, present on the same side as the lesion. In myasthenia gravis the knee jerks and other reflexes tire rapidly in common with voluntary muscular action. The reflexes in hypothyroidism show a normal immediate response but with a delayed return to the resting position, the biceps and ankle jerks especially (*Fig.* 10.55).

### Ankle jerk

If the patient is in bed the knee should be flexed, the hip externally rotated and the foot gently dorsiflexed until the tendo calcaneus (Achillis) is tensed but not overstretched (*Fig.* 10.53). The tendon is then struck with a per-

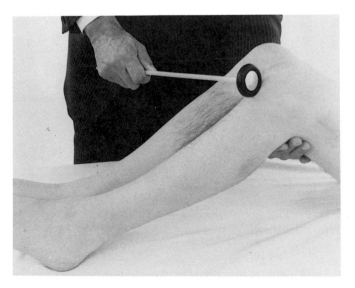

**Fig. 10.51** Knee jerk. The knees are supported and a brisk tap made on each side to compare the response.

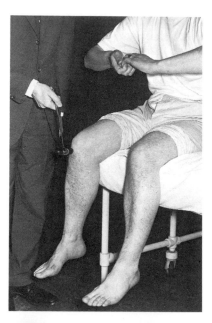

**Fig. 10.52**
Reinforcement of knee jerks.
The patient pulls upon one
hand with the other while the
observer strikes the patellar
tendon.

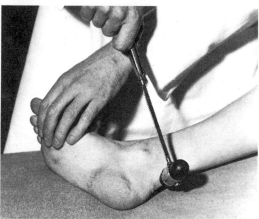

**Fig. 10.53** Ankle jerk. When the patient is unfit to kneel this
test can be carried out in bed.

cussion hammer, each side being tested in quick succession for clear comparison
of the responses. The ambulant patient may kneel (as shown in *Fig.* 10.54). The
result is a brisk plantar flexion of the foot.

### Triceps jerk

The arm is supported at the wrist and flexed to a right-angle. The
triceps tendon is struck just proximal to the point of the elbow (*Fig.* 10.56), and
the resulting contraction of the triceps causes extension at the elbow.

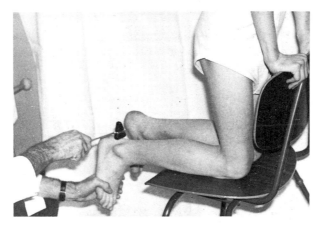

**Fig. 10.54** Ankle jerk. A tap on the tendo calcaneus (Achillis) causes contraction of the gastrocnemius.

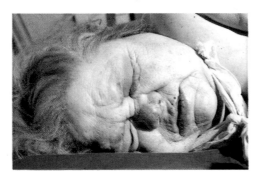

**Fig. 10.55** Hypothyroidism. The biceps, knee and ankle jerks all showed delayed relaxation.

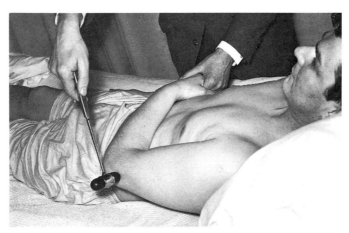

**Fig. 10.56** Triceps jerk. Percussion of the triceps tendon causes contraction of the muscle with extension at the elbow.

### Biceps jerk

The elbow is flexed to a right-angle and the forearm slightly pronated. The thumb is placed over the biceps tendon and struck with a percussion hammer (*Fig.* 10.57). The result is a contraction of the biceps causing flexion and slight supination of the forearm.

### Radial jerk

The elbow is flexed to a right-angle and the forearm placed midway between pronation and supination. The styloid process of the radius is tapped with a percussion hammer (*Fig.* 10.58). The result is a contraction of the brachioradialis causing flexion at the elbow and partial supination of the forearm.

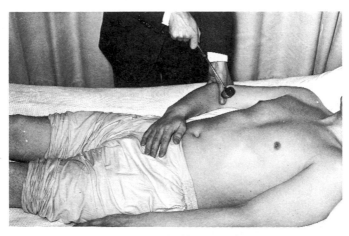

**Fig. 10.57** Biceps jerk. A tap on the biceps tendon causes contraction of the biceps and flexion of the forearm.

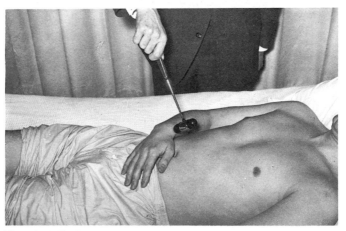

**Fig. 10.58** Radial jerk. A sharp tap on the styloid process of the radius causes flexion at the elbow and partial supination of the forearm.

### Hoffmann's sign

This also indicates increased tendon reflex activity in the hand. The distal phalanx of the middle finger is first flexed and then abruptly released. If the sign is positive the thumb and index finger will then flex and adduct.

### Jaw jerk

The jaw is allowed to relax and the mouth to hang open loosely. The finger is placed on the lower jaw and is struck with the hammer. A brisk response suggests a lesion of both corticopontine (pyramidal) tracts (*Fig.* 10.59).

### Clonus

Closely allied to the tendon reflexes is clonus, a series of involuntary contractions of certain muscles initiated by stretching their tendons. Clonus is usually found when the tendon reflexes are grossly exaggerated and is therefore commoner in organic (upper neuron) than functional nervous disorders. It is of more significance when it is increased by continuing and increasing the stimulus (stretching the tendon) than if it is abolished. The former type is called 'true' or 'inexhaustible' clonus, the latter 'spurious' or 'exhaustible'. In many cases, however, the spurious clonus may become true as the malady progresses. Clonus occurs in two main types in clinical practice: ankle clonus and patellar clonus.

**Ankle clonus** Ankle clonus is elicited by sharply pressing up the foot into the dorsiflexed position (*Fig.* 10.60). This results in contractions of the calf muscle leading to plantar flexion of the foot, and in upper motor neuron disease the contractions usually continue as long as pressure is made. True clonus generally occurs with the foot in plantar flexion and is increased by dorsiflexion of the foot. The spurious forms occur with the foot in any position and tend to diminish and become irregular as the foot is pressed up.

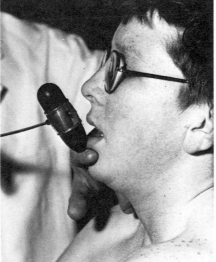

**Fig. 10.59**
Jaw jerk. The finger lies on the lower jaw and is struck with the hammer. A contraction of the masseters may result.

**Patellar clonus** With the leg extended at the knee, the patella is fitted into the angle between the thumb and first finger (*Fig.* 10.61). A sharp downward movement of the hand will induce contractions of the quadriceps which pull the patella upwards and continue so long as pressure is exerted.

## SUPERFICIAL (CUTANEOUS) REFLEXES

These include the plantar responses, abdominal reflexes, cremasteric reflex, ciliospinal reflex and corneal reflex. All consist of a contraction of certain muscles when a particular area is stimulated by stroking or pinching.

### Plantar reflex

If the sole of the foot is stroked firmly with the thumbnail or a key, the great toe becomes plantar flexed, and there is sometimes a contraction of the

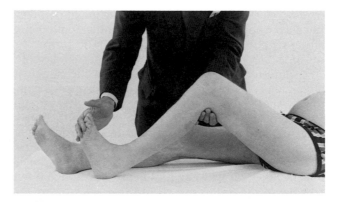

**Fig. 10.60** Ankle clonus. The foot is sharply dorsiflexed. If clonus is present the calf muscles give a series of jerky contractions.

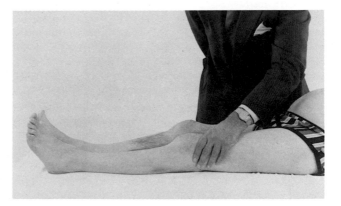

**Fig. 10.61** Patellar clonus. The patella is pressed firmly and sharply downwards. If clonus is present a series of jerky contractions of the quadriceps takes place, continuing while pressure is exerted.

tensor fasciae latae. The stimulus should be applied to the outer half of the sole from the heel to the base of the small toes. This is the normal response which occurs in adults (*Fig.* 10.62). It may be absent without organic disease, especially when the feet are cold or damp, or if there is anaesthesia of the skin or paresis of the relevant muscles.

In infants, the response consists of dorsiflexion of the great toe and occasionally spreading of the small toes in a fan-like manner. In adults such a response is always pathological, and is known as *Babinski's sign* (*Fig.* 10.62). Occasionally a Babinski response may result from stimulation over a wider area, e.g. the leg. If an excessive stimulus is applied, dorsiflexion of the toe may occur as part of a general withdrawal of the foot even in normal people. For this reason, the effect of a gentle stimulus with the thumb alone should always be tried before any form of implement is used.

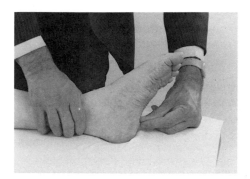 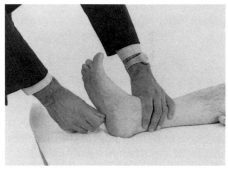

a                                    b

**Fig. 10.62** Plantar reflex. *a*, Normal response. *b*, Babinski's sign.

Babinski's sign indicates that the corticospinal tracts are out of commission. This may be temporary, as in some types of coma and after epileptic fits, but as a permanent phenomenon it is found in such lesions of the upper motor neuron as cerebral vascular disease, disseminated sclerosis and subacute combined degeneration, and it has great significance in distinguishing an organic from a psychoneurotic state, for in the latter it never occurs. Occasionally in cases of paraplegia in extension a crossed response is obtained, namely, a Babinski sign on the stimulated side, and a plantar flexion of the opposite foot.

### Abdominal reflexes

To elicit these reflexes a sharp object, e.g. a metal pencil or key, is drawn firmly but lightly across the abdominal wall, on each side in turn (*Fig.* 10.63). The four quadrants of the abdomen are examined in this way. In a healthy young adult the natural response is a contraction of the underlying abdominal muscles and a deviation of the linea alba to the same side. The response is generally brisker in the upper part of the abdomen (*epigastric reflex*).

In infants the abdominal reflexes are not present, and in adults obesity or laxity of the abdominal wall may abolish them. The abdominal reflexes often 'tire' easily

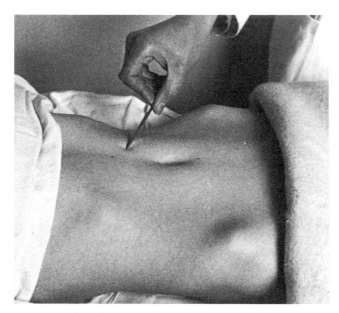

**Fig. 10.63** Abdominal reflex. The skin of the abdomen is lightly stroked with a pencil. Brisk contraction of the underlying abdominal muscles normally occurs.

and may disappear after repeated stimuli. Acute abdominal lesions and sensory loss may also abolish these reflexes, but the most important cause of *absence* or *diminution* is a lesion of the corticospinal system. It is of greater significance, too, if the reflex is lost on one side only (e.g. in hemiplegia). Both the Babinski sign and loss of abdominal reflexes are 'corticospinal' reflexes in which the afferent arc is via a small number of ascending fibres in the corticospinal tracts.

One of the commonest nervous lesions in which the abdominal reflexes are bilaterally lost is disseminated sclerosis.

### Cremasteric reflex

This reflex consists in a retraction of the testicle by the cremaster muscle when the inner side of the thigh is stimulated by stroking the skin or pressure over the subsartorial canal. It is often difficult to elicit in older men, though easy in children. Loss occurs in corticospinal lesions, but is rarely of importance unless unilateral. It is not to be confused with the *dartos reflex* in which the scrotum contracts under the influence of cold.

### Ciliospinal reflex

If the skin of the neck is pinched, the pupil normally dilates. The sympathetic trunk and pathway in the spinal cord must be intact for this reflex to occur, and its abolition therefore suggests a lesion of these. Loss of the ciliospinal reflex is used as a measure of the depth of coma and also as one of the criteria for the diagnosis of 'brain death'.

### Corneal reflex

Light touch with cottonwool on the surface of the eye normally produces blinking in both eyes. This reflex may be bilaterally abolished in coma of any type. Abolition may be confined to one side only. The loss then indicates a lesion either of the efferent limb (7th nerve) or of the afferent sensory limb (5th nerve ophthalmic division). This reflex is important in the early diagnosis of 5th-nerve lesions, testing as it does for anaesthesia of the cornea.

### Pharyngeal reflex

Irritation of the pharynx with a spatula produces contraction of the pharyngeal muscles. This may be absent in hysteria and in 9th-cranial nerve lesions.

### Grasp reflex

When the examiner's finger is drawn across the patient's palm, it may be grasped firmly if there is a lesion of the opposite frontal lobe.

### ORGANIC OR VISCERAL REFLEXES

There are many visceral reflexes but the only ones of prime importance in neurology are those for micturition and defaecation.

### Micturition

This is a reflex act which can be voluntarily controlled to a considerable extent by higher centres in the brain. It is normally initiated by a voluntary effort, but once started becomes a reflex act which is difficult to interrupt. The reflex path is partly through plexuses in the bladder wall and partly in the pelvic plexuses. The innervation of these plexuses is from the sympathetic (from L 2, 3 and 4 segments) and parasympathetic systems (S 2 and 3, nervi erigentes).

The stimulus for this reflex is distension of the bladder with urine. This stimulus passes to the spinal cord by way of the nervi erigentes and rami communicantes. Controlling centres are situated in the spinal cord at various levels, so that, although the reflex arc is left intact, spinal cord and cerebral lesions still result in defects in micturition. In disseminated sclerosis, for example, precipitancy of micturition results from loss of the influence of these controlling centres. The patient cannot control the urgent desire to pass urine.

*Retention* and *incontinence* of urine may occur from interference with consciousness (e.g. cerebral haemorrhage) without affection of the local reflex mechanism, in the spinal cord. When retention has occurred and the distension is sufficiently great, incontinence may result from partial overflow.

In spinal cord lesions with complete paraplegia, similar *retention with overflow* may occur, but it is sometimes followed by *automatic micturition* in which part of the bladder content is discharged at certain fairly fixed intervals.

In all cases in which incontinence occurs it is essential to examine the abdomen for evidence of bladder distension.

In most cases the patient gradually recovers from the bladder effects of lesions of the brain and spinal cord, the bladder becoming capable of expelling larger quantities of urine and the residuum becoming smaller daily. In cauda equina disease, however, the reflex arc is itself interrupted, and the incontinence is therefore prolonged or permanent.

In the male, *impotence* can be a distressing and early symptom of spinal cord diseases which also interfere with micturition.

### Defaecation

The bowel action may be embarrassed, causing constipation (analogous with retention of urine) or incontinence of faeces, especially after purgation (analogous with incontinence of urine).

### Mass reflex

The mass reflex occurs in severe spinal cord lesions. After a period of flaccid paralysis with retention of urine and constipation, there occurs with paraplegia in flexion a periodic involuntary evacuation of the bladder and rectum. On the application of a stimulus (pin-prick or stroking the sole of the foot) to any point below the level of the lesion, especially in the midline of the body, the legs are vigorously drawn up, Babinski's sign occurs, the skin sweats below the lesion, and the bladder is evacuated. This phenomenon is known as the 'mass reflex'.

## ■ CO-ORDINATION

The co-ordination of movement depends among other factors upon the integrity of the sensory paths in the posterior columns and the cerebellum and its tracts, and it is not out of place to consider here the various ways of testing for co-ordination. Lack of proper co-ordination is known as *ataxia*.

In the *arms* the co-ordination of movement may be tested by asking the patient to touch the tip of the nose with the index finger of each hand in turn (*Fig.* 10.64). Tests for co-ordination should be carried out with the eyes open, then closed, to distinguish sensory from motor ataxia (*see below*). The patient should be able to do this accurately both slowly and rapidly. Ataxia of the arms is seen in disseminated sclerosis and other cerebellar lesions.

In the legs ataxia is best observed by watching the patient's attempt to walk (*see* Gaits, pp. 49 and 384–87). In bed the 'heel-to-knee' test (*Fig.* 10.65) may be made. The patient is instructed to touch each knee in turn with the opposite heel and then run it down his shin. The degree of ataxia in the affected limb may be roughly gauged by the clumsiness of the attempt. Ataxia in the legs is well seen in tabes and other lesions (Friedreich's ataxia, subacute combined degeneration) where the posterior columns are diseased. It also results from cerebellar lesions and some forms of peripheral neuropathy.

It is important to note that in the posterior column (sensory) type of ataxia the inco-ordination can be partially corrected by ocular impressions. The ataxia is therefore made worse by closing the eyes. In cerebellar (motor) ataxia, on the contrary, the degree of ataxia is little influenced by ocular impressions. These facts are the basis of *Romberg's sign*. The patient first stands with the eyes open and brings the heels as closely together as possible without losing his balance. The eyes are then closed, and normally the patient sways slightly. In posterior column lesions, he often sways to the extent of falling if unsupported. In sensory ataxia (posterior-column lesions) an error of projection is often present, e.g. when

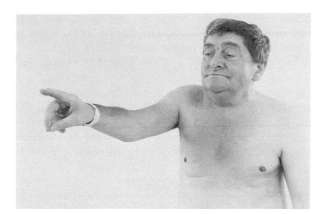

**Fig. 10.64**
Method of testing for ataxia in the arms. This method also demonstrates the presence of any 'intention' tremor.

*a*

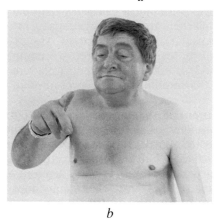

*b*

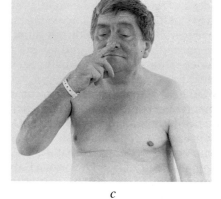

*c*

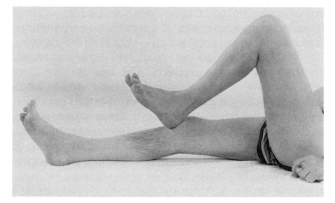

**Fig. 10.65** Testing for ataxia in a recumbent patient. The 'heel-to-knee' test.

the patient attempts to touch the nose with the finger he fails to do so. This differs from the jerky movements of the arm in intention tremor (p. 381), which is essentially a manifestation of cerebellar (motor) ataxia.

Other features of cerebellar ataxia (dysmetria and dysdiadochokinesia) are considered on p. 415.

It must be remembered that the sensory impulses upon which co-ordinated movement depends may be interrupted in the brain itself—for example, in the thalamus or post-central gyrus. Cerebral lesions which injure these parts may therefore result in ataxia. Examples are seen in thalamic tumours or vascular lesions, internal capsular haemorrhage, and tumours of the post-central gyrus.

# ■ LESIONS OF THE UPPER MOTOR NEURON

### Hemiplegia (see also Cerebral Haemorrhage, p. 435)

Vascular lesions are by far the commonest causes of hemiplegia, especially thrombosis of the middle cerebral artery or its branches causing infarction in small (cortical) or larger (internal capsular) areas of the brain. The extent of the paralysis varies with the number of motor fibres affected. In complete hemiplegia the face, arm and leg are paralysed, but the trunk and some cranial muscles escape, at least partially, because they are bilaterally represented in the cortex.

There may be an initial period of cerebral shock in severe cases (especially haemorrhage) in which there is deep unconsciousness, loss of reflexes and conjugate deviation of the eyes away from the lesion. Later, signs of an upper neuron lesion develop. The limbs may at first be flaccid but later spastic, the tendon reflexes increased, clonus may be present, the abdominal reflexes are lost, and the plantar response is extensor (Babinski's sign). These release signs and the paralysis are opposite to the side of the lesion. If the patient recovers partially, contractures may occur and the characteristic posture and gait develop. (*Fig.* 10.48, p. 385, and *Fig.* 10.66.) These have been described.

Whatever the position of the lesion these signs of hemiplegia are the same provided all the corticospinal tract fibres are affected. From the short account of the anatomy of the motor tract given on p. 369 it follows, however, that a complete hemiplegia more frequently results from a small lesion situated in a region where the fibres are closely crowded together, e.g. the internal capsule, crus, pons, or medulla. In the cortex a small lesion results in a more limited paralysis.

Even where the hemiplegia is complete one limb may be more affected than the other. Thus in internal-capsular thrombosis it is common for slight movement to remain in the leg though the arm is devoid of any. That the fibres to the leg are not so completely destroyed is shown by the quicker recovery of this limb. The facial paralysis is only partial and does not include the forehead or eye (cf. Bell's palsy, p. 362) because the occipito-frontalis and orbicularis oculi muscles are supplied by a part of the 7th nerve nucleus which is governed by corticobulbar fibres from both sides of the brain.

**Localization of the lesion** Certain special features help to localize the lesion causing the hemiplegia.

*In the cortex*, as mentioned, monoplegia, or paralysis of an even smaller group

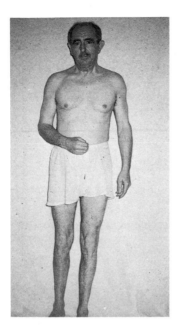

**Fig. 10.66**
Right hemiplegia.

of muscles, is common. Aphasia is a frequent accompaniment if the left side of the brain is affected. Jacksonian fits may occur if the lesion is in or near the cortex, e.g. tumour or subdural haematoma. Of the vascular lesions cerebral thrombosis is the commonest (*see* p. 433).

*In the internal capsule* the hemiplegia is generally complete, and spread of the lesion backwards may result in sensory changes and sometimes homonymous hemianopia on the same side as the paralysis (*See Fig*. 10.38, p. 373)

*In the crus* a form of crossed paralysis may result (Weber's syndrome) in which the 3rd nerve is paralysed on one side and the face, arm and leg on the other (*Fig*. 10.67).

Tumours in the interpeduncular space may have a similar effect by pressure on the crus, but polydipsia and polyuria of hypothalamic origin may also be present.

*In the pons* other types of crossed lesion may occur from involvement of the 6th and 7th nerves at this level. There may be facial paralysis (lower neuron type) on one side and hemiplegia (arm and leg) on the other (*Fig*. 10.68). If the 6th nerve is also affected the external (lateral) rectus will be paralysed on the same side as the 7th. Strictly unilateral lesions of the pons are not common, and hemiplegic signs may therefore be present on both sides in variable degrees. Pinpoint pupils and hyperpyrexia are occasionally seen in cases of pontine haemorrhage. If the medial lemniscus is involved, ataxia and loss of deep sensibility may be present on the opposite side.

Crural and pontine lesions are not common and are generally vascular or neoplastic. In hemiplegia arising from lesions below the pons (7th nucleus) the face is spared.

*In the medulla* crossed paralyses also occur—hemiplegia on one side and paralysis of the 9th, 10th, 11th or 12th nerves on the other. As in pontine lesions the

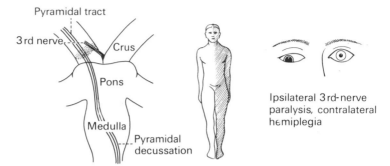

**Fig. 10.67** Weber's syndrome. A lesion in the crus interrupting the pyramidal (corticospinal) tract fibres and simultaneously involving the 3rd nerve. Result: Contralateral paralysis of face, arm and leg (upper neuron type), with ipsilateral 3rd-nerve palsy (lower neuron type). Note the dilated pupil and the eye fixed in the downward and outward position.

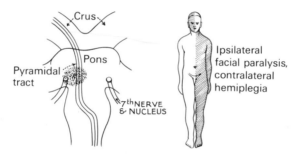

**Fig. 10.68** Pontine crossed paralysis. A lesion in the pons involving the nucleus of the 7th nerve, causing facial paralysis on the same side, and paralysis of the opposite arm and leg.

damage is rarely confined to one side, and frequently extends into the sensory tracts.

A lesion below the decussation of the corticospinal tracts in the lower medulla causes a hemiplegia on the same side. A lesion below the cervical region of the spinal cord will affect the leg alone (*see* Brown-Séquard's Syndrome, p. 425).

### Paraplegia

This word generally means paralysis of both lower limbs, but if the lesion is in the cervical region the arms may also be affected (quadriplegia). The signs are similar to those of hemiplegia, but bilateral (*Fig.* 10.69). The paralysis is generally spastic, though severe lesions of the cord may cause an initial flaccid paralysis from spinal cord shock (*see also* Paraplegia in Flexion and Extension, p. 379); the tendon reflexes are increased; the abdominal reflexes are lost if the lesion is above this reflex arc; Babinski's sign and clonus are present. Another important sign is loss of sphincter control, not generally present if the corticospinal tract is damaged on one side only.

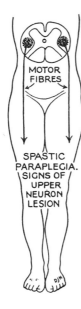

**Fig. 10.69**
Bilateral pyramidal lesions,
e.g. disseminated sclerosis.
For signs of upper neuron
lesion, *see* p. 402.

MOTOR
FIBRES

SPASTIC
PARAPLEGIA.
SIGNS OF
UPPER
NEURON
LESION

Pure forms of spastic paraplegia without sensory changes are sometimes seen in disseminated sclerosis, Little's disease, etc. though even in these other tracts are sometimes affected. Many diseases of the spinal cord are characterized by a combination of spastic paraplegia with sensory changes—for example, compression paraplegia and subacute combined degeneration. They will be described in the discussion of the sensory system.

### Upper motor neuron bulbar paralysis (pseudo-bulbar paralysis)

This term is applied to cases of difficulty in articulation and swallowing, sometimes with facial rigidity, due to *bilateral* involvement of the corticospinal fibres to the cranial nerve nuclei. It is usually due to bilateral cerebral thrombosis affecting the internal capsular region. Mild bilateral hemiplegic signs are present together with the bulbar symptoms and generally some emotional instability. The jaw jerk is increased, a sign which helps to differentiate this syndrome from Parkinsonism.

The history is one of hemiplegia, often slight on one side, followed after an interval (sometimes months or years) by similar affection of the opposite side. The first 'stroke' does not interfere with bulbar activities as the cortical control of these is bilateral.

### ■ LESIONS OF THE LOWER MOTOR NEURON

The lower neuron may be injured or diseased in the cranial nerve nuclei or spinal anterior horn cells, in the anterior nerve roots, or in the nerves themselves.

The commonest acute lesion of the anterior horn cells is poliomyelitis (infantile paralysis). A chronic degeneration of the anterior horn cells also occurs as a part of motor neuron disease (progressive muscular atrophy).

The anterior nerve roots may be damaged by trauma, especially that associated with cervical spondylosis, and more rarely vascular, inflammatory and neoplastic lesions. The effects are similar to and frequently indistinguishable from disease of the anterior horn cells.

Lesions of the peripheral nerves are generally due to trauma, inflammation and various toxic or metabolic disorders (neuropathies). The results depend upon the distribution of the nerve and the position in which it is affected. When the nerve is purely motor (e.g. the long thoracic nerve to the serratus anterior) paralysis of the muscles supplied results; but as the majority of nerves are 'mixed', i.e. contain both motor and sensory fibres, muscular paralysis is frequently accompanied by sensory changes.

Some examples of lower neuron lesions may now be considered in more detail.

### Lesions of the anterior horn cells and of the bulbar nuclei

**Acute poliomyelitis** (*Infantile paralysis*) This disease is commonest in children and young adults, but has become less frequent since the introduction of preventive inoculation. It is infectious (virus) in origin, and the onset is therefore like other febrile illnesses, with which it is not uncommonly confused unless or until paralytic symptoms appear.

Pain in the back and tenderness of the limbs are suggestive early symptoms. Fever is often accompanied by signs of meningeal irritation (*see* p. 433). In a few days a *flaccid paralysis* occurs and establishes the diagnosis. It is generally maximal at the onset, but occasionally extends with a new bout of fever. The extent is variable. Sometimes only a few muscles are affected; sometimes the greater part of all the limbs and trunk may be involved. The distribution of paralysis corresponds with the affected segments of the spinal cord (*see* table on p. 375). Involvement at the cervical and thoracic levels may lead to respiratory failure due to phrenic and intercostal nerve paralysis. The muscles most commonly singled out are those of the lower limbs, especially the extensors of the thigh, tibialis anterior, peronei and extensors of the feet and toes.

The signs of a lower neuron lesion are present: rapid wasting of the paralysed muscles (*Fig.* 10.70), loss of tendon reflexes, flaccidity and trophic changes in the skin. Although acute poliomyelitis is now rare in the developed countries, it remains the commonest cause in adult life of a wasted and shortened limb.

**Motor neuron disease** This is a progressive degenerative condition of middle or later life which may affect both upper and lower motor neurons. i.e. the corticospinal tracts, anterior horn cells and motor nuclei of the brainstem. Lower motor neuron signs are found mainly in the arms and consist of weakness, wasting and fasciculation especially in the small muscles of the hand (*see Fig.* 10.40, p.378), where there may be a 'claw' deformity (*see Fig.* 10.45, p. 383). The tendon reflexes in the arms may be either diminished or increased according to whether the lower or upper neuron lesion predominates. In the legs, the tendon reflexes are usually exaggerated and the plantar responses extensor. Involvement of medullary nuclei may lead to bulbar paralysis (*see below*). The absence of sensory symptoms and signs helps to distinguish this condition from syringomyelia and cord compression.

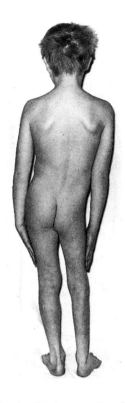

**Fig. 10.70**
Poliomyelitis, showing
wasting and shortening of the
right leg with compensatory
tilting of the pelvis.

**Bulbar paralysis** Reference has been made to this as a manifestation of motor neuron disease.

The principal symptoms are increasing difficulty in articulation due to paresis of the tongue (12th nucleus), difficulty in swallowing from paresis of the soft palate and pharynx, regurgitation of fluids through the nose and nasal voice (10th and 9th nuclei). The tongue wastes, shows fasciculation, and its movement is more and more limited. The larynx may also be involved. (*See also* Cranial Nerves, p. 342). The process is essentially a chronic one, and death usually results from an inhalation pneumonia consequent upon the swallowing defect.

More rarely, bulbar paralysis of this type may be an acute process due to acute poliomyelitis, encephalitis or to vascular lesions. It may also be imitated by a peripheral neuropathy affecting the 9th, 10th and 12th cranial nerves. In myasthenia gravis bulbar symptoms are present but improve after a rest, only to recur after use of the affected muscles.

### Lesions of the anterior nerve roots

The anterior nerve roots contain autonomic preganglionic fibres and motor fibres which are distributed to the muscles in a segmental fashion so closely resembling that of the anterior horn cells as to make a diagnosis between a lesion of one or the other impossible unless other signs of spinal cord disease (e.g. corticospinal tract signs) are present.

The commonest lesions of the anterior nerve roots are traumatic, e.g. brachial plexus injuries, and the student's knowledge of anatomy has a direct practical application in such cases. It is not possible here to deal with the many varieties of traumatic lesions of the anterior nerve roots or the peripheral nerves. One example of a lesion of the anterior nerve roots may, however, serve as an illustration: the obstetrical palsy of Erb–Duchenne type.

**Erb–Duchenne paralysis** In this condition the 5th cervical anterior nerve root is torn at birth. The result is a paralysis of the muscles governed by this segment— the deltoid, brachioradialis and biceps. From action of the unopposed muscles the hand and arm are held in the characteristic position. The arm is adducted and extended at the elbow, and the forearm pronated, giving the 'waiter's hand' position.

No lesion of an individual nerve could produce such a combination of muscular paralyses, and the cause can be narrowed down to a lesion of the anterior horn cells or the corresponding nerve root of the 5th cervical segment. The characteristics of a lower neuron lesion will be present, and the absence of sensory changes will further exclude a peripheral nerve lesion.

## Lesions of the peripheral nerves

**Traumatic lesions** Here again the student must be prepared to work out on anatomical grounds the nerve or nerves affected. The problem is made easier by the combination of muscular paralysis and anaesthesia corresponding with the distribution of an individual nerve. The paralysis, again, is of the lower neuron type, and in the area supplied by the sensory fibres of the nerve all types of sensation are lost.

As an example of a peripheral nerve lesion paralysis of the radial nerve may be taken.

*Radial nerve paralysis* This is of particular interest to the physician, as not only is the radial the nerve most commonly injured, but it is sometimes affected in neuropathies.

The nerve, including its posterior interosseous branch, has a large motor distribution, comprising the triceps, brachioradialis, extensor carpi radialis longus and brevis and extensor digitorum. When it is injured high up (for example, in 'crutch paralysis' or 'Saturday night paralysis' due to pressure on some hard object during alcoholic stupor) these muscles are paralysed in varying degrees. The main result is wrist-drop, i.e. an inability to use the extensors of the wrist, and weakness of the extensors of the digits. In cases of lead palsy a peculiar feature is the escape of the brachioradialis from the general paralysis of muscles supplied by the radial.

The sensory changes are limited owing to overlap with other nerves. Generally the anaesthesia is confined to a small area on the back of the thumb and the skin between this and the index finger.

**Entrapment syndromes** Constriction or entrapment of a peripheral nerve may give rise to pain and paraesthesiae as well as objective motor and sensory changes in the distribution of the nerve. The three nerves most prone to such constriction are the median nerve in the carpal tunnel at the wrist, the ulnar nerve between the two heads of the flexor carpi ulnaris at the elbow and the lateral cutaneous nerve of the thigh as it passes behind the inguinal ligament.

The *carpal tunnel syndrome* occurs especially in middle-aged women doing heavy manual work. It may also complicate pregnancy, rheumatoid arthritis and hypothyroidism. The typical story is of severe pain and paraesthesiae, which may involve the whole arm as well as the hand, waking the patient from sleep. In the morning, the hand feels stiff and swollen and paraesthesiae may recur throughout the day. There may be few objective signs of a median nerve lesion. *Ulnar nerve constriction* is less common but occurs more often in men. There is a slowly progressive ulnar nerve palsy, sensory symptoms preceding motor effects. *Meralgia paraesthetica* is the name given to the burning pain, paraesthesiae and sensory loss over the lateral aspect of the thigh which results from entrapment of the lateral cutaneous nerve, usually in obese men.

**Peripheral neuritis and neuropathies** Many cases formerly regarded as neuritis do not justify the term as they are not inflammatory in origin. For those which do not fall under this heading the term *neuropathy* is preferable.

*Neuritis* Examples of this are: .

1. Lesions of the main nerve trunks as in leprosy (*Fig.* 10.71). There is an actual inflammatory change in the nerves and sensory manifestations, notably anaesthesia, are present. Similar changes may occur locally when nerves are involved in a septic area.

2. Acute polyneuritis (Guillain–Barré Syndrome). Although this commonly follows virus infection, it is probably due to a non-infective inflammatory reaction in the peripheral nerves. The onset is usually sudden with a symmetrical paresis which starts in the legs but may rapidly ascend to affect the arms, the respiratory musculature and the cranial nerves. Paraesthesiae occur, but objective sensory changes are usually minimal. There is a lower motor neuron type of paresis with

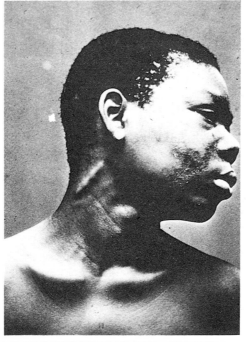

**Fig. 10.71**
Leprosy: visible enlargement of the great auricular nerve.

flaccidity and absent tendon reflexes. Unless the patient succumbs to respiratory failure, recovery is usually complete within a few months.

3. A type of shoulder-girdle neuritis (neuralgic amyotrophy) may occur after inoculation. It causes pain in the distribution of the 5th and 6th cervical nerve roots and there is usually weakness and wasting of the muscles. This is thought to be inflammatory but may be imitated in older people by a neuropathy due to cervical spondylosis.

*Polyneuropathies* Many diseases can result in peripheral nerve changes. They include infections such as diphtheria in which the organism remains localized to the throat, but the toxins affect the nerves. Poisons have a similar effect, e.g. arsenic, lead and carbon tetrachloride used in industry, isoniazid and nitrofurantoin used in treatment. Among important metabolic causes may be mentioned diabetes (*Fig.* 10.72), uraemia, amyloid disease and porphyria. Deficiency diseases which are responsible include beriberi, pellagra and probably chronic alcoholism which leads to vitamin deficiency. Deficiency of vitamin $B_{12}$ can cause a peripheral neuropathy as well as degeneration of the cord. The condition is not uncommon in malignant diseases, but the mechanism is more obscure.

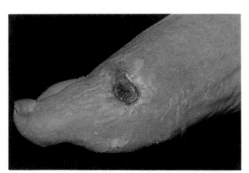

**Fig. 10.72**
Painless trophic ulcer in a diabetic with polyneuritis.

Most varieties of neuritis and neuropathy show the signs of lower neuron involvement together with sensory changes, but in some the motor signs predominate (e.g. lead poisoning) and in others there may be sensory loss alone (e.g. certain malignant neuropathies). The degree and distribution of the signs vary much in the individual case and help in deciding the aetiology. The causal agency may also be suspected by associated non-neurological signs, e.g. alcoholism, exposure to poisons, diabetes and diphtheria.

### ■ LESIONS OF THE MUSCLES: THE MYOPATHIES

A few diseases apparently have their pathological seat in the muscles themselves, the motor neurons, both upper and lower, remaining intact. These diseases are often characterized by muscular weakness, and their diagnosis is therefore made during the examination of the motor system. The same applies to certain diseases in which there is some disorder of transmission of impulses at the myoneural junctions, viz. myasthenia gravis, and also to the phenomenon of myotonia which consists of difficulty in relaxing muscles.

### Muscular dystrophies

Muscular atrophy due to primary changes in the muscles, as distinct from neural muscular atrophy, occurs in certain families. This familial nature of the dystrophies is all-important in diagnosis. They usually appear in childhood or, in some forms, in adolescence. In many cases, alongside of the wasting of certain groups of muscles, there is apparent hypertrophy of others, really due to overgrowth of fat and connective tissue.

Various types of dystrophy are described, according to the groups of muscles affected, the age of onset and the mode of inheritance.

**Duchenne type** This is inherited by boys as a sex-linked recessive characteristic. It presents in early childhood and is usually fatal in adolescence. The *atrophy* is seen especially in the latissimus dorsi and lower halves of the pectorals, but the biceps, peronei and hamstrings are also affected. Winging of the scapulae results from wasting of the serratus anterior. Lordosis is common owing to wasting of the flexors of the thighs. By contrast with these wasted muscles, those of the calves and buttocks and the deltoids and spinati are enlarged owing to pseudohypertrophy. The gait is waddling and the classic method of rising from the supine to the erect posture is described on p. 387. In this and other forms of muscular dystrophies, the serum creatine kinase (a muscle enzyme) is characteristically raised.

**Facio-scapulo-humeral type** This starts at about the same age as, or somewhat older than the Duchenne type. The distribution of muscles affected is indicated by the name. The facial weakness causes a characteristic myopathic facies with drooping of the lower lip and wasting of the facial muscles (*Fig.* 10.73*a*). The shoulder-girdle muscles (especially trapezius and serratus anterior) and the muscles of the upper arm (biceps, triceps and pectorals) are involved, causing drooping of the shoulders and winging of the scapulae (*Fig.* 10.73*b*).

**Limb girdle type** This manifests later than the other kinds, usually in adolescence. It is inherited as an autosomal recessive and therefore affects both sexes. The biceps, triceps, brachioradialis, and to a lesser extent the quadriceps and glutei, are the paretic muscles.

**Dystrophia myotonica** This condition is transmitted by dominant inheritance and usually presents in adult life. There is diffuse muscle weakness and wasting but involvement of the facial muscles with ptosis is a characteristic feature. Myotonia consists of a failure of muscle relaxation after voluntary contraction. When the patient grips the examiner's hand, he is unable to release it. This phenomenon is also seen in myotonia congenita (Thomsen's disease) which may be associated with other congenital anomalies including baldness, cataract, testicular atrophy and dementia.

### Myasthenia gravis

This is a disease in which there is muscle weakness, without wasting, due to a failure of normal neuromuscular transmission. The muscles tire easily, especially towards the end of the day. Any muscle group can be involved but those supplied by the cranial nerves are commonly affected first so that the patient complains of ptosis, diplopia, dysarthria, dysphagia or difficulty in chewing or holding up the head. Simple tests for muscle fatigue will demonstrate the patient's inability to sustain activities such as opening and shutting the eyes or mouth,

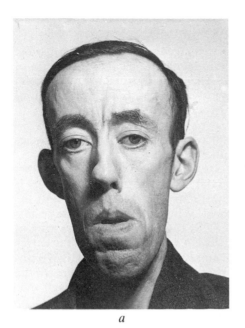
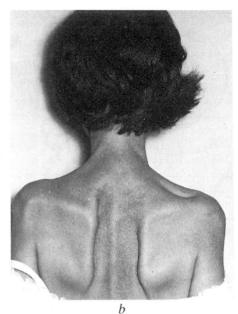

a          b

**Fig. 10.73** *a,* myopathic facies. The loose part of the lips is due to weakness of the orbicularis oris. *b,* muscular dystrophy. Shoulder girdle distribution. Note winging of scapula.

clenching and unclenching the fist or raising the head from the pillow. The diagnosis can be established by intravenous injection of edrophonium chloride (Tensilon) which results in a rapid, dramatic but transient improvement in muscle power (*see Fig.* 10.74).

### Acquired myopathies

In this group, the weakness and wasting mainly affect proximal limb muscles. The commoner causes are carcinoma, collagen disorders such as polymyositis, and endocrine conditions, including diabetes (*Fig.* 10.75), thyrotoxicosis and corticosteroid therapy. Some of these diseases, notably thyrotoxicosis and carcinoma, may also be accompanied by a myasthenic syndrome.

### ■    LESIONS OF THE EXTRAPYRAMIDAL SYSTEM

### Parkinsonism

This disease is a good example of a degenerative process affecting the basal ganglia (corpus striatum). It appears insidiously in elderly persons who at first may complain only of a vague tiredness or stiffness of the limbs with difficulty in the performance of fine movements. Relatives may notice that the patient has been slowing up and the whole illness is often attributed by patient and doctor alike to 'rheumatism' or 'old age'. Like hypothyroidism (with which

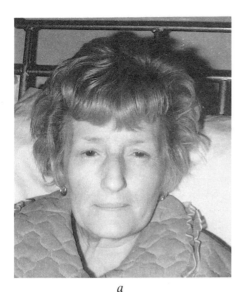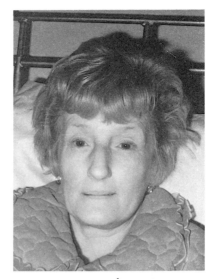

*a*                                                    *b*

**Fig. 10.74**  *a*, Myasthenia gravis. *b*, Same patient after injection of edrophonium chloride.

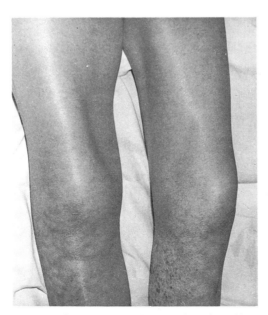

**Fig. 10.75** Diabetic myopathy: wasting of quadriceps.

early Parkinsonism may be confused), Parkinsonism is usually not recognized until some years after its onset. Early diagnosis depends more upon general inspection of the patient's posture, gait and facies than on a detailed neurological examination. Parkinsonism is characterized by three principal signs, which depend on disordered function in the extrapyramidal system. These are: (1) Poverty of movement (akinesia); (2) Muscular rigidity; (3) Tremors.

The chief disability arises from a complex disturbance in which voluntary movements are slowed (bradykinesia) or absent altogether (akinesia). This, combined with muscular rigidity, causes difficulty in carrying out everyday activities such as washing, dressing and writing. The gait is shuffling, and the patient appears to hurry in the direction he is going (festination), or if gently pushed backwards may continue in this direction (retropulsion), gathering speed and tending to fall unless stopped. The patient does not swing his arms when walking, and in turning round does so 'by numbers'. The attitude is one of flexion, the head depressed on the chest, the shoulders bowed, the knees and elbows slightly bent (*see Fig.* 10.47). The rigidity of the facial muscles gives a characteristic immobility to the face which is known as the 'Parkinsonian facies' (*Fig.* 10.76). The expression is fixed and staring; blinking is infrequent, the patient smiles little or not at all; the mouth is often slightly open and saliva dribbles away. The voice is monotonous and later dysarthria and dysphagia may result from rigidity of the bulbar muscles.

The tremor is not always present, but in many cases is the first sign observed. It is described as 'pill-rolling' owing to the characteristic movement of the thumb and index finger. Later the tremor extends to the whole hand, to the leg on the same side and finally to other parts of the body. Both rigidity and tremor may for a long time be unilateral. It may be momentarily controlled by an effort of will, or by muscular movement, only to return when these cease. The combination of tremor and increased muscle tone give rise to the typical 'cog-wheel' rigidity; this can best be elicited by passive flexion and extension of the elbow.

Encephalitis lethargica was a common cause of Parkinsonism, but is no longer so. Some cases are of unknown aetiology, though bearing some resemblance to the postencephalitic syndrome. Others can be associated with cerebral arterio-

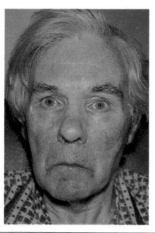

**Fig. 10.76**
Parkinsonian facies. Note fixed stare and dribbling which has caused angular stomatitis.

sclerosis, with manganese poisoning or with disturbance of copper metabolism in Wilson's disease. Parkinsonism is observed as a reversible side-effect of phenothiazine tranquillizers.

■      **LESIONS OF THE CEREBELLUM**

Cerebellar lesions may involve the vermis as in medulloblastoma or ependymoma in children. The early sign is ataxia of gait alone. As the tumour spreads other features due to involvement of adjacent structures become apparent.

More commonly, the lesion involves the lateral lobe, as in otitic abscess, and produces a variety of signs which are due mainly to abnormalities of tone and postural fixation; not only are the muscles in action affected but also those passively maintaining the background of correct posture. It is important to note that the signs of unilateral cerebellar disease are on the same side of the body as the lesion. The signs are as follows:

**Loss of muscle tone** (*Hypotonia*) Hypotonia is conspicuous only in acute cerebellar lesions. The limbs are unduly flaccid and can be moved through unusually large ranges of movement. The hypotonia is generally accompanied by slight weakness, because perfect muscular action is impossible with atonic muscles. Hypotonia also explains the swinging or 'pendular' response when the knee jerk is elicited with the legs hanging freely (*see Fig.* 10.52, p. 392).

**Muscular inco-ordination** This is seen in the ataxic (drunken) gait so often present. The patient tends to fall to the affected side. Ataxia in the arms may be demonstrated by asking the patient to make a fist and then to pronate and supinate the forearms rapidly. On the affected side this cannot be properly accomplished (*dysdiadochokinesia*). Intention tremor is another example. When the patient attempts to touch the nose with the finger, the arm and hand become increasingly shaky until the nose is reached (*see Fig.* 10.64, p. 401). The precision of movement which depends upon the appreciation of the force and rate of muscular contraction is also lost. This is known as *dysmetria*.

**Ocular disturbances** The commonest is *nystagmus* (oscillations of the eyeball – *see* p. 366), usually lateral, but sometimes rotary. Nystagmus is again a defect of postural fixation and can be regarded as an intention tremor of the orbital muscles. Occasionally *skew deviation* is observed, one eye being turned upwards and outwards, the other downwards and inwards.

**Altered postures** The position of the head is sometimes altered. It is retracted, with the face turned upwards towards the lesion. When the middle lobe is affected a position may be assumed similar to that of meningeal disease – the head retracted, the back arched, and the legs extended. The natural tendency of the patient to lean towards the side of the lesion may be overcorrected, producing an abnormal attitude.

These signs of cerebellar disease are present chiefly on the side of the lesion. Signs may be present on the opposite side due to involvement of surrounding structures. This is particularly so in tumour. The 6th nerve, owing to its propinquity, frequently suffers in cerebellar tumours, with consequent paralysis of the lateral (external) rectus (*see also* Cranial Nerves, p. 355).

**Speech defects** These generally take the form of 'staccato' speech, in which each syllable is pronounced as though it was a word. Here the muscles of articulation are affected by the defect of postural fixation.

In tumours of the cerebellum the general signs of increased intracranial pressure are more marked than in supratentorial lesions.

## ■ THE SENSORY SYSTEM

### ANATOMICAL AND PHYSIOLOGICAL CONSIDERATIONS

As in the case of the motor system the fibres conveying sensation run in relays, but the neurons have a more complex course and are more numerous.

From the peripheral nerves they enter the spinal cord through the posterior nerve roots. In the cord they dissociate to run in different tracts, some ending in the cord itself, some in the gracile and cuneate nuclei of the medulla, some proceeding to the thalamus, and some passing directly to the cerebellum, their impulses thus not reaching consciousness, but supplying proprioceptive information to this region of the brain. From the thalamus a last relay conveys the sensory impulses to the post-central area of the cerebral cortex.

The path taken by the different types of sensation is of great importance in clinical neurology.

### Path in the peripheral nerves

All types of sensation are conveyed by the peripheral nerves, but they arise from special end-organs in the skin, muscles and tendons. The modes of sensibility include cutaneous sensations, i.e. light touch, cold, warmth and pain, and deep impressions (kinaesthetic sensation) such as painful and painless pressure, postural sensibility and vibration sense. There are no nerves that are specially for discrimination and localization, though the end-organs may afford some localizing facilities (*Fig.* 10.77).

### Path in the posterior nerve roots

From the peripheral nerves the various types of sensation enter the cord through the posterior nerve roots, in which the fibres are arranged in segmental fashion similar to the motor fibres in the anterior nerve roots (*Fig.* 10.78). Lesions in the posterior roots are not common but must be considered when segmental anaesthesia is present.

### Path in the spinal cord

In this part of their course the fibres of sensation are grouped entirely differently from the arrangement in the peripheral nerves.

*Touch* fibres cross to the opposite side soon after their entry and run in the anterior spinothalamic tracts (lateral columns). Some also pass up the posterior columns crossing to enter the anterior spinothalmic tract at successive levels up to the gracile and cuneate nuclei in the medulla. A lesion in the lateral column will thus result in partial loss of tactile sensation (and loss of pain and temperature) on the opposite side below the level of the lesion, together, of course, with motor paralysis on the same side of the type already discussed.

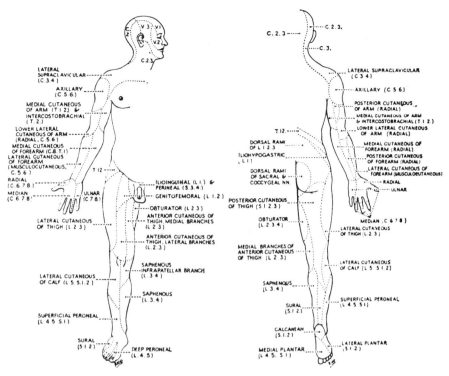

**Fig. 10.77** The distribution of sensory nerves in the skin.

*Pain and temperature* sensibility is conveyed by fibres which cross after traversing a few segments of the cord above their point of entrance. In crossing they pass closely in front of the central canal and ascend the opposite lateral spinothalamic tract to the thalamus. A lesion near the central canal (e.g. syringomyelia or intramedullary tumour) will involve these fibres and cause a limited loss of pain and temperature sense corresponding to the affected segments. Touch is affected to a much smaller extent, initially at least, because of the double pathway in the cord ('dissociated sensory loss').

*Deep sensibility* fibres pass up the posterior columns to the gracile and cuneate nuclei before crossing to the opposite side. Lesions of the posterior columns therefore result in loss of the kinaesthetic or proprioceptive sensations (deep pressure; muscle joint and tendon position; vibration sense) on the same side as the lesion. Some loss of touch also occurs.

### Paths in the medulla and brain

Leaving the spinal cord the sensory paths are continued in the following manner. *Touch* fibres pass through the medulla, pons and crus in the formatio reticularis, ending in the thalamus. *Pain and temperature* fibres run to the outer side of the medulla separate from the tactile fibres, but in the pons and crus the touch, pain, and temperature paths approximate and pass upwards to the

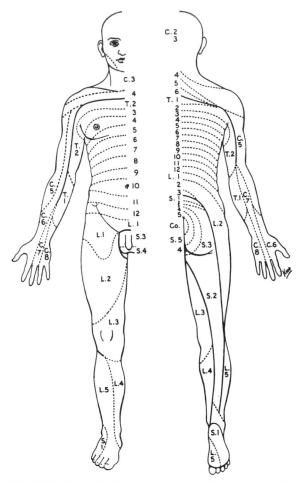

**Fig. 10.78** The radicular sensory areas of the human body.

thalamus. *Proprioceptive* sensations differ from pain, temperature and part of touch, the fibres of which have already crossed in the cord, by continuing uncrossed until they reach the medial lemniscus, where the superior sensory decussation takes place (*Fig.* 10.79).

From these anatomical and physiological data will be seen that *dissociated anaesthesia*, i.e. loss of some types of sensation, with preservation of others, is most likely to occur in cord lesions, less commonly in midbrain lesions, but very rarely in lesions of the peripheral nerves.

### The thalamus

This large basal ganglion is the final cell-station for many types of sensation before these are passed along new relays of fibres to the cerebral cortex. The ventromedial part of the thalamus is responsible for this sensory function;

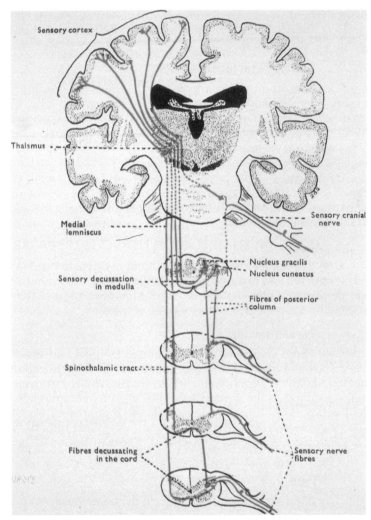

**Fig. 10.79** The sensory pathways.

the ventrolateral part is functionally related to the extrapyramidal motor system. The sensations received in the thalamus are crude perceptions of pain and temperature (but not touch), gross joint movements, or merely a sense of comfort or distress or a general 'sense of awareness'.

The results of a thalamic lesion are:

Hemianaesthesia, excessive sensibility to painful stimuli, spontaneous pains, and misinterpretation of other stimuli (e.g. light touch or tickling may give an unpleasant sensation), possibly ataxia and choreiform movements from concurrent involvement of the corpus striatum. These signs are present on the side opposite to the lesion.

Lesions of the thalamus are commonly vascular or neoplastic. If vascular, they are rarely confined to the thalamus but involve the internal capsule, so that hemiparesis is also present.

### The parietal lobes

Sensory fibres pass from the thalamus via the internal capsule to the sensory cortex behind the central sulcus in the parietal lobe. Complex forms of sensation are appreciated in the parietal lobes and lesions may give rise to spatial disorientation, astereognosis and agnosia (sensory suppression) (*see* p. 424). *Apraxia* may also occur, i.e. the inability to perform a particular movement although the patient is aware of what he wishes to do and has no paralysis preventing him from doing it. This can be tested by asking the patient to use a key or pencil.

The parietal lobes, together with the frontal lobes, are also concerned with higher intellectual functions.

## SENSORY SYMPTOMS IN NERVOUS DISEASES

The subjective sensations commonly experienced in disease of the nervous system fall into two groups: (1) *Paraesthesiae*; (2) *Pain*. Certain phenomena are described under the objective examination, though they may well be appreciated by the patient, i.e. anaesthesia or ataxia.

### Paraesthesiae

These consist of such sensations as 'pins and needles', pricking, numbness and band-like sensations around the trunk. They are common as transient phenomena when the peripheral nerves are stretched or subjected to pressure. A familiar example is the paraesthesia produced by compression of the lateral popliteal nerve after sitting too long with the legs crossed. Equally they may herald serious disease of the nervous system (e.g. spinal tumour, subacute combined degeneration, disseminated sclerosis). The distribution of the paraesthesiae has localizing value.

### Pain

Impulses interpreted as pain in the consciousness are carried by the nervous system whatever their origin may be, but the description of pain as a symptom of visceral disease is considered under the various systems and on pp. 7–10. Special types of pain associated with lesions of the nervous system need mention here.

**Peripheral nerve pain** This may occur in various forms of injury, neuritis and neuropathy. Sensory loss accompanied by pain follows the distribution of the nerve and may be associated with motor changes.

Sometimes pain occurs alone, i.e. without motor or sensory changes, and this may be called *neuralgia*. In time, however, objective changes indicating involvement of the nerves may appear. For example, sciatica is neuralgic pain referred to the muscles supplied by the sciatic nerve, but sooner or later it is usual for some objective signs to appear such as pain on stretching the nerve or tenderness over its course. There may also be loss of the ankle jerk on the affected side. Disc lesions are held to be responsible for many cases, but pelvic examination is

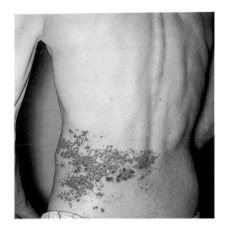

**Fig. 10.80**
Herpes zoster (shingles). The vesicles in this case are haemorrhagic.

necessary to exclude the presence of neoplasms. Another example is the neuralgia preceding, or more commonly following, herpes zoster. (*See also* Trigeminal Neuralgia, p. 360.)

**Root pains** These are often of a neuralgic type but are characteristically increased by coughing and sneezing. They follow the distribution of the particular root or roots affected, and may at first be unaccompanied by objective evidence of root irritation. It is therefore of great importance to ascertain the exact distribution of pains in the trunk. Examples may be seen in the girdle pains of tabes and the half-girdle pains of herpes zoster, a virus infection of the posterior-root ganglia associated with a vesicular rash followed by scarring and sensory loss in the same area as the pain (*Fig.* 10.80). Cervical and lumbar root pains are distributed to the appropriate limb and are most often due to spondylosis with disc protrusions. Tumours arising from the meninges of the cord produce pain of a root type, at first confined to one side, later spreading to the other. The 'lightning pains' of tabes are an example of a root pain in the limbs.

**Causalgia** This is an unusual type of burning pain, generally occurring after limb injuries in cases where the nerve damage is comparatively slight.

**Visceral pains** Excluding pains due to visceral disease, pains of a visceral type may occur in the well-known *visceral crises* of tabes. The commonest of these is the gastric crisis, in which epigastric pain and vomiting may erroneously suggest a diagnosis of gastric ulcer.

*Headache and Thalamic Pain* are considered elsewhere (pp. 7–10).

### PHYSICAL SIGNS: EXAMINATION OF THE SENSORY SYSTEM

In all neurological cases a thorough investigation of the perceptions of sensations is valuable, and in many diagnosis depends chiefly upon this. (*See Fig.* 10.81.)

The examination must test *tactile sensation and discrimination, deep sensibility, perception of pain and temperature, joint and vibration sense, co-ordination of movement and stereognosis.*

When the exact localization of the lesion is of direct therapeutic importance,

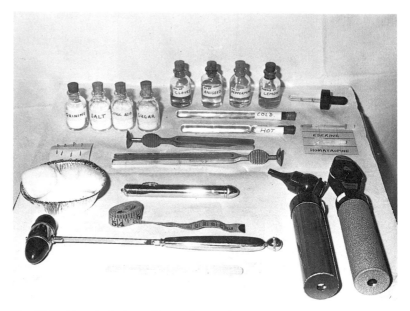

**Fig. 10.81** Neurological tray. The equipment for neurological examination includes: (1) Substances for testing taste and smell; (2) Hot and cold test tubes; (3) Tuning-forks of high and low frequency; (4) Cottonwool; (5) Pins; (6) Ophthalmoscope with homatropine and eserine eye drops; (7) Auroscope; (8) Pocket torch; (9) Tendon hammer; (10) Tape measure; (11) Spatula.

the areas of disturbed sensibility should be carefully charted (simple line drawings of the body are readily obtainable) (cf. *Figs*. 10.77, 10.78). This is the more important as it enables the observer to appreciate changes in the distribution of anaesthesiae, etc., which may take place from time to time. The recognition of a sensory 'level' is of particular relevance to the diagnosis and localization of spinal cord compression. The appropriate stimulus (touch, prick, vibration, etc.) is applied at about one-inch intervals down each side of the trunk in turn, both front and back. The spinous processes of the vertebrae may be used for testing vibration sense. Particular attention is paid to the 'saddle' area of the buttocks and perineum where sensory loss may be the only sign of a cauda equina lesion. Sensory levels and areas of sensory loss may be lightly marked with a skin pencil prior to recording on a chart.

### Tactile sensation

This is best tested by gently touching the skin with a wisp of cotton-wool; the patient's eyes should be covered. If an area of *anaesthesia* is found, it should be carefully compared with the corresponding area on the opposite limb or part of the body. The anaesthesia may be graded as slight (*hypoaesthesia*) when sensation is merely dulled, or complete when it is entirely absent. If the touch is more acutely felt than normal, *hyperaesthesia* is said to be present. If it is felt as a perverted sensation, e.g. tingling or pain, the term *paraesthesia* or *dysaesthesia* describes it.

### Tactile discrimination

This is tested by determining at what distance apart two points of a compass can be distinguished as separate entities. This varies greatly in different parts of the body. It corresponds with the richness of touch spots which are numerous on the tongue and nose so that the points of the compass can be distinguished a few millimetres apart, whereas on the lower part of the back they may need to be separated by several inches.

Tactile discrimination is less sensitive in cortical lesions.

### Deep sensibility (*Pressure pain*)

This may be tested by firm pressure with a blunt object such as a pencil, or by pinching the muscles, tendons, etc. Testicular pain on squeezing is another form of pressure pain, often absent in tabes.

This type of sensation is often retained when cutaneous sensibility is lost.

### Pain

Pain sensibility may be tested by pricking with a pin; heavy pressure must be avoided, otherwise pressure pain may be induced.

The patient's expression should be noted and compared with his statement about the sensation and the time relationship between the stimulus and the response noted. The term *analgesia* signifies absence of the sense of pain, and in dissociated 'anaesthesia' the part may be analgesic without being anaesthetic.

### Temperature discrimination

Two test tubes of water, cold and warm (not hot), may be conveniently used. They should be interchanged frequently so that the patient cannot guess which is being used.

### Sensations of joint movement and posture

The joint must be moved passively, making sure that the muscles to it are completely relaxed. In the case of the great toe, for example, the patient should know when it is extended or flexed without moving it himself (*Fig.* 10.82). When the limb (especially the upper) is put in a certain position it should be possible for the patient to put the opposite limb in a similar position.

### Vibration sense

This is tested by placing a tuning-fork of low pitch over the superficial bones, e.g. tibia or phalanges. The patient is normally conscious of a vibratory tremor, not merely the touch of the fork.

### Stereognosis

This requires not only an appreciation of the form of the object but of its weight and texture. It may be tested by asking the patient to identify familiar objects such as a key, a coin or a pencil. Impairment of such appreciation results from lesions in the higher parts of the sensory system, e.g. in the parietal lobes.

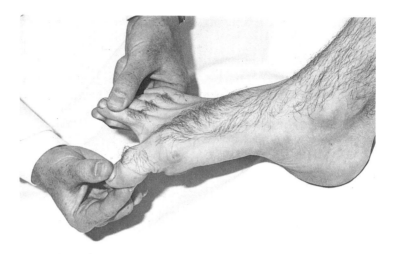

**Fig. 10.82** Toe position sense. The patient should recognize that the toe is in the flexed position. To prevent him from obtaining this information by the sense of touch, the other toes are kept well away from the toe which is moved.

With certain lesions *sensory suppression* is found. This means that when touch or pin-prick is tested on either side of the body independently, sensation is normal, but when the two sides are tested simultaneously the sensation is appreciated on the normal side only.

## ILLUSTRATIVE LESIONS OF THE SENSORY NEURONS

A few diseases affect chiefly the sensory neurons but many involve concurrently the motor neurons. As lesions of the motor neurons have already received attention, it will be convenient to use as illustrations some diseases in which sensory and motor lesions are combined, but in which the sensory changes are more notable.

Lesions of the sensory neurons have a similar causation to those of the motor system (*see* Table 10.7, p. 439).

**Localization** The localization of a lesion of the sensory neurons depends partly on the distribution of the disturbance of sensation and partly on its type. This has been partially discussed in the sections on anatomy and physiology, and may be recapitulated here.

From an anatomical point of view lesions of the peripheral *nerves* result in anaesthesia corresponding to the distribution of the sensory fibres (*see Fig.* 10.77); segmental anaesthesia results from *root* lesions (*see Fig.* 10.78). Complete transverse lesions of the *spinal cord* cause anaesthesia in the limbs and trunk below the level of the lesion. Unilateral lesions result in the dissociation of anaesthesia found in the Brown-Séquard syndrome (opposite). Lesions of the *brainstem* may also result in dissociation, some types of sensation being lost on the same side of the body, some on the opposite side. Lesions of the *thalamus*, *internal capsule* or *cortex* result in hemi-anaesthesia affecting the face, arm and leg on the opposite side of the body.

As regards the type of anaesthesia, all varieties of sensation may be lost in peripheral nerve lesions and complete transverse lesions of the spinal cord although, in the former case, some sensations may be affected more than others. *Dissociated anaesthesia*, e.g. abolition of pain and temperature sense with preservation of touch sensibility, may result from lesions in the grey matter of the cord near the central canal. Such a lesion may occur in syringomyelia and intramedullary tumours which interrupt the pain and temperature fibres as they cross over from one side to the other.

Dissociated anaesthesia also results from brainstem lesions (particularly the medulla), as in syringomyelia of these parts, or thrombosis of the posterior inferior cerebellar artery.

The loss of proprioceptive sensations (joint movement, vibration sense, etc.), with little or no loss of tactile, thermal or pain sensibility, is characteristic of lesions of the posterior columns (tabes, subacute combined degeneration) or of their continuation fibres to the medulla.

When anaesthesia is central in origin (thalamus, internal capsule and cortex) it is rarely so complete as in peripheral lesions, and it affects the distal parts of the limbs more than the proximal. It is further characteristic of thalamic lesions that the response to sensory stimulation is exaggerated and frequently perverted (touch may produce an unpleasant sensation almost amounting to pain). Spontaneous pain may also occur. Such symptoms may be thought to be hysterical. In lesions of the sensory cortex the higher types of sensation are impaired (astereognosis) (*see also* p. 423).

### Brown-Séquard Syndrome (*Fig.* 10.83)

Although not common, this phenomenon is an excellent illustration of one type of dissociated anaesthesia. The lesion consists of a hemisection of

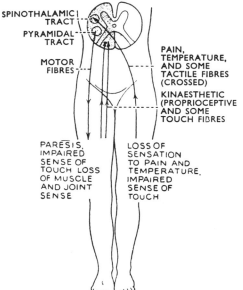

**Fig. 10.83**
Brown-Séquard syndrome. Hemisection of the cord. As touch has a double pathway, it may be impaired on each side, as shown in the diagram, or may be preserved on both sides.

the cord and is usually traumatic (e.g. stab wound), though tumours and other conditions occasionally produce the same effect.

On the side of the lesion the sensations from tendons, muscles, and joints, vibration sense and tactile discrimination are lost. On the opposite side pain and temperature sense are abolished and to a lesser extent touch. In addition, motor and vasomotor signs are added: on the side of the lesion there is paralysis of the upper neuron type, and signs of vasomotor paresis. A limited lower neuron paralysis may also be present, corresponding with the segments of the cord affected.

### Syringomyelia

This condition results from obstruction to the flow of cerebrospinal fluid between the spinal subarachnoid space and the cisterna magna or through the foramina in the roof of the fourth ventricle. The commonest cause of obstruction is the Chiari malformation in which a tongue of cerebellum projects down through the foramen magnum, but arachnoid adhesions following meningitis may be responsible in some cases. The resulting distension of the central canal or perivascular spaces in the spinal cord interrupts the pain and temperature fibres crossing here but only affects part of the touch fibres, those in the posterior columns remaining intact. Pain and temperature sense are therefore lost while common touch and postural sensibility are preserved. When the spinothalamic tract is interrupted there is loss of sensation below the level of the lesion. When segmental fibres only are involved, there is a lower as well as an upper limit to the area of anaesthesia; this is referred to as *suspended anaesthesia*. Injuries due to the non-appreciation of pain and heat may first call attention to the disease (*Fig.* 10.84). Charcot's joints (*see* p. 335) may occur in the upper limbs in chronic cases.

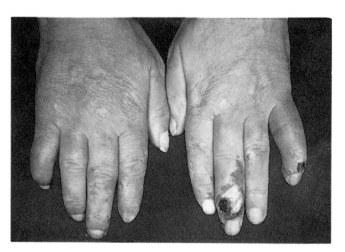

**Fig. 10.84** Syringomyelia, showing burns and whitlows. Note also the resorption of the terminal phalanges (especially the right hand) and the puffy appearance of the hands (the 'succulent' hand).

Motor signs are also generally present. If the lesion extends into the anterior horn cells there will be a lower neuron type of paralysis corresponding with the spinal segments affected. As these are usually the lower cervical and upper dorsal segments, the paralysis affects the small muscles of the hand, as in motor neuron disease.

Involvement of the lateral columns often gives upper neuron signs on one or both sides, but the degree of paralysis is rarely great. Less often, the posterior columns are damaged, with corresponding loss of deep sensibility, etc. Signs of involvement of these long tracts are found only below the level of the lesion and are thus evident in the legs rather than the arms. A rare type of syringomyelia affects the brainstem—*syringobulbia*. Here the bulbar nuclei are affected, and dissociated anaesthesia may be present in the face.

### Tabes dorsalis (*Locomotor ataxia*) (Fig. 10.85)

This disease is an example of a degenerative lesion resulting from syphilis. It is now uncommon but illustrates well the results of involvement of the sensory neurons (principally) and is largely confined to the posterior nerve roots and the posterior columns of the spinal cord. The disease also implicates the cranial nerves in most cases and thus provides valuable confirmatory clinical signs. Both the symptoms and physical signs are mainly sensory.

Among early symptoms must be mentioned pains. These may be of the 'lightning' variety—hot, sharp pains generally in the limbs striking them at right-angles, or 'girdle pains' due to the root changes. Other subjective sensations are a feeling of walking on air or cottonwool (due to light anaesthesia of the soles of the feet), and the band-like sensation experienced around the chest (cuirass sensation) which corresponds with an area of analgesia. Interference with the vesical and rectal reflexes (tabes affects especially the lumbar and sacral roots and segments

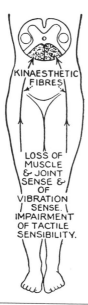

**Fig. 10.85**
Tabes. Lesion of the posterior columns. The lumbar and sacral segments are generally affected.

of the cord) may result in difficulty in beginning micturition, often with retention. More rarely defects in the bowel action result. Usually much later the patient may complain of unsteadiness in walking, especially in the dark, or a tendency to fall when he stands with the eyes closed as may occur when washing the face. These symptoms are due to the ataxia which develops from loss of proprioceptive (kinaesthetic) sensations. The visceral crises (gastric, laryngeal, renal and cardiac) are analogous to the lightning pains, consisting of sharp pain simulating that due to visceral disease, sometimes accompanied by other visceral symptoms. They often occur early in the disease, sometimes leading to an erroneous diagnosis. The commonest is the gastric crisis in which abdominal pain, vomiting and skin hyperaesthesia are usually found, imitating an acute abdominal catastrophe.

The physical signs result partly from the damage to the posterior nerve roots and posterior columns and partly from cranial nerve involvement. Loss of tendon reflexes due to interruption of the sensory limb of the reflex arc is exemplified by the absent knee and ankle jerks (reflex centres in the lumbosacral region). Ankle jerks are generally lost much earlier than the knee jerks. Areas of anaesthesia and even more commonly analgesia occur on the trunk and limbs. Analgesia may also be found on the nose and lips, though common touch is preserved. Deep sensibility is impaired and a particular sign of this is delayed pain on squeezing the tendo calcaneus (Achillis). The ulnar nerve when rolled under the fingers at the elbow is also frequently analgesic. Ataxia is not usually an early sign, but before it results in the characteristic gait (*see* p. 386) it can be demonstrated by Romberg's sign. Cranial-nerve signs are often early manifestations of tabes. The more important are the Argyll Robertson pupil, optic atrophy and ptosis, the last being partly responsible for the 'tabetic facies'.

Lastly, in tabes, trophic disorders may occur in the limb's, causing perforating ulcers and arthropathies (Charcot joints, *see* p. 335). The exact mechanism by which these are produced is not fully understood, but the loss of sensations from the parts is undoubtedly an important factor.

### Compression of the spinal cord (*see also* Cauda Equina Lesions)

Compression of the cord illustrates a combination of motor and sensory phenomena varying in type and degree according to the nature of the compressive lesion. A number of causes may be responsible, e.g. fractured spine, cervical spondylosis, Paget's disease, extramedullary tumours, malignant disease and so forth. As in many diseases the symptoms vary with the rapidity with which the compression occurs. In sudden catastrophes, such as fracture of the spine, immediate paralysis and loss of sensation below the level of the lesion results. When the compression is more slowly produced as by tumour, there are often pains in the limbs or around the trunk due to root irritation. These are increased by sneezing, coughing and movements of the spine and often precede other signs. Later the general symptoms consist of progressive paraplegia with characteristic upper motor neuron signs together with sensory loss, sphincter paralysis and impotence. The level of the spinal compression can be located by finding paralysis, sensory loss and altered reflexes at or below the affected segment of the cord. As previously described, the finding of a level below which power or sensation is impaired is of the great importance in determining the site of a spinal lesion. It must be remembered, however, that spinal nerves supply the skin and muscles ('dermatomes' and 'myotomes') of the trunk at a level two or three vertebrae lower than the vertebral level at which they arise (*Fig.* 10.86). Certain infective and metastatic lesions can be located by finding tenderness on pressure over the affected vertebra.

Useful evidence of compression is also obtained by examination of the cerebro-spinal fluid. The protein is greatly increased without any cellular increase and

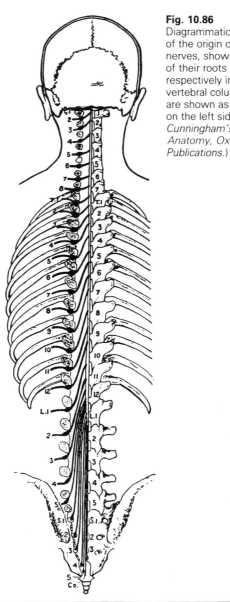

**Fig. 10.86**
Diagrammatic representation of the origin of the spinal nerves, showing the position of their roots and ganglia respectively in relation to the vertebral column. The nerves are shown as thick black lines on the left side. (*From Cunningham's 'Textbook of Anatomy, Oxford Medical Publications.*)

occasionally is so great that spontaneous coagulation occurs, and the fluid may assume a yellow colour, *xanthochromia*. The fluid removed from above the level of the obstruction, e.g. by cisternal puncture, remains normal. Queckenstedt's test, i.e. pressure on the jugular veins, fails to cause the normal rise of pressure noted at lumbar puncture.

Certain types of intramedullary tumour do not produce these compression symptoms but tend to imitate other centrally situated lesions of the spinal cord such as syringomyelia.

### Cauda equina lesions

These result in combined motor and sensory symptoms varying considerably in distribution according to the particular nerve roots affected.

Their characteristic features are a saddle-shaped area of anaesthesia over the genitalia, perineum and buttocks, with disturbances of micturition and defaecation—especially retention of urine—and motor paralysis of the lower neuron type affecting all or several groups of muscles in the lower limbs. Both the anaesthesia and muscular paralysis have a root distribution; so also has pain if present.

### Subacute combined degeneration

The degeneration of the spinal cord which occurs in cases of vitamin $B_{12}$ deficiency is another example of combined motor and sensory lesions of the cord, but in this instance there is usually a peripheral neuropathy as well and sometimes a psychosis due to cerebral cortical degeneration. Anaemia is usually absent but sternal puncture may reveal a megaloblastic marrow, and the diagnosis is supported by the finding of a reduced serum level of vitamin $B_{12}$. (*See also* p. 304.)

Symptoms of a peripheral neuropathy usually occur first (numbness or tingling in the hands and feet), followed later by unsteadiness of gait, ultimately resulting in gross ataxia due to degeneration of the posterior columns. Vibration sense is also lost. Simultaneously the pyramidal tracts are affected with a consequent spastic paraplegia and other signs of upper motor neuron disease. In severe cases, and in the terminal stages, the increased tendon reflexes may become diminished or lost and the paralysis flaccid. Disturbances of micturition and defaecation and trophic changes in the skin, may occur, as in other spinal cord diseases.

### Friedreich's ataxia

This disease also illustrates the effects of a simultaneous involvement of motor and sensory tracts. It is familial, being transmitted by recessive autosomal inheritance, and usually becomes manifest in childhood.

The posterior columns and cerebellar tracts are affected, causing ataxia both of the arms and legs. Other cerebellar signs include nystagmus, head tremor and scanning speech. Affection of the corticospinal tracts gives signs of an upper motor neuron lesion, especially Babinski's sign and spasticity. The tendon reflexes are, however, lost owing to an interruption of the sensory limb of the reflex arc in the posterior nerve root. There are often congenital skeletal deformities, especially pes cavus and scoliosis.

Other types of familial ataxia are described bearing a close resemblance to Friedreich's disease.

## MENINGES

The meninges form a continuous membrane over the whole brain and extend down to cover the spinal cord. The pia and arachnoid are in close contact in most places, and between them circulates the cerebrospinal fluid, which is more plentiful in the 'cisterns', where the pia and arachnoid separate from one another to accommodate it. The pia-arachnoid follows the convolutions of the brain closely and carries the blood vessels in its substance.

These facts explain the necessity for considering the meninges, both cerebral and spinal, as a whole, and of remembering that some of the symptoms and signs in meningeal disease may be due to spread of the disease process from or into the brain itself and to involvement of the cranial nerves which are partly or completely ensheathed by the meninges.

Whatever the cause of meningeal irritation, the symptoms and signs are similar. They will be modified by the part of the membranes which are most affected, e.g. cerebral or spinal; by the actual pathology, e.g. inflammation or haemorrhage; and by the rapidity with which the membranes are affected. They may be conveniently grouped as follows.

**1. Symptoms and signs of increased intracranial pressure** (*see* p. 405) Headache, vomiting and sometimes papillocdema may result from the increased tension on the meninges by the accumulating cerebrospinal fluid between the pia and arachnoid, and also from hydrocephalus if adhesions or exudate have obstructed the free circulation of the fluid. The headache is frequently referred to the nape of the neck and may be very severe. Vomiting may be of the cerebral type.

**2. Essential signs of meningeal irritation** The characteristic phenomenon of neck rigidity occurs early and later changes to definite head retraction (*Fig.* 10.87). To test neck rigidity the observer attempts passively to flex the head

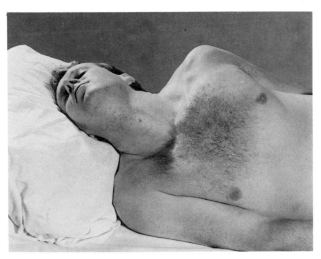

**Fig. 10.87** Head retraction. A sign of meningeal irritation.

on the chest and with his other hand notes the tautness of the neck muscles. When the spinal meninges are much affected, particularly in infants, the phenomenon of opisthotonos may be seen. The body is then arched backwards and held rigidly. This sign is but one example of the generalized muscular rigidity which occurs in meningeal irritation.

Two special signs depend upon traction of the inflamed meninges and spinal nerves.

*Kernig's sign*: The hip is flexed to about 90° and any attempt then to straighten the knee results in pain and spasm in the hamstrings (*Fig.* 10.88).

*Brudzinski's sign*: The head is flexed on the chest, which causes the lower limbs to be drawn up. The sign is valuable if it is suspected that the head retraction (which relieves tension on the spinal nerves) is partly voluntary.

**3. Signs of brain involvement** Some spread of the disease process may take place to the brain itself or the meningeal infection may have arisen in the brain. As examples of the resulting signs may be mentioned motor phenomena such as fits and paresis, mental disturbances and so forth.

**4. Signs of cranial nerve involvement** These are found in chronic forms of basal meningitis but only rarely in acute disease unless treatment has been delayed or ineffective. The oculomotor, 7th and 8th nerves are most commonly affected.

**5. Changes in the cerebrospinal fluid** Early lumbar puncture is necessary so that the cerebrospinal fluid can be examined and an accurate diagnosis made.

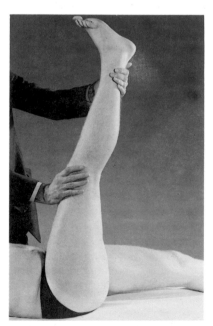 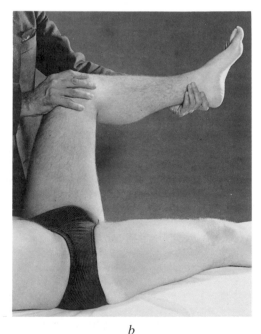

*a*      *b*

**Fig. 10.88** Kernig's sign. *a*, Negative response. The leg can be well extended. *b*, Positive response. The leg cannot be extended to more than a right-angle when the thigh is well flexed on the abdomen.

### Meningitis

This may be caused by the meningococcus, by the tubercle bacillus, by the pneumococcus and other cocci, and by virus infections. *Haemophilus influenzae* is an important cause in children while in diabetic, leukaemic and other immunosuppressed patients, a variety of micro-organisms including fungi can produce meningitis. Whichever organism is responsible, the results are similar, though special clinical signs may help in distinguishing one type from another. Tuberculous meningitis is often suggested by a long prodromal period and by the discovery of other tuberculous lesions. Cerebrospinal fever (meningococcal meningitis) is rapid in onset, often found in epidemics and sometimes accompanied by a petechial or roseolar rash, which has given it the name 'spotted fever'. Pneumococcal meningitis is a likely diagnosis if signs of pneumonia are found, or in cases of pneumococcal otitis media. It may also be a primary infection. Direct extension of sepsis from the skull bones, e.g. osteomyelitis resulting from chronic sinus infection or mastoiditis, and trauma, account for some cases. *Viral meningitis* is accompanied by changes in the cerebrospinal fluid similar to those of polio-encephalitis. The term *meningismus* is given to a condition of meningeal irritability due to toxaemia without any actual inflammation of the meninges. It occurs especially in pneumonia and is most common in children. The headache is said to cease when delirium begins, whereas in meningitis it continues.

The diagnosis not only of the type of meningitis, but of the disease itself, is not complete without examination of the cerebrospinal fluid.

Meningitis is an inflammatory disease and fever is a symptom. It is variable in degree, and the pulse rate may be proportionately increased at first, but later tends to become slower owing to the increase in intracranial pressure.

### THE CEREBRAL VESSELS

Atheroma may affect the cerebral arteries or the extracranial arteries which feed them. Thus the supply of blood to the brain may be interrupted both within and without the skull. This is of importance because of the difficulty it causes in topographical diagnosis which may be essential from the point of view of treatment.

The flow of blood may be greatly reduced by conditions which cause a fall of blood pressure, as in shock or haemorrhage. Similar effects are caused by external pressure upon the neck arteries, e.g. vertebral artery compression in cases of cervical spondylosis.

The amount of damage resulting from brain infarction after vascular occlusion depends upon the site of the occlusion and the adequacy of collateral circulation through the circle of Willis. Infarction is especially likely to follow the occlusion of small end arteries, such as the perforating vessels supplying the internal capsule. Atheroma is particularly common in the middle cerebral artery, but changes in the carotid, basilar and vertebral arteries are certainly important contributory causes. Similarly, haemorrhages may arise from an atheromatous cerebral artery, and emboli may occur in mitral disease, atrial fibrillation, bacterial endocarditis and cardiac infarction. Atheromatous plaques may be responsible for microemboli from extracranial arteries.

It is therefore necessary in a case of 'stroke' that the condition of the arteries arising from the arch of the aorta and those in the circle of Willis and in the cerebral vessels proper should be considered as a whole. Information about the arteries in the neck may be obtained by careful palpation of the carotid vessels, by auscultation to search for any unusual murmurs, and, if necessary, by the use of arteriography.

Subject to the conception that any change in the flow of blood through the extracranial vessels will modify the results of changes in the cerebral vessels themselves, the following comments may be made.

| Table 10.5 | **Common features of cerebrovascular disorders producing stroke** | | | | |
|---|---|---|---|---|---|
| | *Onset* | *Course* | *Loss of consciousness* | *Associated findings* | *CSF* |
| Intracerebral haemorrhage | During activity Headache | Minutes to hemiplegia | Rapid coma | Hypertensive retinopathy and cardiomegaly Bleeding diathesis | Bloody |
| Cerebral thrombosis | At rest Variable onset | Minutes to hours to hemiplegia | Unusual | Atherosclerosis and cardiovascular disease | Clear |
| Cerebral embolism | Instantaneous | Rapid recovery | Possible | Cardiac arrhythmia Mitral stenosis Myocardial infarction Carotid murmur | Clear |
| Subarachnoid haemorrhage | Sudden headache | May relapse early | Common | Hypertension Neck stiffness Subhyloid haemor- rhage | Bloody |
| Subdural haemorrhage | Gradual Preceding trauma | Days Weeks Months | Eventually | Headache, vomiting Confusion Papilloedema Bradycardia | Xantho- chromia |

**The middle cerebral artery** The middle cerebral artery supplies the lateral aspects of the anterior two-thirds of the brain, including the internal capsule. This is the commonest site for cerebral thrombosis and usually results in hemiplegia and hemianaesthesia (cortical type), on the opposite side, particularly in the face, tongue and upper limb. Aphasia of various types is also common and may occur alone. Hemianopia due to involvement of the optic radiation in the internal capsule may also occur.

**The anterior cerebral artery** The anterior cerebral artery supplies the medial aspects of the anterior two-thirds of the brain. Motor and sensory impairment are more marked in the lower limb than in the arm and may be accompanied by mental deterioration.

**Posterior cerebral artery** The posterior cerebral artery mainly supplies the occipital pole of the brain, and occlusion results in contralateral hemianopia.

**Carotid artery** This may be the site of stenosis which interferes with the blood supply to the intracranial vessels. Any insufficiency of this kind may make lesions, for example, in the middle cerebral, of much more serious significance. The suspicion of a carotid artery stenosis should lead to careful examination of the neck for the pulsation (inequality or absence) of the carotid vessels or presence of a systolic murmur over the bifurcation of the carotid. Fleeting episodes of ischaemia due either to micro-emboli or diminished perfusion may affect the territory supplied by the carotid. The most characteristic of these is *amaurosis fugax*, or transient blindness, due to impared circulation through the retinal artery.

**Vertebrobasilar system** Partial occlusion may occur without symptoms if the circulation in the carotid artery and the circle of Willis is adequate. Transient ischaemic attacks from vertebrobasilar insufficiency are common and may consist of vertigo, migraine-like visual disturbances, facial paraesthesiae, dysphasia, hemiparesis, hemianaesthesia or 'drop' attacks in which the patient suddenly falls without loss of consciousness. These may be provoked by vertebral artery compression on extending or turning the head, especially when there is cervical spondylosis. Another less common cause is stenosis of the subclavian artery proximal to the origin of the vertebral artery producing reversal of flow in the latter when the arm is in use (*'subclavian steal'*).

Infarction of brain within the territory supplied by the vertebrobasilar system (brainstem, cerebellum and occipital pole) can produce a variety of syndromes in which the most constant features are vertigo, ipsilateral cerebellar and cranial nerve signs (5th–10th) with contralateral spinothalamic and pyramidal tract signs.

## Intracranial haemorrhage (*see* Table 10.5)

The site and therefore the clinical features of intracranial haemorrhage depend to some extent upon the cause. Intracerebral haemorrhage is usually due to atheroma and (or) hypertension, subarachnoid haemorrhage to aneurysm and subdural or extradural haemorrhage to trauma.

**Intracerebral haemorrhage** Generally involves the internal capsule (middle cerebral) and usually causes abrupt loss of consciousness with hemiplegia, but these may be preceded by intense headache and vomiting. The subjects commonly have hypertension as well as cerebral arteriosclerosis. Blood may appear in the cerebrospinal fluid and cause neck rigidity. Thrombosis also occurs within the same vascular territory but is less likely to be associated with coma, has a better recovery prospect and often a more limited paralysis, because branches of the middle cerebral rather than the main stem may be picked out. Cerebral embolism may occur in the young (mitral stenosis with atrial fibrillation or subacute bacterial endocarditis) or older persons with myocardial infarction. Hemiparesis occurs, rarely associated with unconsciousness, and usually suddenly on the dislodgement of the embolus.

**Subarachnoid haemorrhage** The usual cause is the leakage or rupture of a congenital aneurysm on the cerebral arterial circle of Willis or less commonly an angioma. Sometimes in older persons a degenerate artery bursts, or trauma may be responsible. Hypertension is a common precipitating cause. The clinical manifestations vary. Meningeal symptoms—slowly or suddenly produced—include head retraction, neck rigidity, Kernig's sign, pyrexia and other signs which may lead to a wrong diagnosis of meningitis. A systolic murmur arising from an aneurysm or angioma may be heard on auscultation over the skull or the closed eye.

The truth is established on lumbar puncture when pure blood or heavily blood-stained fluid is withdrawn. After settling, the supernatant fluid remains straw-coloured, thus distinguishing the blood from that due to imperfect lumbar puncture. The blood is evenly mixed throughout the fluid, whereas in the case of a 'traumatic tap' the first sample obtained is usually more heavily stained than subsequent samples.

In a patient who survives the first haemorrhage the aneurysm becomes lined with clot. This tends to be removed after a few days so that a second bleed commonly occurs about 10 days after the first. This fact is relevant to surgical treatment of the aneurysm which should be attempted within 10 days of the original haemorrhage.

**Subdural haemorrhage** Sometimes a comparatively minor injury to the skull may result in a gradual leakage from the cortical veins into the subdural space, and a haematoma is formed causing pressure symptoms; it may therefore be confused with cerebral tumour unless the history of trauma is elicited. The symptoms manifest themselves in a few days, weeks or months after the injury, and

| Table 10.6 | **A routine for recording examination of the nervous system** |
|---|---|
| Cerebral dominance | Left- or right-handed |
| Mental state | Orientation, memory, intelligence, grasp of information, behaviour, mood, talk, delusions, hallucinations, insight |
| Speech | Dysarthria, dysphasia, stuttering |
| Stance and gait | Romberg's test |
| Skull and spine | Congenital or acquired deformities. Bruits. Symmetry of development |
| Cranial nerves | 1 Recognize test odours with either nostril<br>2 Visual acuity: near and distance vision<br>Visual fields; scotomas<br>Optic disc and retinae<br>3, 4, 6 Enophthalmos or exophthalmos. Ptosis<br>Pupils equal, central, circular and regular<br>Pupils react to light, direct and consensual and to convergence<br>External ocular movements. Nystagmus<br>5 Corneal reflexes. Facial sensation<br>Jaw opens centrally; normal power<br>Jaw jerk<br>7 Facial asymmetry or weakness (upper and lower divisions)<br>8 Hears whispered voice at 3 ft, either AC>BC; Weber's test not lateralized<br>9, 10 Palate elevation; gag reflex; cough and voice<br>11 Sternomastoids and trapezius: weakness, wasting or fasciculation<br>12 Tongue: wasting, fasciculation, protrusion (central or elevated) |

concussion may not have occurred. Headache, vomiting, drowsiness, mental confusion and bradycardia are common, but subject to remarkable fluctuation, seldom seen to the same extent in tumour. Papilloedema of moderate degree may develop. Variable changes in the pupillary, tendon and superficial reflexes result, hemiplegia may develop, and drowsiness changes to stupor or, later, coma and death, if unrelieved.

## ■ THE DIAGNOSIS OF DISEASES OF THE NERVOUS SYSTEM

### The anatomical diagnosis

Diagnosis may often be achieved with more precision in diseases of the nervous system than in other parts of the body.

The reason for this is the fact that disturbances of function are closely related to the anatomical site of the lesion. This is well illustrated in the examples already given of affections of the motor and sensory tracts in the spinal cord, of the

| | |
|---|---|
| *Motor system* | Posture |
| | Muscle bulk |
| | Fasciculation |
| | Tone |
| | Voluntary movements—power |
| |     fine movements |
| |     akinesia |
| |     bradykinesia |
| | Co-ordination |
| | Involuntary movements—tremor |
| |     chorea |
| |     athetosis |
| | Tendon reflexes |
| | Superficial reflexes |
| | Plantar responses (Babinski sign) |
| *Sensory system* | Light touch   (cottonwool) |
| | Pain  (sharp pin) |
| | Temperature  (hot and cold tubes) |
| | Joint position sense |
| | Vibration sense (128 Hz) |
| | 2-point discrimination  (compasses) |
| *Peripheral nerves* | Palpation |
| | Response to percussion |
| *Autonomic system* | Sweating on peripheries |
| | Blood pressure control—postural hypotension |
| | Heart-rate control—Valsalva manoeuvre |

localizing value of the abolition of tendon reflexes and the modification of reflexes, as in the case of Babinski's sign. It has been seen how a combination of signs may lead to a topographical diagnosis of such diseases as motor neuron disease, subacute combined degeneration, neuropathies and myopathies.

Similarly, damage to the motor system in the brain may result in characteristic patterns as in the complete hemiplegia of an internal capsular lesion. Special functions of other parts of the brain may be lost or altered and cause impairment of intellect, memory and personality when the frontal lobes are affected.

Involvement of cranial nerves may have great localizing value if associated with other neurological signs, but not if the nerve alone is involved because of the long course of certain cranial nerves.

By contrast with examination of other systems, e.g. the heart, the nervous system stands almost alone in enabling the patient to co-operate fully in the diagnosis and displaying the higher faculties of the brain in speech, thought, memory and reasoning.

### The aetiological diagnosis

This has a close bearing on the anatomical diagnosis, for it is known that certain types of pathological process repeatedly occur in the same site.

The virus of poliomyelitis has a selective affinity for the anterior horn cells, the virus of herpes zoster favours the posterior nerve root, and deficiency of vitamin $B_{12}$ leads to degenerative changes in the peripheral nerves, posterior column and pyramidal tracts—to give only a few examples (*see Table* 10.7).

It sometimes happens, therefore, that the anatomical picture of the lesion suggests its pathology.

The medulloblastoma of childhood is an example. This tumour brings headache, vomiting, papilloedema and other signs associated with an expanding lesion within the skull, but cranial nerve lesions, especially oculomotor pareses, are common, and there is some inco-ordination of movement of a cerebellar type. Such features in a young child indicating an involvement of the brainstem, cerebellum and cervical cord are rarely caused by anything other than medulloblastoma, though tubercular meningitis has certain symptoms and signs in common.

Time relationships are also closely bound up with aetiology. Trauma often causes instantaneous effects, as does haemorrhage into the brain or spinal cord.

Inflammatory lesions develop in a matter of days, while neoplastic conditions may take weeks or months, and degenerative processes may require months to years before revealing a diagnosable clinical picture.

The aetiology in neurological disease does not differ in principle from the causes at work in other parts of the body, but emphasis can be placed upon certain causes which are common.

Some examples are seen in the table on the facing page. The special investigations must be interpreted in the light of the clinical picture.

### ■ ILLUSTRATIVE DISEASES

In conclusion, three common diseases of the nervous system will be described to illustrate some important principles in neurological diagnosis. *Epilepsy* is a paroxysmal disorder of cerebral function, and the patient may be in

| Table 10.7 | **Some common diseases of the nervous system** | |
|---|---|---|
| *Disease* | *Parts selected* | *Causative agent or explanation* |
| **Developmental** | | |
| Syringomyelia | Central cervical cord: spinothalamic fibres and anterior horn cells | Possibly due to congenital defect of upper cervical spine and foramen magnum |
| **Genetic** | | |
| Myopathies | Muscles | Variable hereditary factors |
| Friedreich's ataxia | Pyramidal tracts Posterior columns Cerebellar tracts | A heredo-familial disorder |
| **Trauma** | | |
| | Brain Spinal cord Cranial and spinal nerves | Fractures and concussion |
| **Vascular** | | |
| Haemorrhage | Pyramidal tract, especially in the | Hypertension |
| Thrombosis | internal capsule and motor | Atheroma |
| Embolism | cortex Cranial nerve nuclei Less commonly the spinal cord | Mitral stenosis (embolism) |
| **Inflammatory** | | |
| Poliomyelitis | Anterior horn cells | Virus infection |
| Meningitis | Cerebral and spinal meninges | Coccal, TB and virus infections |
| Syphilis: Tabes | Posterior columns Posterior nerve roots Optic and oculomotor nerves | Spirochaete infection |
| GPI | Cerebral cortex: pyramidal and mental changes | Spirochaete infection |
| **'Idiopathic'** | | |
| Disseminated sclerosis | Pyramidal tracts Optic and oculomotor nerves Cerebellum Posterior columns | Demyelinating process |
| Motor neuron disease | Pyramidal tracts Anterior horn cells Cranial nerve nuclei (9–12) | Unknown |
| **Deficiency, toxic and biochemical** | | |
| Subacute combined degeneration of cord | Pyramidal tracts Posterior columns Peripheral nerves | Vitamin $B_{12}$ deficiency |
| Peripheral neuropathy | Peripheral nerves | Vitamin B deficiency (e.g. beriberi) Diabetes Carcinoma Alcohol Drugs (e.g. nitrofurantoin isoniazid) Lead and other toxins |
| Liver–brain disorders | Lenticular degeneration Phenylketonuria (mental deficiency in infants) | Defect in copper metabolism Defect in enzymes in liver |

perfect health at other times. Diagnosis depends upon an accurate account of the attack and a careful physical examination to exclude the early signs of a focal cause. A *space-occupying lesion* such as tumour exemplifies an organic and progressive focal process which may sometimes be precisely localized by clinical examination based on a knowledge of the functional anatomy of the nervous system. *Multiple sclerosis* is characterized by episodes of neurological disturbance which may be scattered over a long period of time and accompanied by multifocal signs. Special investigations are of little value, and diagnosis may sometimes rest upon the history alone.

## EPILEPSY

Epilepsy consists of a recurrent transient disturbance of cerebral function usually accompanied by an abnormal and excessive discharge from cerebral neurons. Epilepsy is classified as 'idiopathic' or 'symptomatic' according to whether a specific cause can be found. The causes include high fever in children, cerebrovascular disease in the elderly, trauma, tumour, metabolic disorders such as uraemia and the withdrawal of alcohol or sedative drugs. A familial incidence is common especially in the idiopathic form.

Epilepsy may manifest itself as generalized convulsions (*grand mal*), minor momentary attacks (*petit mal*, myoclonic, etc.) and focal epilepsy (psychomotor, Jacksonian).

### Generalized convulsions (grand mal)

The fits of epilepsy follow, in classic cases, such a definite sequence of events as to make their recognition easy. The events are: (1) The aura; (2) The cry; (3) The tonic stage; (4) The clonic stage; (5) Postepileptic phenomena. Usually there is no apparent precipitating cause, but occasionally the attack seems to result from some specific sensory stimulus or emotion, such as music or flickering light.

1. *The aura*: This is a warning occurring a short time before the fit. It usually takes the form of a peculiar subjective phenomenon, e.g. tingling in one hand, queer sensations in the epigastrium, sense of constriction around the leg, visual or auditory sensations. The aura is generally constant for the same individual. It is important, though difficult, to distinguish an aura of motor character (trivial twitchings followed by other phenomena) from true Jacksonian or focal epilepsy.

2. *The cry*: As the patient falls to the ground the respiratory muscles are in a state of tonic spasm and a grunting cry is emitted. The patient is unaware of this as he falls unconscious.

3. *The tonic stage*: The muscles of the whole body are in tonic contraction. The body is therefore rigid, the hands and jaws clenched. The cessation of respiratory movements causes cyanosis and engorgement of veins in the neck. Occasionally the muscular involvement is unequal, twisting the body to one side. This stage lasts about half a minute and passes into—

4. *The clonic stage*: Clonic movements affect the whole body almost instantaneously. The limbs are alternately flexed and extended, and the movements rapidly increase in excursion and then diminish in intensity and frequency. The convulsions last about three minutes. During them the patient may injure himself by the champing movements of the jaw (laceration of the tongue, injury to the

teeth, frothy and often blood-stained saliva on the lips) or by contact with surrounding hard or dangerous objects. During the clonic stage incontinence of urine and more rarely of faeces also occurs.

5. *Postepileptic phenomena*: Following the clonic stage, coma of short duration occurs during which the tendon reflexes are abolished and the plantar responses are extensor. The pupils are dilated and the corneal reflexes absent. There may be a slight rise in temperature, more pronounced if a succession of fits occurs—status epilepticus. Usually the patient passes from coma into a natural sleep which lasts for several hours and from which he awakes with a headache. More rarely *post-epileptic automatism* results: the patient may perform acts (e.g. undressing or walking) of which he afterwards has no recollection. In some cases 'psychic equivalents' of epilepsy may be found—e.g. complete change in personality and habit and liability to criminal acts of which the patient later has no knowledge.

### Minor momentary attacks

**Petit mal** This is a term used to describe transient 'absence' attacks in children, accompanied by a diagnostic 3 per second 'spike and dome' pattern in the electroencephalograph (*see Fig.* 10.94). There is a sudden interruption of activity lasting only a few seconds with blankness of expression, perhaps a momentary twitching of the face or limbs, but the child rarely falls, objects held are seldom dropped and incontinence is unusual. A family history is common and most cases are 'idiopathic'.

**Myoclonic seizures** These consist of violent jerking movements usually of one or both arms. Other transient motor forms of epilepsy in children include sudden bowing of the head (*Salaam attacks*) and *akinetic seizures*, in which the child suddenly falls to the ground without loss of consciousness.

### Focal epilepsy

**Psychomotor epilepsy** This is the commonest form of seizure in which the symptoms arise from one particular focus in the brain, in this case the temporal lobe. This focus may be an identifiable structural lesion, especially in adults, but many cases are idiopathic. Sensory hallucinations, especially of taste and smell, are accompanied by mental and emotional phenomena including 'dreamy' states, which may be pleasant or otherwise, and a sensation known as *déjà vu*, in which surroundings or events seem strangely familiar. The motor features of temporal lobe epilepsy consist of purposive but inappropriate movements which include smacking the lips, chewing, muttering or more complex activities such as undressing. The patient may also display anger, laughter and other motor manifestations of the emotional disturbance. These attacks may be distinguished from *petit mal* and other forms of minor epilepsy by the fact that movements are co-ordinated rather than clonic and last for minutes rather than seconds.

**Jacksonian epilepsy** This was first described by the pioneer neurologist Hughlings Jackson. It generally consists of a localized fit without loss of consciousness. The convulsive movements usually start in the same group of muscles and extend in a 'march'. Thus twitchings may be observed in the right hand followed by movements of the arm and shoulder-girdle, and then of the whole of the right side, sometimes spreading to the left. Occasionally the attack ends in generalized convulsions, in which case consciousness may be lost. Such a history suggests an irritative lesion of the brain such as tumour or trauma, though the story in these two examples will be quite different.

The physical examination in cases of Jacksonian epilepsy is more likely to yield signs than in the case of the idiopathic variety, though not always so. The commonest sign is a hemiparesis (Todd's paralysis), which may last for several hours after an attack. The attacks are not always motor in character but may be sensory with visual, auditory or other sensory phenomena.

The electroencephalogram (EEG) has proved the clear vision of Hughlings Jackson when he defined epilepsy as an excessive, sudden and unruly discharge of neuronal cells. For during the attacks distinctive waves appear, indicating that there is a dysrhythmia of the electrical potentials of the brain, due in its turn to physicochemical changes (*see Fig.* 10.94). These may be congenital, but it is not surprising that one or more of the several factors causing symptomatic epilepsy may modify the physicochemical state of the brain.

### Observation and causation of epileptic fits

It is useful to provide the nursing staff or relatives with a questionnaire to cover the points described in the various forms of epilepsy. Often the patient has no knowledge of the attack unless there has been injury or incontinence. This particularly applies to nocturnal attacks. Sometimes he feels ill afterwards or behaves strangely and knows that something has happened, but generally one must depend upon information provided by an intelligent observer.

True *petit mal* is usually idiopathic and Jacksonian fits are usually symptomatic, but in every case of epilepsy a careful search must be made for an organic cause by thorough general and neurological examination and by appropriate investigations (*see* p. 416). Hypertrophy of the gums (*Fig.* 10.89) and megaloblastic anaemia may be found in epileptic patients who are taking phenytoin sodium.

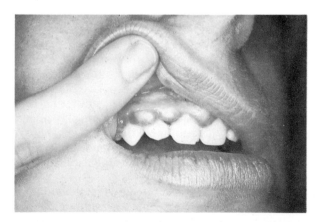

**Fig. 10.89** Gum hypertrophy in a patient taking phenytoin sodium for epilepsy. The patient, a female, also had megaloblastic anaemia due to folic acid deficiency. (*See also* p. 300.)

### Hysterical fits

These can usually be distinguished from epilepsy, though *petit mal* may cause difficulties. They are commoner in women. Hysterical 'convulsions' are so violent as to be obvious purposeful struggling. Incontinence and injury do not occur for they are too unpleasant, but manifestations such as shutting the eyes against resistance and persistent general rigidity or movements all increase if the patient feels that she is attracting attention. It is important to note that hysterical fits may be a manifestation of organic brain disease and are not uncommon in epileptic subjects.

### Narcolepsy and cataplexy

These rare conditions, which usually occur together, resemble epilepsy in that they each consist of a paroxysmal but transient disturbance of cerebral function. The cause is unknown and is not associated with structural disease of the brain. Narcolepsy is characterized by bouts of uncontrollable sleep from which the patient can easily be roused. In cataplexy, there are abrupt but momentary episodes of muscular weakness usually precipitated by emotion such as laughter. Other features of this syndrome are hypnagogic hallucinations (vivid dreams on first falling to sleep) and sleep paralysis (inability to move on first waking).

### SPACE-OCCUPYING LESIONS

The recognition and localization of an intracranial space-occupying lesion is of the greatest importance, because the condition can often be relieved and sometimes cured by surgical treatment. Examples of such lesions include tumour, abscess, cyst, haematoma and aneurysm. The two principal manifestations are increased intracranial pressure and focal signs.

### Symptoms and signs of increased intracranial pressure

Whatever the cause of a rise of intracranial pressure, certain common symptoms and signs result. The most important of these are headache, vomiting, papilloedema, disturbances of cerebration, fits, bradycardia and respiratory arrhythmias.

**Headache** This symptom is considered on pp. 10–12 as it results from many conditions not primarily affecting the nervous system. As a feature of increased intracranial pressure it may occur in paroxysms of great severity, often with periods of freedom, be mild or even absent. The headache is usually maximal in the early morning, sometimes waking the patient, and then improves after he gets up from bed. It is sometimes over the site of a tumour, but more often it is generalized.

**Vomiting** Typical cerebral vomiting is not preceded by nausea and is sometimes projectile in character. This is often seen in meningitis. In children especially, the gastric contents may be ejected quite forcibly through the mouth. Vomiting due to increased intracranial pressure is, however, not commonly of this cerebral type. It may resemble other forms of sickness preceded by nausea. Vomiting is a late sign of raised intracranial pressure and is usually associated with severe headache.

**Papilloedema** (*Choked disc*) (*Fig.* 10.90) This is the sign of greatest importance

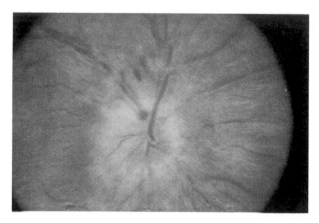

**Fig. 10.90** Papilloedema.

in the diagnosis of increased intracranial pressure, though it does not correlate well with the level of the pressure and may take several days to develop. The patient may complain of impaired vision, which is confirmed by the discovery of enlargement of the blind spot and contraction of the periphery of the visual field. In many cases no subjective visual changes are present, emphasizing the necessity of examining the retina in all neurological cases. The objective sign consists in swelling of the optic nerve head to an extent of several dioptres. (*See also* The 2nd Cranial Nerve, p. 343 *et seq.*)

**Mental changes** Mental confusion and apathy are common but late signs in most cases of increased intracranial pressure (*see* Cerebration and Consciousness, *above*) and stupor or coma follow in severe unrelieved cases.

**Fits** (*see also* pp. 15, 441) It is important to remember that generalized convulsions resembling idiopathic epilepsy are a commoner manifestation of increased intracranial pressure than localized fits. Fits occurring first in middle life should emphasize the necessity of excluding organic cerebral disease.

**Bradycardia** The general rise of intracranial pressure in time causes slowing of the heart rate owing to its effect on the vagal centres in the medulla; a grave sign of most value when the normal heart rate for the individual is known.

**Respiratory arrhythmias** Increasing intracranial pressure impairs the cerebral circulation including that of the medulla with involvement of the activities of the respiratory centre. This may result in abnormalities of the rate or rhythm of respiration such as Cheyne–Stokes breathing (*see* p. 169).

### Focal Signs (*Table* 10.8)

It is important to localize a space-occupying lesion as accurately as possible, because upon this will depend the success of any operative treatment. The earlier the anatomical diagnosis can be made, the more likely is the treatment to be successful, not only because the encroachment of even a simple tumour upon the brain substance is attended by grave results, which increase the longer the tumour remains, but also because the slight localizing signs of the early stages are often masked by increasing intracranial pressure. Moreover, the disturbances

| Table 10.8 | Localizing focal signs in the cerebrum |
| --- | --- |
| *Site* | *Symptoms and Signs* |
| Frontal lobe | Personality change, facetiousness<br>Anosmia<br>Optic atrophy and papilloedema |
| Pre-central gyrus | Focal convulsions and hemiparesis |
| Parietal lobe | Spatial disorientation, astereognosis, alexia,<br>homonymous hemianopia |
| Temporal lobe | Psychomotor convulsions<br>Memory and emotional disturbances<br>Sensory aphasia<br>Homonymous hemianopia |
| Occipital lobe | Homonymous hemianopia<br>Papilloedema |
| Cerebellum | Disturbances of equilibrium and tone<br>Papilloedema |
| Pituitary | Bitemporal hemianopia |

of consciousness which have been mentioned (impairment of intellect and increasing stupor) soon render the patient unable to help in the diagnosis of the condition by his accurate history.

This preamble emphasizes the necessity for paying due attention to the slightest focal signs in the early stages of intracranial disease. These signs depend upon the abolition or alteration in function of the various parts of the brain and the cranial nerves which proceed from it. Some areas—for example, the motor area—have well-defined functions, the loss or alteration of which will almost certainly occur when a lesion affects them. Others—for instance, the frontal lobes—may be the seat of gross changes without symptoms or signs of real localizing value. In this connection it is well to note that supratentorial tumours are relatively silent, while below the tentorium lesions generally produce early focal signs.

Those focal signs which appear earliest are of greatest value, for they are more likely to be due to the original lesion. The same signs appearing later may merely result from secondary changes in the neighbourhood of the lesion, e.g. meningitis or thrombosis, or from displacement of intracranial structures by rising pressure.

Local signs are of even greater value than general ones in the diagnosis of cerebral lesions, for whereas such signs as headache, vomiting and retinopathies may be caused by hypertension, blood diseases and other conditions, local signs such as paresis or disturbances of sensation indicate a local lesion. Sometimes a combination of signs is known to be associated with a particular type of tumour. For example, a medulloblastoma is the commonest cerebral tumour of childhood and causes a combination of signs, indicating both the position of the tumour in the vermis and surrounding structures and its pathology. Local signs may now be discussed in more detail and grouped according to the various parts of the brain affected.

*Mental disorder* should draw attention to the frontal, parietal or temporal lobes. Frontal tumours may reach a considerable size and produce no focal signs other than personality changes, sometimes with loss of inhibitions and urinary incontinence. Temporal lobe lesions cause impairment of memory and emotional disorders (*see also under* Epilepsy, p 440), while parietal lesions are characteristically associated with spatial disorientation (*see also* p. 420). It should be noted that any tumour interfering with the circulation of the CSF (especially in the posterior fossa) may cause intellectual impairment secondary to hydrocephalus.

*Motor phenomena* such as Jacksonian fits and paresis point to lesions in the precentral gyrus and the neighbouring subcortical regions. Paralysis with involvement of the cranial nerves suggests lesions in the midbrain—crura, pons or medulla. They are more fully described under the motor system, p. 402 *et seq.*

*Cortical sensory disturbances*, i.e. astereognosis, loss of point discrimination and of the perception of small variations in temperature, suggest a lesion of the parietal lobe.

*Aphasia* may suggest temporal lobe involvement if of the auditory type, a lesion of areas 18 or 19 when visual, or an affection of Broca's centre (area 44) in the inferior frontal gyrus, when essentially motor (*see Figs.* 10.36, 10.37). Aphasia is a sign which must be used with caution for localizing purposes, owing to the difficulty in analysing different types.

*Perversions of smell*, when local nasal causes have been excluded, may throw suspicion on the uncus.

*Hemianopia*, especially homonymous and quadrantic types, is found in lesions of the optic radiation and area 17 of the occipital cortex (*see Figs.* 10.2, 10.37). Bitemporal hemianopia suggests a tumour in the region of the pituitary.

*Cranial-nerve palsies* are sometimes of localizing value and are particularly found when the tumour is situated at the base of the brain, though when not accompanied by other neurological signs they may be due to lesions involving only the nucleus or its nerve.

*Disturbances of equilibrium and muscle tone* are the most important symptoms suggestive of cerebellar tumours.

It must not be forgotten that the functions of several adjacent areas may be affected successively as the tumour grows, so that new signs continue to appear. An important example is the acoustic neuroma which usually presents with unilateral nerve deafness followed in succession by signs of vestibular nerve damage (absent caloric reaction), signs of trigeminal involvement (absent corneal reflex), facial paresis, cerebellar ataxia and contralateral pyramidal tract signs from medullary compression. This tumour may be associated with generalized neurofibromatosis (*Fig.* 10.91). The possibility of tumour should be considered when any localizing signs are present, especially when these appear gradually over a period of some months. If signs of increased intracranial pressure (*see* p. 443) occur concurrently, the diagnosis becomes more certain. The reverse, however, is commonly the case, namely, the signs of increased intracranial pressure occur early and the localizing signs only later. In such cases the careful exclusion of other diseases causing the triad of headache, vomiting and papilloedema may establish a diagnosis of tumour, but its position may remain uncertain. Of the general signs, it is to be noted that papilloedema and vomiting are often more pronounced in subtentorial than supratentorial tumours.

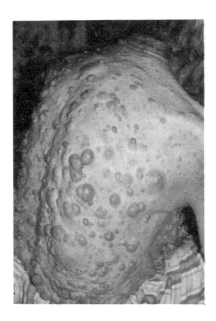

**Fig. 10.91**
Neurofibromatosis (von Recklinghausen's disease). This condition is sometimes associated with an acoustic nerve tumour.

In the diagnosis of the nature of a tumour the patient's age takes a prominent part. Carcinoma, which is always secondary, is naturally found in older people. A primary focus should be sought. One of the commonest is carcinoma of the bronchus. Among primary tumours an important distinction is to be made between intracerebral and extracerebral growths. The former include various forms of glioma which replace brain tissue, while the extracerebral varieties, e.g. meningioma and pituitary tumours, cause special pressure effects and are in general more amenable to treatment. Whatever the nature of the tumour the signs of increased intracranial pressure will depend largely on whether it obstructs the free circulation of cerebrospinal fluid and how rapidly it grows.

## MULTIPLE SCLEROSIS (DISSEMINATED SCLEROSIS)

This is one of the commonest organic nervous diseases. It affects both sexes, usually between the ages of 20 and 40 years, and is generally insidious in its onset. Its progress is marked by remissions in which the symptoms and signs may disappear partially or entirely.

Among early symptoms may be mentioned transient pareses, paraesthesiae (subjective sensory phenomena, *see* p. 420), disturbances of micturition and ocular symptoms. The ocular manifestations, which include diplopia and blurring of vision, are perhaps most characteristic. Blurring of vision may occur for a few days to a few weeks, indicating a retrobulbar neuritis, and may precede cord symptoms by months or years. It is often followed by a degree of optic atrophy, especially noticeable in the temporal halves of the optic discs. In a developed case, spastic paraplegia is the commonest clinical picture. But as the name of the disease indicates, the lesions are scattered, and before a diagnosis of disseminated sclerosis is justifiable, the paraplegia must be accompanied by signs of damage to other parts of the nervous system. The triad of symptoms described by Charcot, nystagmus, staccato speech and 'intention' tremor, is by no means commonly found, but one of the triad with signs of a spastic paraplegia may suggest disseminated sclerosis, indicating patches of sclerosis in the cerebellum and corticospinal systems. Both nystagmus and staccato speech are defects of postural fixation (tone) due to cerebral involvement.

Evidence of sclerotic patches in the posterior columns or cerebellar pathways is to be found in ataxia, a common symptom. Loss of vibration sensation and of sense of position are more rarely found on objective examination. Damage to other sensory tracts may result in various anaesthesiae and paraesthesiae.

## ■ SPECIAL INVESTIGATIONS

### Cerebrospinal fluid

This is secreted by the cells of the choroid plexus and absorbed via the arachnoid villi into the dural sinuses and spinal veins.

The information which it gives in diseases of the nervous system includes:

1. The pressure.
2. The presence of blood and turbidity from increased cellular content, observable by the naked eye.
3. The cell content, microscopically.
4. The chemical content.
5. The Wassermann reaction.

1. The normal pressure, when measured at lumbar puncture in the lateral recumbent position, with the patient completely relaxed, varies between 100 and 180 mmH$_2$O. The fluid is contained in the ventricular system which has foramina communicating with the subarachnoid space. Any condition which causes a rise of intracranial pressure, e.g. tumour or abscess, may at first be compensated for by displacement of the fluid. As this runs into the sheath of the optic nerve it may cause papilloedema, and when it affects the posterior fossa of the skull there may be crowding of the cerebellum and medulla into the foramen magnum. This process is easily aggravated by lumbar puncture and may cause serious ischaemia of the medulla which can be fatal. By these pressure effects the escape of the cerebrospinal fluid into the spinal theca and its absorption from this part of the subarachnoid space are prevented. A failure of absorption in the ventricles also occurs if the foramina are blocked, and hydrocephalus may result. See also Queckenstedt's test (p. 430).

2. The presence of blood in considerable quantities may be noted in subarachnoid haemorrhage (p. 435), or the fluid may be yellow due to altered blood from an earlier bleed ('xanthochromia'). The fluid may be turbid if there is a large number of cells, as in certain types of coccal meningitis.

3. An increase of cells occurs as in the case of infections in other parts of the body. These cells are usually polymorphonuclear leucocytes in coccal infections and certain other acute infections, or lymphocytes when the infection is more chronic. When the cells are increased, a specific organism, e.g. the meningococcus or tubercle bacillus, may be identified immediately on microscopy or only after

culture. Cellular changes may, however, occur in certain nervous diseases in which no organism is present.

4. The chemical constituents of the cerebrospinal fluid are not dissimilar from those in plasma, except for a much lower protein content. There is an increase in protein and a decrease in sugar and chlorides in many types of meningitis. Gross increase in the protein content is seen when the free flow of the cerebrospinal fluid is prevented by blockage of the theca in cases of spinal-cord tumour (Froin's syndrome). A very high protein level may also occur with certain forms of cerebral tumour and peripheral neuropathy.

The normal values of the main constituents of the cerebrospinal fluid and the changes commonly found in disease of the central nervous system are set out in *Table* 10.9.

### Radiology

A plain radiograph of the *skull* may show evidence of fractures; raised intracranial pressure ('beaten silver' appearance of the vault and erosion

| Table 10.9 | **The cerebrospinal fluid in health and disease** | | | | |
|---|---|---|---|---|---|
| | *Appearance* | *Pressure* (mm CSF) | *Cells* (per mm³) | *Protein* (mg/100 ml) | *Other* |
| *Normal* | Clear Colourless | 100–180 | 0–5 Lymphocytes | 15–45 | glucose (3·3–4·4 mmol/l |
| *Traumatic* | Bloody at first | 100–180 | Red blood cells | Elevated 4 mg per 5000 red blood cells | Supernatant clear |
| *Subarachnoid haemorrhage* | Bloody throughout | Raised | Red blood cells | As above | Supernatant xanthochromic |
| *Purulent meningitis* | Turbid | Raised | Polymorphs 100–5000 | 100–400 | Glucose low, organisms on smear |
| *Viral meningitis* | Clear to opalescent | Normal | Lymphocytes 20–2000 | 150 | Sterile |
| *Tuberculous meningitis* | Clear to cloudy | Raised | Lymphocytes up to 500 | 80–400 | Glucose low, organisms on smear or culture |
| *Neurosyphilis* | Clear | Normal | Lymphocytes up to 50 | Up to 100 | Positive antibody titres |
| *Multiple sclerosis* | Clear | Normal | Normal or up to 20 lymphocytes | Normal up to 120 | Raised γ-**globulins** |
| *Spinal tumour with block* | Yellow xantho-chromia | Normal or low | Normal or up to 20 lymphocytes | 200–600 | May coagulate |

of the clinoid processes); bone destruction by tumour or infection (e.g. of sinuses or mastoid cells); expansion of the pituitary fossa or of the various neural foramina (e.g. optic and auditory) due to tumours; calcification within tumours or vascular lesions such as aneurysm and angioma.

*Arteriograms* are radiographs of the cervical and cerebral vessels taken after the intra-arterial injection of a radio-opaque contrast material. They may be used to locate and display cerebral aneurysms and obstruction or displacement of arteries.

*Pneumoencephalography* consists of injecting air into the spinal subarachnoid space (or directly into the ventricular system) to outline the cerebral ventricles. Radiographs may then help to demonstrate cerebral atrophy, distension or displacement of the ventricles and the site of obstruction to the flow of CSF.

*Myelography* is used to determine the level of a lesion compressing the spinal cord. A radio-opaque dye is injected into the lumbar subarachnoid space, and radiographs are taken with the patient tilted so that the dye can move up or down the spinal canal. (*Fig.* 10.92.)

### Computerized axial tomography

This technique has largely replaced the more invasive methods already mentioned for the location of intracranial lesions. X-rays penetrate the head from different angles, and by a process of triangulation the exact density of each point is obtained from the hindrance to the X-ray beams. A series of cross-

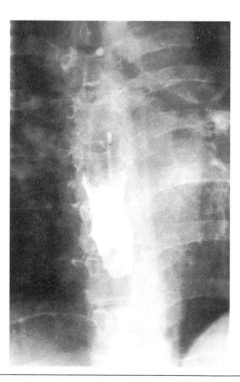

**Fig. 10.92**
Myelogram. Opaque oil in the spinal theca demonstrating an obstruction to the flow due to a large tumour of the meninges.

sections of the brain is mapped out by a computer, and the various tissues, both normal and abnormal, are clearly distinguished by the difference in their densities (*see Fig.* 10.93).

### Isotope brain scan

Certain radioactive substances (e.g. technetium isotopes) are selectively localized in tumours and other lesions of the brain, especially those near the surface. This local concentration of the isotope can be detected by means of a scintillation scanner and displayed on suitable paper or film.

### Electroencephalography

The rhythmical activity of the cortical neurons is recorded by the electroencephalograph.

Departures from normal may be seen in many brain disorders, notably epilepsy but also in some cerebral tumours and occasionally in certain metabolic and psychiatric diseases. (*Fig.* 10.94.)

The electroencephalogram is a valuable aid in neurological diagnosis, even in localization of the lesion as in tumour, but needs special skill in its interpretation and close correlation with the clinical findings.

### Electromyography, muscle biopsy and nerve conduction studies

The records of electrical variations made by insertion of a needle into muscle can give important information in various rare muscular diseases: myopathies, neuropathies and myasthenia. It may also indicate the presence or absence of muscular contraction where this is clinically abolished, as in traumatic lesions of nerves.

Muscle biopsy can be a similar aid to diagnosis.

Nerve conduction is determined by measuring the time taken for a stimulus to travel from one point on the nerve to another. This technique may be helpful in the assessment of peripheral nerve lesions (*see Fig.* 10.95.)

---

### ■ THE DIAGNOSIS OF PSYCHIATRIC DISORDERS

---

It is now established that much disability arises from causes other than physical disease. The physiological somatic responses to emotion, together with the unpleasant feelings associated with conflict, provide the basis for many symptoms and complaints of patients in medical practice. These, together with problems of personality disorder and the effects on personality of physical disease, comprise the basic substance of psychiatric practice.

The individual personality is unique and develops as a result of the interreaction over the years between genetic constitution and environmental influences. The latter include physical disease and injuries. Disorders of personality may, therefore, arise through inherited genetic influences (e.g. many instances of subnormality; some forms of dementia—Huntington's chorea); physical diseases, especially those affecting the central nervous system (the organic psychoses—delirium, dementia); and as a result of conflict either in the individual himself or

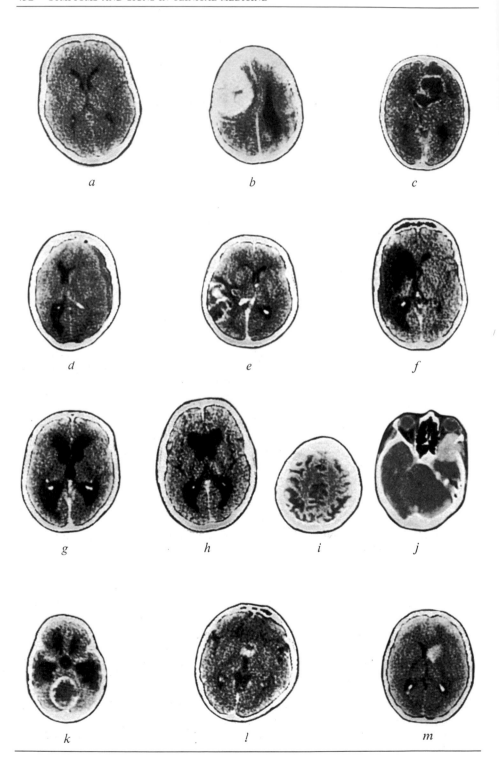

*a*

*b*

*c*

*d*

*e*

*f*

*g*

*h*

*i*

*j*

*k*

*l*

*m*

**Fig. 10.93** Computerized tomographic (CT) scans of the brain and head (EMI Mk I and Mk II Head Scanners were used).

*a,* Normal scan of young adult. The third and lateral ventricles are seen, and there is some differentiation between the white and grey matter.

*b,* Large meningioma indenting the convexity of the left hemisphere in the fronto-parietal region. Note obliteration of the upper part of the left lateral ventricle, and distortion of the falx cerebri towards the right.

*c,* Multi-loculated abscess in the frontal region. Note that the frontal horns of the lateral ventricles are almost obliterated. This child, who was admitted in a comatose condition, made a good recovery.

*d,* Right subdural haematoma, 3 weeks after a mild injury. Note that the altered blood shows as a dark crescent between the skull and the cerebral hemisphere. Note also the right-to-left displacement of the ventricles and distortion of the right lateral ventricle.

*e,* Left parietal glioblastoma multiforme. Note patchy light (higher density) and dark (lower density) regions within the tumour, and the dark zone surrounding the medial aspect of the lesion which represents oedema in the adjacent brain, particularly the white matter.

*f,* Healed infarct in the left middle cerebral territory. The low density (dark) infarcted brain is hard to distinguish from the lateral ventricle nearby. Note enlargement of the left lateral ventricle compared with that on the right, because of shrinkage of the infarct during healing.

*g,* Hydrocephalus due to obstruction to CSF flow through the posterior fossa. Symmetrically enlarged third and lateral ventricles are seen. The white dots on either side are caused by physiological calcification in the choroid plexus of each lateral ventricle.

*h,* Cerebral atrophy. Compare with *g.* In this case the sylvian fissures and the cortical sulci are more easily seen than usual, because they are widened. In obstructive hydrocephalus they are less well seen, and are often not visible at all.

*i,* Wide cortical sulci at the vertex give clear evidence of cortical atrophy.

*j,* A metastasis from thyroid carcinoma is shown invading the right orbit, causing proptosis. It is also invading the right temporal lobe, and has destroyed part of the sphenoid wing, between the orbit and middle cranial fossa.

*k,* A juvenile cerebellar astrocytoma is shown as a light ring of abnormal tissue with a cystic space (dark) occupying the central portion of the tumour. Note the dilated third ventricle, and the dilated frontal and temporal horns of the lateral ventricles, because CSF flow is obstructed by the mass in the posterior fossa.

*l,* A scan taken through the suprasellar region, below the lateral ventricles, shows a pituitary adenoma rising up in the midline to encroach on the anterior part of the third ventricle. The irregular dark markings laterally are the sylvian fissures, rather wider than usual, because of coincidental cerebral atrophy.

*m,* A haematoma, which resulted from a spontaneous intracerebral haemorrhage, is shown as a light zone in the region of the right internal capsule. The frontal horn of the right lateral ventricle is obliterated by pressure from the haematoma. The patient suffered from left hemiparesis, but made a good recovery.

(By courtesy of Dr L. G. Brock, Consultant Neuroradiologist, Liverpool Regional Department of Medical and Surgical Neurology.)

between the individual and his environment (the neuroses). Additionally, there may be failure of personality maturation, and this may be one of the main factors in the psychopathic state. Finally, there are groups of illnesses, as yet not clearly identified on an aetiological basis, but which appear to be, in part at least, genetically determined and are described under the terms 'affective illness' and 'schizophrenia'. In formulating a diagnosis in psychiatric disorder it must be continually borne in mind that such a disorder may coexist with organic disease. In other instances organic and psychiatric disorders may be inter-related. Emotional and other stress may aggravate organic diseases or, alternatively, physical disease itself may play a large part in the development of the psychiatric disorder, e.g.

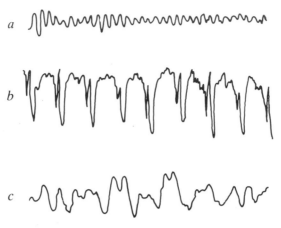

**Fig. 10.94** Electroencephalogram. *a*, Normal record (alpha waves). *b*, *Petit mal* epilepsy (spike and dome pattern). *c*, Slow activity (delta waves): this can be generalized, as in epilepsy, or localized to one part of the brain, e.g. cerebral tumour.

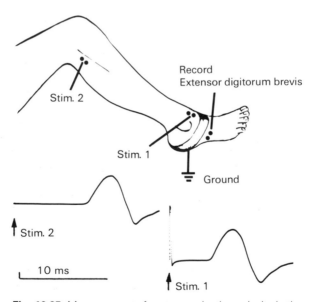

**Fig. 10.95** Measurement of motor conduction velocity in the lateral popliteal nerve. The anterior tibial branch is stimulated at the ankle (stim. 1) and the response recorded. The nerve is then stimulated at the head of the fibula (stim. 2) and the response is recorded. The time from the stimulus to the onset of the muscle potential is measured from each trace and the difference represents the time taken for the impulse to pass down the nerve between the two stimulus points.

toxic states, cerebrovascular disease, altering the pattern of other psychiatric syndromes.

### Psychiatric history taking

History taking, important in the investigation of all patients, may be crucial in the investigation of patients suffering from the psychiatric disorders. The technique of the psychiatric interview may well determine not only the diagnosis of a psychiatric illness but also its therapeutic outcome. Any skilled interviewer will help a patient to reveal not only elements of his history but also his general attitude, personality and mental state. The relationship that develops between doctor and patient during the initial interview may become the predominant factor in his subsequent treatment. The treatment role of the initial interview must be ever-present in the mind of the examiner.

History taking, in the main, follows the outline already given (*see* Chapter 1). *Complaints* should be elicited in detail. Open-ended questions are particularly valuable in the first instance. They enable the patient to reveal not only symptoms but frequently his attitude to them and belief as to their origin. Although multiple complaints at first sight may appear misleading, their multiplicity can direct one's attention to the possibility of a psychological disorder, especially when such symptoms involve many systems. If the examiner regularly ensures that all symptoms are detailed in the first instance, then he is in the position later to recognize the emergence of fresh symptoms as a sign that treatment is not progressing satisfactorily. When discussing the *history of the present illness*, dates should always be included. These may subsequently be correlated with factors in the personal history. Equally, when detailing the *past medical history*, psychiatric symptoms and disorders require special attention, and the symptoms' duration, place and nature of treatment are noted. The *family history* should include descriptions of personality, education, social class, attitudes, religion and emotional stability of relatives, quite apart from noting such conditions as alcoholism, suicides and mental illness. In this area relationships between relatives and the home atmosphere can be recorded. The *personal history* requires to be investigated in great detail. It should be a biography of the patient with details not only of early development, childhood, schooling, work, marriage, etc. but also include details of psychosexual development, habits and interests. Additionally, details of *personality prior to illness*, mood, character, standards, energy, ambition and tendency to fantasy should also be noted. Much tact will be required in eliciting this information. Whilst giving the patient maximum freedom the time should not be wasted by allowing him to drift into irrelevancy as a means of directing attention away from important topics.

In many instances it will be necessary to obtain a history from a relative or other person. This especially applies to psychotic states. In obtaining this information one should be careful not to make the patient resentful or suspicious by giving the impression that the relative's word is being taken before his own.

### Examination of mental state

Whilst it is convenient to describe a patient's mental state systematically, the examination should proceed in as informal a manner as possible. Much of what follows will reveal itself as the patient's identification and history is obtained, with only the occasional question required to amplify specific points as they occur.

**General behaviour** Under this heading the patient's appearance of health, dress, general awareness of his surroundings and response to the examination should be described. Note should be made as to whether there is over- or under-activity, excessive tension or agitation, and special mannerisms and gestures. Occasionally, behaviour modified by hallucinatory experiences can be observed.

**Talk** Conversation may be spontaneous or only in reply to questions. Coherence and relevance of replies should be noted.

**Mood** Does the patient appear sad or elated? Is he fearful or over-anxious and is his mood appropriate or incongruous?

**Thought** Thought processes may be faster or slower than usual and may flow easily or be interrupted (thought blocking).

*Content of thought* This includes details of problems, preoccupations, misinterpretations such as giving special or false meaning to trivial events and delusions. The precise nature of delusions and also of hallucinations (auditory, visual, tactile, etc.) should be recorded. Compulsive phenomena, including obsessions, should be enquired about and special fears also noted. Morbid thoughts and especially thoughts of self-injury must be closely, but tactfully, investigated in every depressed patient.

**Intellectual resources** This includes a patient's orientation in time, place and person. His memory for recent and remote events and his ability for immediate recall emerge usually from the history without any special tests being made. Attention, equally, can be assessed and concentration evaluated. The serial subtraction of 7 from 100 can give an objective assessment of this. Finally, in this section, the patient's general information will give an assessment of his education. His level of intelligence will usually emerge as a result of his school, academic and work record, but this can also be investigated by special tests.

**Insight and judgement** The patient's awareness of his problems and appreciation of his illness require careful assessment. These factors may well determine his ability to co-operate with treatment.

A complete physical examination is essential in every patient suffering from a psychiatric disorder. Further physical studies, including radiological tests, blood examination, electroencephalography or serology may be necessary. Tests of thyroid and other endocrine disorders are frequently indicated.

Special psychological tests of intellect (Terman and Merrill in children, Wechsler in adults), memory (Bender) and personality (Rorschach, Thematic Aperception Test) are available and may give valuable information.

## ■ CLASSIFICATION OF PSYCHIATRIC DISORDERS

### The neuroses

In these conditions the patient's ability to function is reduced, but his symptoms are, in the main, exaggerations or prolongations of normal reactions to stress. His symptoms are frequently understandable reactions to anxiety or conflict and may be either psychological or physical.

**Anxiety states** Anxiety and fear with the physiological components of these emotions provide the main basis of symptoms. Many such patients exhibit a constitutional liability to react excessively to stresses of many kinds—business, domestic, etc. Others of more normal constitution develop similar symptoms, but only under severe stress. Physical symptoms include sweating, palpitations, tremor, giddiness, dyspepsia, anorexia, diarrhoea, frequency of micturition. Sleep is delayed and interrupted. Mental symptoms include impaired concentration, irritability, noise sensitivity and depression. Abnormal fears—claustrophobia or fear of closed spaces, agoraphobia or fear of open spaces—may seriously limit the patient's freedom of action.

**Hysteria** In this condition physical or mental symptoms provide a partial solution, albeit an unsatisfactory one, to a conflict situation. Symptoms in hysteria always involve the patient in some gain. Whereas the malingerer consciously feigns illness, the hysterical patient is partially or completely unaware of the motivation behind the symptom. Symptoms may be physical—paralysis, aphonia, sensory loss including deafness or blindness, etc.; or mental—amnesia, fugues, 'emotional storms', etc. Patients suffering from hysteria frequently show a recognizable lack of concern for what appears to be a serious disorder—*belle indifference*.

**Obsessional disorders** An obsession is a persistent thought or compulsion to action, arising against the patient's will and from which the patient cannot free himself, but which he recognizes as being senseless. In severe forms the life of a patient may be interfered with to a considerable degree. Many individuals with obsessional features in their personality are capable of high quality work of great accuracy and care but may develop anxiety if asked to work under pressure when they cannot check their work or do it to their own satisfaction.

## The psychoses

In the psychoses the patient's whole personality is distorted and he may not be able to distinguish fantasy from reality. Judgement may be grossly impaired. The patient's symptoms and behaviour are not understandable in terms of normal experience.

**Affective disorders** These disorders manifest essentially as change of mood. There may be elevation of mood (elation) with acceleration of thought and action. These features provide the essential basis for the symptoms of a mania. Alternatively, there may be a lowering of mood (depression) with retardation of thought and movement. This is the depressive phase. The illness tends to be a recurrent one and may manifest itself only in attacks of mania or depression, but frequently the patient suffers at different times from both of these states. Each attack usually has a good prognosis and remissions may be complete. The depressive phase carries with it a serious risk of suicide.

**Schizophrenia** Under this term is included a group of illnesses manifested by disorders of thought, perception, emotion and behaviour. Symptoms include delusions, hallucinations (especially of hearing), emotional incongruity and blunting, and a tendency to impulsive and erratic behaviour, which the patient explains in terms of his thought disorder. In young patients deterioration of personality may occur. In older patients the personality may be fairly well maintained, but there is a greater tendency to the development of systematized delusions (paraphrenia, paranoia).

**Organic** These psychotic disorders arise as a result of organic disease affecting the brain. Acute organic illness produces acute psychiatric disorder—delirium; subacute organic disease produces the dysmnesic syndrome or Korsakoff state; chronic organic disease causes dementia. Acute and subacute disease may lead to dementia as an end state.

*Delirium* An acute psychosis manifested by clouding of consciousness, restlessness, and an affect of fear and visual hallucinations, usually of a threatening nature. The latter may precipitate impulsive behaviour, in which the patient attempts to escape his persecutors. Insomnia is a prominent feature. Delirium may occur in the serious acute infections—pneumonia, meningitis, in hypoxia, and may also result from intoxication, e.g. alcohol.

*Dysmnesic syndrome:* A subacute psychosis manifested by progressive amnesia and a tendency to confabulation. Originally described in association with polyneuritis due to alcoholism, i.e. Korsakoff's psychosis, a dysmnesic syndrome may follow delirium from any cause.

*Dementia:* A chronic psychosis manifested by progressive intellectual failure, characterized by loss of memory for recent events whilst memory for remote events is maintained. Associated with the intellectual impairment there is emotional lability; and patients tend to become careless of dress, their behaviour shows a lack of normal restraints and inhibitions. As dementia progresses the patient ceases to be able to care for him or herself and may become incontinent. Dementia results from arteriosclerosis or other causes of cerebral degenerative change. In middle age the condition is termed 'presenile dementia'.

### Psychopathic personality

These individuals exhibit a persistent tendency since childhood or adolescence to behave in an abnormal manner and whilst not psychotic or subnormal appear to be unable to learn from experience. They are frequently involved in asocial or antisocial behaviour. They may commit serious crimes, after which they show little remorse or regret. Many sex offenders and drug addicts fall within this group.

### Subnormality

This implies subnormality of intelligence, which may occur in various degrees. The most severe—the severely subnormal—are incapable of living an independent existence. The milder subnormal group may be capable of being educated or working under sheltered conditions. Subnormality may result from genetic causes, e.g. mongolism, or be secondary to organic cerebral disease occurring in childhood or early adolescence.

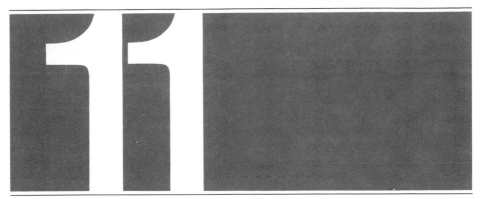

# The endocrine system

## ■ INTRODUCTION

The endocrine system comprises various tissues secreting hormones which are conveyed by the circulation to distant organs. In general, the time scale over which hormones act is generally longer than that for the nervous system, the other major controller of body function. However, the ability to measure the minute concentrations of hormones using only small blood samples has caused a revision of certain older ideas, such as the relative constancy of hormone secretion. Indeed, many hormones are characterized by the notably pulsatile nature of their secretion. Nevertheless, it is true to say that hormones can have both rapid metabolic effects, as exemplified by adrenaline, and long-term effects on processes such as growth and sexual development. Many hormones exert multiple actions, spanning both rapid and prolonged activities, for example, insulin.

Although individual endocrine glands have certain specific functions, they also operate through their relationship with others. This applies particularly to the pituitary, which exercises control over other glands through its trophic hormones. The pituitary is, in turn, influenced by the secretions from these other members of the system, which provide 'feedback' regulatory signals that are of primary importance in maintaining homeostasis.

Whereas most hormones are secreted from condensed collections of cells termed endocrine glands, the large number of gut hormones are usually secreted from cells scattered over great lengths of the gastrointestinal tract. Nevertheless, excess gut hormone hypersecretion is usually caused by localized, albeit sometimes multiple, endocrine tumours. In consequence of the small size of endocrine glands (and usually also their tumours) as well as the potency of their secretions, an endocrine disorder shows itself more often in the functional and morphological changes wrought by the abnormal state of hormone output rather than in local signs arising from the affected organ itself.

Hormonal dysfunction may also be secondary to disease in organs other than the endocrine glands. Examples include hyperaldosteronism secondary to cardiac failure, hyperparathyroidism in renal failure and the 'ectopic' production of hormones from several tumours, notably ACTH and vasopressin from small cell carcinomas of the lung.

The diagnostic approach to endocrine disorders can be considered in two stages. The first is an evaluation of hormonal status, which is essentially a physiological assessment, and the second is an effort to define precisely the nature of any underlying pathological process. Both approaches involve clinical skills of history and examination, backed up by an array of investigations involving hormone measurements in blood, urine (less frequently nowadays) and occasionally saliva, as well as various radiological, ultrasound and radio-isotopic imaging techniques. The complexity of these investigations lies outside the scope of this chapter but certain principles will be mentioned and it should be recognized that with their aid, documentation of endocrine status and pathology can often be made with a precision unrivalled in many other areas of modern medical practice.

## ■ LOCAL STRUCTURAL EFFECTS

It must again be stressed that an endocrine disorder can exist without any detectable clinical abnormality in the vicinity of the diseased gland.

The *thyroid* is the most accessible gland but is not usually visible or palpable. Any enlargement of the thyroid is termed a goitre without any implication of cause. (*Fig.* 11.1). To inspect the thyroid, it is best to give the patient water to sip as normally the thyroid is freely mobile but invested in fascia attached to the larynx which moves up on swallowing. Swallowing may disclose unsuspected enlargement of the thyroid, especially if a significant portion is restrosternal. Retrosternal goitre may impede venous return from the head which is more obvious when both arms are raised.

Palpation of the thyroid is performed by standing behind the patient, gently encircling the neck from each side with the hands and localizing the cricoid cartilage below the thyroid cartilage. The middle fingers are then largely used to palpate, starting medially below the cricoid cartilage where the isthmus generally crosses the trachea and up at the sides for the thyroid lobes. Texture and symmetry

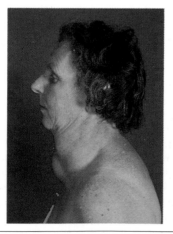

**Fig. 11.1**
Goitre.

are noted and the patient is asked to swallow in order to assess size and mobility. The thyroid is usually asymmetrical with the right lobe slightly larger and this pattern often persists with diffuse enlargement of the gland. Localized lumps or nodules should be individually defined. When attempting this, it is helpful to place one hand on the top of the patient's head to 'steer' it downwards, forwards and rotated away from the side being palpated in order to relax the sternomastoid on that side. This provides visual access to localized lesions. Palpation continues with checking for tracheal deviation or local lymphadenopathy.

Thyroid cysts occasionally transilluminate. The vascularity of the thyroid is increased in thyrotoxicosis and may cause a palpable thrill or audible bruit. The latter is heard when the patient stops breathing (*Fig.* 11.2). It is localized, sometimes loud and may be predominantly systolic or continue throughout the cardiac cycle. A thyroid bruit should not be confused with carotid bruits, conducted aortic murmurs or venous hums; these last are easily abolished by momentary light occlusion of jugular venous return. Goitres may compress the trachea to cause dyspnoea and stridor while invasive carcinomas may also result in dysphagia, change of voice and pain, which can radiate to the ear.

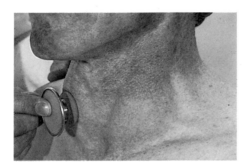

**Fig. 11.2**
Auscultation of the thyroid.

The *testes* are also readily amenable to clinical examination. It is often helpful to estimate the size of each testis. This is most accurately done using Prader's orchidometer, when each testis is matched most closely with one of a series of calibrated ellipsoids (*Fig.* 11.3). These were originally devised for assessing testicular development through puberty, but it is also useful to quantitate testicular shrinkage, which commonly occurs with damage to seminiferous tubules, as these constitute 95 per cent of testicular volume. Any abnormality of testicular position, consistency and associated structures such as epididymis and vas deferens, or of venous drainage causing varicocele, should be recorded. *Ovaries* are far less accessible but cystic or generalized enlargement may be detectable per vaginam on bimanual examination.

The *pituitary gland* is normally seated within the aptly named sella turcica (Turkish saddle) or pituitary fossa, on the superior surface of the sphenoid. These close confines, together with effects on important neighbouring structures, are responsible for the local symptoms and signs of expanding pituitary lesions. These include headache, usually attributed to pressure on the diaphragma sellae, and the important consequences of impingement on the optic chiasma. Chiasmal com-

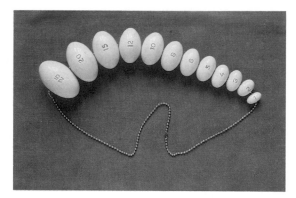

**Fig. 11.3** Prader's orchidometer.

pression from below will initially affect the lowermost decussating fibres causing upper, outer field defects. With increasing involvement, the field loss progresses to cause the classical bitemporal hemianopia. It is important to recognize that the optic chiasma occupies variable positions in different individuals and that tumour growth is more often than not asymmetrical, so that variation from the classical patterns of field loss is common. In keeping with the general principle of physical examination that subtle abnormalities are best elicited by using the minimal effective stimulus, it is often helpful to use a red hat pin (having established whether the patient has normal colour vision) to examine the peripheral visual fields. The pin should be slowly brought in from the periphery along each diagonal in a plane midway between the patient and the observer, while asking the patient to cover one eye and fix on the eye of the tester. The patient is asked to state immediately the pin is recognizably red. If there appears to be a hemianopia, its border can be mapped by bringing the pin horizontally across the visual field, starting out in the blind area and gradually working down the whole field. In this way, more reproducible information can be obtained than with crude finger wagging—since the retina is especially attuned to detecting movement that would still be recognized when colour vision is impaired.

Although pituitary tumours may raise intracranial pressure if they extend significantly above the sella turcica, it is exceptional for them to cause papilloedema. Instead, long-standing chiasmal compression causes optic atrophy, recognized by pallor of the discs on examining the fundi with an ophthalmoscope. Such changes may be associated with diminished visual acuity but, even in cases where surgery has successfully restored acuity and fields, the pallor tends to persist.

Despite lack of bony lateral walls to the pituitary fossa, invasion of the cavernous sinuses on either side is fortunately very rare but, when it occurs, may cause diplopia and ophthalmoplegia, especially through involvement of the oculomotor or third cranial nerve. Downward invasion is more frequent; the tumour may enter and fill the sphenoid air sinus and even very rarely erode into the nose, causing leakage of cerebrospinal fluid or rhinorrhoea.

# ■ GENERAL FUNCTIONAL EFFECTS

Because of the close integration between different parts of the system, the functional or metabolic features of endocrine disorder cannot always be attributed to disease of one particular gland. With experience, the major site of disturbance can readily be identified, however, and a detailed analysis of the contribution of different hormones to various metabolic processes is not warranted. This section will be confined to consideration of abnormalities of growth and development and those areas of metabolic disorder which can lead to critical illness and where the contribution of the endocrine system may not always be immediately obvious.

## Abnormalities of growth

Disorders of endocrine function can have profound effects on body form, size, proportion and development. These are most clearly seen in children and adolescents, but are by no means confined to the young. Assessment of growth can be made by height measurements and comparison with expected findings given by standard charts, with appropriate allowances for parental height (*see* Chapter 13). Marked differences from the normal age-related distribution may be associated with discrepancies between the chronological age and skeletal development as assessed radiologically by the 'bone age', in which relevant areas, especially the hand and wrist, are examined for epiphyseal fusion, which tends to follow a characteristic age-related pattern. Various endocrine conditions can delay or even halt growth. These aspects of Turner's syndrome and hypothyroidism are dealt with in Chapter 13.

Growth hormone deficiency is often apparent within the first year of life but is frequently missed to the detriment of the child, as the potential for 'catch-up' growth diminishes with increasing delay in treatment. Affected children are very short and chubby due to excessive subcutaneous fat, and boys may have a micropenis. Corticosteroid excess can also decelerate growth and induce obesity, in contrast to the simply obese child who normally has accelerated skeletal growth. Poorly controlled diabetes mellitus may retard growth.

Growth acceleration in childhood may result from hyperthyroidism or any cause of excessive sex steroid secretion, including the various causes of true precocious puberty. The latter group will have stunted ultimate height since premature epiphyseal fusion follows the early accelerated growth. On the other hand, the delay of puberty may prolong skeletal growth, especially of the long bones. This feature of hypogonadism leads to eunuchoid proportions in which the long limbs cause the span to exceed the total height by 5 cm or more—since the additional lengths of both arms are added (measurement in series) but not in the legs (measurement in parallel). Interestingly, this skeletal pattern is frequently seen during childhood in Klinefelter's syndrome—a condition of supernumerary X chromosomes, associated with gonadal failure (*Fig.* 11.4). The early skeletal changes are probably genetic rather than endocrine in origin.

## Water and electrolyte metabolism

It is essential to recognize the factors responsible for the separate

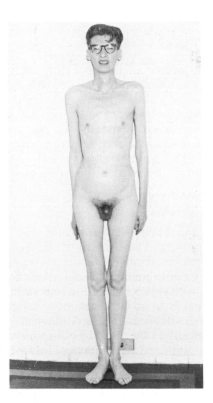

**Fig. 11.4**
Klinefelter's syndrome in a man aged 50. Note the youthful appearance, small genitalia, feminine hair escutcheon and pelvic contour and the long, thin limbs.

regulation of body water and salts which in health are closely controlled. Disproportionate loss of water can occur in various ways, including impairment of vasopressin (antidiuretic hormone, ADH) secretion (cranial diabetes insipidus) or action (nephrogenic diabetes insipidus). It can also follow excessive osmotic load, as in uncontrolled diabetes mellitus. Excessive water retention is seen with inappropriate ADH secretion, which may result from a variety of intracranial or intrathoracic diseases and leads to stimulation of pathways activating hypothalamic release of ADH from the posterior pituitary gland. Some tumours, especially of the bronchus, have a propensity to secrete ADH: so-called ectopic hormone production.

Sodium retention is largely controlled by aldosterone. With increased aldosterone secretion there is normally concomitant potassium loss. It should also be recognized that hydrocortisone (cortisol) has some mineralocorticoid activity which may be significant in states of marked cortisol hypersecretion or Cushing's syndrome. Adrenal insufficiency can lead to excessive sodium loss with ensuing dehydration and postural hypotension manifesting as dizziness or syncope on standing. As mentioned above, salt and water metabolism and the hormones involved in their regulation may be disturbed by a variety of cardiac, renal, gut and hepatic disorders as well as drugs.

# ■ ENDOCRINE ASSESSMENT

Questions of endocrine dysfunction generally revolve about hyper- or hypofunction of specific glands with the consequent clinical sequelae. In many more advanced cases spot diagnoses are possible owing to pathognomonic facies, but the attachment of a label is not enough. Thus in the conditions which readily fall into this situation, such as hypothyroidism, hyperthyroidism, acromegaly, Cushing's syndrome, to name but a few, it is essential to document in as quantitative fashion as possible the degree of local and systemic involvement, before embarking on the sometimes difficult further task of precise aetiological diagnosis.

# ■ ILLUSTRATIVE DISEASES

## THYROID DISEASE

### Thyroid status

The clinical assessment begins with assigning patients into one of these categories: hyper-, eu- and hypo-thyroid. It should be noted that most thyroid diseases are more common in women than men.

**Hyperthyroidism** The clinical features of marked thyroid overactivity are termed thyrotoxicosis. Milder degrees of hyperthyroidism do not have all the 'toxic' aspects and may only be confirmed after biochemical investigation, instigated on the basis of one or two suspicious signs. Important features in the history include heat intolerance and excessive sweating; increased irritability and emotional lability; palpitations, dyspnoea, tremor and weakness; weight loss despite a good or enhanced appetite; increased frequency of bowel action; menstrual disturbance of any type, frequently with scanty periods; excessive thirst. The general appearance is often pathognomonic, with the patient frequently unable to sit still, pouring the history out and looking anxious or startled. Even on a cold day the patient may wear only light clothing. The hands may display a fine tremor which is best appreciated by placing a piece of paper on the outstretched hands (*see Fig.* 10.44, p. 381) and have a characteristically 'velvety' feel due to their hyperaemia and perspiration. There is usually a tachycardia which persists during sleep, and a full volume to the pulse which is detectable through the palm while clasping the flexor aspect of the forearm. Atrial fibrillation is common especially in the older patient.

Hyperthyroidism due to any cause may cause two eye signs arising from the sympathetic component of the innervation of levator palpebris superioris: lid retraction and lid lag. In lid retraction, a rim of white sclera is seen above the iris when the patient is at rest and looks ahead. To elicit lid lag (von Graefe's sign), the observer moves his finger slowly downwards from above the seated patient, who is asked to watch the finger all the way without moving the head (which is best held steady by the observer's other hand); the upper eyelid is then seen to lag behind the eyeball. (*Fig.* 11.5). Weakness of proximal muscles is common in hyperthyroidism, often only mild, but detectable on asking the patient to rise from a squatting position, holding the back vertical and using only quadriceps to elevate the trunk.

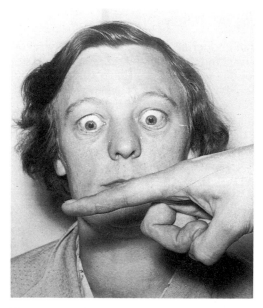

**Fig. 11.5** Von Graefe's sign, lid lag. Although the lower margin of the iris is level with the lower eyelid, the upper eyelid has not moved downwards. The finger has been moved slowly from the level of the hair to its present position.

Hyperthyroidism may be much more difficult to detect in the elderly in whom the disease may have a particular impact on the cardiovascular system. Osteoporosis may also occur with vertebral collapse. In some elderly patients, an apathetic form of the disease is seen with anorexia, marked weight loss, atrial fibrillation, cardiac failure, ptosis and deeply hollowed temporal fossae (*Fig.* 11.6). On the other hand, some young thyrotoxics develop such ravenous appetites that, despite their increased metabolic rate, they actually gain weight. Rare complications include thyroid crisis, in which hyperpyrexia, psychosis and cardiac decompensation occur. Some oriental races are liable to develop hypokalaemic paralysis when thyrotoxic.

**Hypothyroidism** This characteristically creeps on insidiously. It is more commonly met with in the elderly (congenital hypothyroidism is dealt with in Chapter 13). In the older patient, the neurological system may be most profoundly affected with non-specific features of lethargy, loss of concentration and memory. Cold intolerance is a frequent complaint, as are paraesthesiae especially in the distribution of the median nerve in the hand due to carpal tunnel compression. Deafness and unsteadiness may occur, as well as aches and pains in muscles and joints. Cardiovascular symptoms are also common, including angina and intermittent claudication, both of which may improve strikingly on cautious replacement therapy, suggesting a biochemical as well as structural cause of tissue anoxia. Weight gain is frequently attributed to hypothyroidism but is rarely massive. Constipation is common.

Hypothyroidism is a good example of a disease in which 'the wood may be missed for the trees' as the overall first impression is often more telling than the individual items (*Fig.* 11.7). There is a general slowness and sluggish response to questions. The voice may be husky with a changed timbre rather than deep, and this feature may have been commented on by people telephoning the patient. The skin is dry and cold and the face puffy with periorbital oedema—often with great bags under the eyes (*Fig.* 11.8). By contrast, the loss of outer eyebrows is

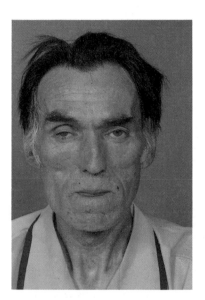

**Fig. 11.6**
Ptosis with hollowed cheeks
and temporal fossae:
'apathetic' hyperthyroidism.

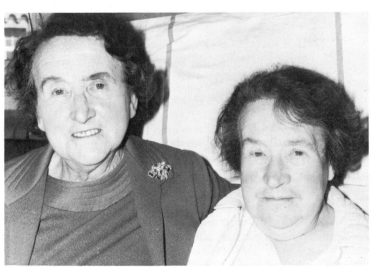

**Fig. 11.7** Hypothyroidism in identical twins, one (*left*) treated
and the other (*right*) untreated.

far less useful a sign than the myth retold in countless textbooks would suggest. Non-pitting myxoedema is only seen in advanced cases. The pulse is characteristically slow. Examination of the tendon jerks is especially useful, as they almost invariably have a slow relaxation phase or, as they have been vividly described, are 'hung-up'. In the clinic, this sign is best elicited in the ankle reflex with the patient kneeling on a chair. Some grossly hypothyroid patients have cerebellar dysfunction especially affecting the trunk and causing difficulty with balance. Occasional patients have serous fluid accumulations, especially in the pericardium, but rarely ascites and hydrocele. Hypothyroidism can be difficult to diagnose in young women who may present with menorrhagia, infertility or recurrent abortion. Galactorrhoea occasionally also occurs as a presenting feature (*Fig*. 11.9). The elderly are prone to hypothermia, intestinal obstruction from paralytic ileus and occasionally psychosis (myxoedema madness).

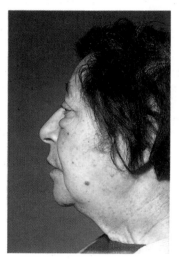 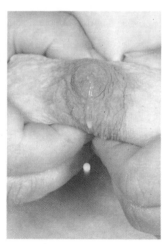

**Fig. 11.8**
Hypothyroidism: infra-orbital myxoedema.

**Fig. 11.9**
Galactorrhoea in hypothyroidism.

### Aetiological diagnosis

The majority of thyroid disease has an autoimmune basis and this should be suspected especially when another autoimmune disease such as pernicious anaemia is present. Vitiligo (*see Fig*. 3.19) is also not uncommon in patients with autoimmune thyroid disease.

**Hyperthyroidism** Autoimmunity causing thyrotoxicosis is called Grave's disease. In such patients extrathyroid manifestations are commonly found, especially in the eyes. The best known sign is exophthalmos (or proptosis) where the increase in orbital contents pushes the eyeball forwards. This can be observed by looking from above the patient while gently sweeping the brows and soft tissues backwards and observing whether the cornea can be seen (Nfziger's sign).

This can be quantitated using Hertel's exophthalmometer but this requires skill for safe use and reproducible measurement.

Even more common is the complaint of grittiness in the eyes. It is important to see whether the eyelids fail to close completely at rest (lagophthalmos) as this puts the cornea at risk of ulceration by abrasion during sleep. The eyes are often asymmetrically involved and indeed one side may be the sole abnormality in some patients who are clinically euthyroid (dysthyroid eye disease). The ocular muscles may become infiltrated, thickened and weakened, leading to diplopia and ocular pareses, especially failure of upward gaze—which again may be strikingly obvious only unilaterally.

The ocular manifestations include conjunctival oedema (chemosis) and an oedematous angry inflammation—so-called malignant exophthalmos: a rather poorly defined term (*Fig.* 11.10). Rarely optic nerve compression leads to impairment of sight. It must be recognized that the state of the eyes in Graves's disease is independent of thyroid status and may suddenly worsen when the patient is euthyroid or even hypothyroid. Other extrathyroidal signs are less common but include pre-tibial myxoedema, where a plaque-like infiltration of the skin over the shin and sometimes encircling the calf or extending on to the foot, occurs. This has a characteristic sudden beginning or edge, easily felt on running the thumbnail along the skin. It is usually red, coarsely pitted and often bears black thick hairs and is cosmetically disfiguring. In some patients the fingers have an appearance very similar to clubbing – thyroid acropachy – in which a lace-like periosteal appearance may be seen on a radiograph. Splenomegaly and fat deposition over the angles of the jaws are occasionally found.

In Graves's disease the thyroid varies from the impalpable (especially in the elderly) to the diffusely large and vascular in which a bruit is of especial significance. Other forms of hyperthyroidism occur as toxic multinodular goitre in

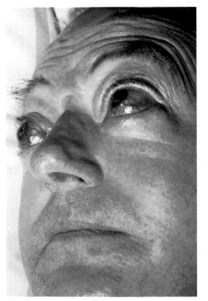

**Fig. 11.10**
Exophthalmos with chemosis and congestion of conjunctival vessels. A case of hyperthyroidism.

which the extrathyroid signs of Graves's disease are absent and the disease is usually milder; the goitre may be vast with great retrosternal extension and tracheal compression (*see Fig*. 11.1). A solitary nodule may become autonomously overactive and if this reaches hyperthyroid levels, will suppress the remaining normal gland (Plummer's disease).

**Hypothyroidism** With most causes of primary thyroid failure the thyroid becomes a shrunken fibrous ghost, which is impalpable. In some cases, the thyroid enlarges due to autoimmune thyroiditis – Hashimoto's disease. This is partly a response to the rise in thyroid stimulating hormone secretion evoked as thyroid reserve fails; the gland is characteristically diffusely enlarged and very firm. Thyroid hormone replacement generally leads to shrinkage of the gland. Ablative therapy of thyrotoxicosis—whether by surgery or radio-iodine—is an increasingly common cause of hypothyroidism. Late treatment of cretinism will be detected by the neurological sequelae, especially a low IQ and short stature. Secondary hypothyroidism due to deficiency of thyroid stimulating hormone usually has other features of pituitary failure.

## PITUITARY DISEASE

Normal pituitary function is regulated by the overlying hypothalamus. Control of the anterior pituitary gland is mediated humorally by factors liberated from the median eminence into the hypothalamo–hypophyseal portal blood supply. The posterior pituitary gland is an evagination of the brain; its hormones are synthesized in the magnocellular neurons of the hypothalamus and travel down their axons to be liberated into the venous drainage of the posterior lobe of the pituitary.

### Functional diagnosis

**Hypopituitarism** Total loss of pituitary function is rare. Lesser degrees often develop along a characteristic path of anterior pituitary deficiency. Gonadotrophin deficiency develops early, manifesting in women as an ovulatory infertility, amenorrhoea, loss of libido, superficial dyspareunia due to vaginal dryness and, in the long-term, osteoporosis: all due to secondary ovarian failure. Men become impotent, lose libido and fertility; the androgen loss is accompanied by poor muscular development. Hypogonadism in both sexes is associated with loss of secondary sexual hair. Men's beards may become softer and require less frequent shaving. These changes vary markedly in degree in patients with hypopituitarism.

Gonadotrophin deficiency in childhood is undetectable except for failure of phallic growth but later may appear as delayed puberty in either sex and eunuchoidal proportions due to delayed epiphyseal fusion (*see above*). Hypogonadism of any cause leads to finely wrinkled skin, especially on the face, with lines spreading up from the upper lip.

Deficiency of growth hormone makes for extra thinning of the skin, which also may be markedly pale (*see below*). Growth hormone loss tends to occur early but is unimportant clinically in adults, other than making for increased liability to hypoglycaemia. This feature is more marked in growth hormone deficient children, where, however, the overwhelming impact is on growth (*see above* and Chapter 13).

ACTH and TSH secretion are generally preserved until much later. ACTH deficiency has two distinct effects. The first is due to loss of the skin pigmentation, which results from its extra-adrenal action (it is now known that separate melanocyte-stimulating hormones are not secreted in man); skin pallor is therefore disproportionate to mucous membrane pallor since the degree of anaemia that may accompany hypopituitarism is usually quite modest. The second effect of loss of ACTH is glucocorticoid deficiency, with general asthenia, hypotension and impaired response to stresses such as fever or trauma. Nausea and vomiting may occur but salt loss is mild, though water overload may be severe. TSH deficiency leads to all the changes of hypothyroidism but is frequently milder than that due to primary thyroid failure. Prolactin deficiency is very rare and its sole unequivocal effect is to render lactation impossible.

Of the two posterior pituitary hormones, only loss of vasopressin or antidiuretic hormone (ADH) is clinically important. This leads to diabetes insipidus with failure to concentrate the urine and liability to marked dehydration. It should be noted that the concomitant presence of adrenocortical insufficiency may mask the ADH deficiency, which only appears on glucocorticoid replacement therapy. The polyuria of absolute ADH deficiency is more marked than virtually any other polyuric state, but minor degrees are less easily recognized.

**Hyperpituitarism** Prolactin is the pituitary hormone most frequently secreted in excessive amounts. It causes hypogonadism in both sexes. In women this may range from primary amenorrhoea to anovulatory infertility. In men it causes striking loss of sexual function due to diminished libido and sexual impotence—often to a much greater degree than the associated hypogonadism. Inappropriate lactation or galactorrhoea occurs in up to half hyperprolactinaemic women if sought for diligently (*Fig.* 11.9). A small amount of galactorrhoea may be found in hyperprolactinaemic men, in whom there is frequently little or no palpable enlargement of breast tissue.

Growth hormone hypersecretion in adult life (following epiphyseal closure) causes acromegaly. Here there are changes in bones, viscera and soft tissues leading to pathognomonic features (*Fig.* 11.11). The skull vault thickens with marked supraorbital and occipital bossing. The mandible enlarges, causing the lower teeth to jut in front of the upper, with an increase in interdental spacing (*Fig.* 11.12). The bony changes affect also the hands, vertebrae and ribs. The hands and feet enlarge, due especially to soft tissue growth with consequent increase in ring and shoe sizes, often dating back several decades by the time the diagnosis is finally made—a testament to the slow and gradual changes that can sometimes be recognized by a series of dated photographs. The skin becomes increasingly sweaty and greasy, with occasional pigmentation, small skin tags or even papillomata. The enlarged nose, coarse features and thick lined skin gives a readily recognized facies (*Fig.* 11.13). The thickened soft tissues in the upper airways may cause snoring and enlargement of the tongue and larynx with deepening of the voice. About a quarter of acromegalics have nodular enlarged thyroid glands, and a similar proportion are hypertensive; a few are diabetic and many develop the carpal tunnel syndrome. Long-standing acromegaly causes severe osteoarthrosis. The rare occurrence of growth hormone secretion earlier in life leads to pituitary gigantism.

ACTH hypersecretion leads to Cushing's disease—the features of which are

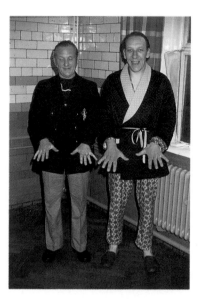

**Fig. 11.11**
Identical twins: one with acromegaly.

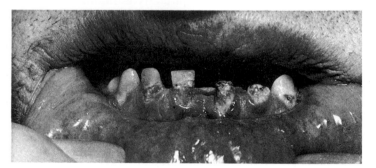

**Fig. 11.12** Acromegaly: separation of the teeth.

described below under 'Adrenals'. Primary overproduction of TSH and gonado-trophins, whilst being recognized more frequently nowadays, are still very unusual.

The overproduction of ADH is described above, and may cause severe or even lethal cerebral complications, including coma and fits, due to water retention.

### Aetiological diagnosis

Hypopituitarism most frequently results from a pituitary tumour. This may cause headaches or visual field defects and can be confirmed by appropriate radiological investigation. Hypersecreting tumours, however, are often small and present a purely endocrine picture. They are characterized by their hormone products, and terms such as chromophobe, eosinophil and basophil adenoma are obsolete. Large hypersecreting tumours may have any of the space-

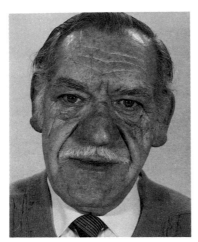

**Fig. 11.13**
Acromegaly: note enlarged nose and ears and prominent lower jaw.

occupying features of large non-functioning tumours, including the suppression of other pituitary functions.

Hyperprolactinaemia can result not only from prolactin secreting tumours but also from impairment of the hypothalamic influence, which in this case is inhibitory. Posterior pituitary failure—diabetes insipidus—is almost invariably the consequence of hypothalamic disease or at least high stalk section by tumour or trauma. The formerly common state of post partum pituitary necrosis, usually associated with a hypotensive episode caused by haemorrhage (Sheehan's syndrome), has been virtually abolished by improved obstetric practice. It is one of the few causes of hypoprolactinaemia.

## ADRENAL CORTICAL DISEASES

The groups of hormones produced by the adrenal cortex are the glucocorticoids, mineralocorticoids and androgens. Destructive processes of the glands may lead to diminished production of all hormones. Congenital enzyme deficiencies can lead to mixed pictures of hormone deficiency and excess, while hormone hypersecretion may involve one or more groups.

### Functional diagnosis

**Hypoadrenalism** The majority of causes of primary adrenal insuffiency, or Addison's disease, act over a long time scale but often the diagnosis is not made until very late. The progress can be viewed in successive stages. The initial phase is one of progressive lethargy, anorexia and nausea, particularly in the morning, weight loss and symptoms of postural hypotension—dizziness on standing. Women may become amenorrhoeic and lose pubic hair. Later, there may be vomiting, diarrhoea or abdominal pain. The final stage is adrenal crisis which is often precipitated by an inadequate response to the stress of an intercurrent illness, especially gastroenteritis. The crisis is characterized by circulatory collapse, severe vomiting and pre-renal uraemia. Throughout the illness the falling cortisol levels lead to increasing levels of ACTH secretion which is responsible for the characteristic pigmentation especially on exposed areas, surfaces subject to friction (*Fig.* 11.14), recent scars, palmar creases and knuckles (*Fig.* 11.15) and gingival and buccal mucosae (*Fig.* 11.16). Very rarely septicaemia causes acute adrenal failure (Waterhouse–Friderichsen syndrome).

### Hyperadrenalism

*Cushing's syndrome* This is the result of excess of cortisol (hydrocortisone) or synthetic glucocorticoids. The commonly stressed features of truncal obesity with relatively thin legs, mooning and reddening of the face, hirsutes (most cases are women), 'buffalo hump', mild diabetes and hypertension are not always present. More useful are signs suggestive of protein wasting, clinically apparent in three main tissues: skin, muscle and bone. The skin becomes thin and fragile, bruises spontaneously (*Fig.* 11.17) and the weakened collagen tears in stretched areas giving livid, thin, purple striae (*Fig.* 11.18) which are readily distinguishable from those seen following childbearing, or in some adolescents who gain weight rapidly. Proximal muscle weakness is the rule and wasting commonplace (*Fig.* 11.19). This is best shown by asking the patient to rise from squatting. Osteoporosis may cause vertebral collapse with the appearance of horizontal creases and loss of height as well as neurological sequelae. Cortisol excess may lead to aseptic necrosis of the femoral neck.

*Virilization* This may result from adrenal or ovarian androgen hypersecretion.

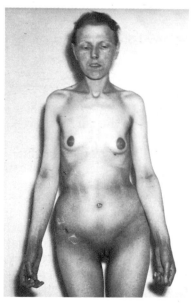

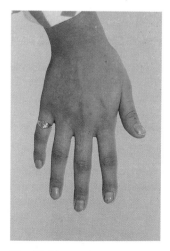

**Fig. 11.14**
Addison's disease, showing pigmentation specially marked over areas of friction.

**Fig. 11.15**
Addisons's disease: pigmentation of the knuckles.

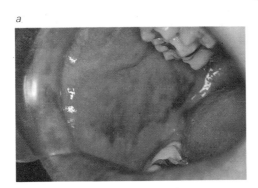
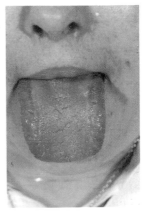

*a*

**Fig. 11.16** Addison's disease: buccal pigmentation; *a*, cheek; *b*, tongue.

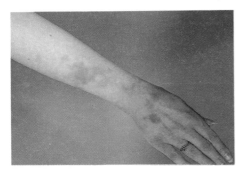
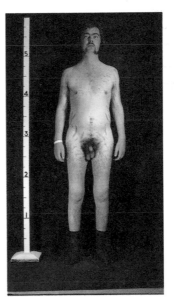

**Fig. 11.17** Cushing's syndrome: spontaneous bruising.

**Fig. 11.18** Cushing's syndrome: purple striae.

The clinical features include hirsutes (hair growth on face and body of women in excess of racial norms), acne, greasiness of the skin, clitoral enlargement, enhanced muscularity, loss of the female pattern of fat deposition, temporal recession of head hair and deepening of the voice.

*Conn's syndrome* Primary hyperaldosteronism may have no signs other than hypertension. Oedema does not occur. Muscle weakness and tetany may be present.

### Aetiological diagnosis

The commonest cause of Addison's disease is auto-immune adrenalitis and this may be associated with vitiligo and other auto-immune disorders. Tuberculosis is today a relatively less frequent cause.

Cushing's syndrome is most commonly due to pituitary ACTH excess (Cushing's disease). This may rarely cause sufficient ACTH to pigment the skin (*Fig. 11.20*). Of the numerous tumours capable of ectopic ACTH secretion, bronchial small cell carcinomas are the commonest. The ACTH excess may be so high that a distinct syndrome arises of pigmentation, severe wasting, weakness and oedema due to hypokalaemic alkalosis from the massive hypercortisolaemia and diabetes but without the classical stigmata of long-standing Cushing's syndrome. Adrenal tumours hypersecreting cortisol autonomously may be benign adenomas, usually small, or carcinomas, often large and even palpable. The differential diagnosis of the underlying cause of Cushing's syndrome is a difficult and specialized matter relying heavily on biochemical and imaging techniques.

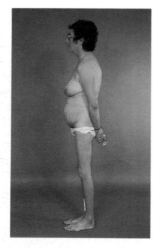 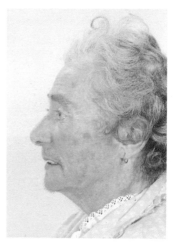

**Fig. 11.19**
Cushing's syndrome: wasting especially of thighs; note also the abdominal striae.

**Fig. 11.20**
Cushing's syndrome: hirsutes and pigmentation.

## ADRENAL MEDULLA

Loss of adrenal medullary tissue is without significant clinical consequences. Hypersecretion of adrenal catecholamines occurs from phaeochromocytomas, tumours which are most often intra-adrenal, single and benign. They cause symptoms of sweating, trembling and fear associated with pallor and episodic hypertension, sometimes followed by hypotension especially on standing and with intervening normal or raised blood pressure. Hypertensive crises are usually spontaneous but can follow pressure, hence abdominal palpation should be especially gentle when phaeochromocytoma is suspected. This tumour may occur together with medullary cell carcinoma of the thyroid.

### GONADAL DEFECTS

Hypogonadism has been described under the heading of hypopituitarism. There are many causes of primary hypogonadism in men, ranging from Klinefelter's syndrome (*see Fig.* 11.4) to myotonic dystrophy, but in most cases the cause remains unknown and simple testicular atrophy will be found. A history of cryptorchidism, testicular torsion or mumps in postpubertal life may be significant. Hypogonadism may be the consequence of diseases such as hepatic cirrhosis and haemachromatosis ('bronzed diabetes'). It may frequently be associated with features of feminization such as gynaecomastia (true, palpable, sometimes tender breast tissue—to be distinguished from excess fat) and a female fat pattern (*Fig.* 11.21). This is common in Klinefelter's syndrome, cirrhosis and spironolactone therapy. In women there are less frequently diagnostic stigmata of the cause of ovarian failure. A notable exception is Turner's syndrome, with amenorrhoea, short stature, widely spaced nipples, puffy hands and feet, often present from birth, nail defects and webbing of the neck (*Fig.* 11.22).

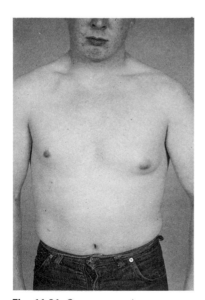

**Fig. 11.21** Gynaecomastia.

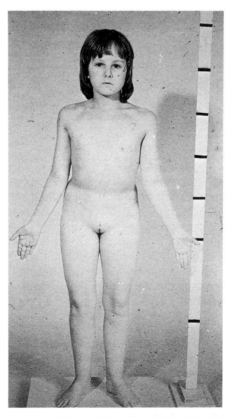

**Fig. 11.22**
A woman of 22 years with Turner's syndrome. Note the broad chest, short neck, lack of pubic hair and child-like appearance.

## PARATHYROID DISEASE

### Functional diagnosis

**Hypoparathyroidism** In this condition, hypocalcaemia causes tetany, convulsions, psychiatric disorder and ectodermal changes; also cataract and nail dysplasias, often with moniliasis. Tetany may present as painful carpopedal spasms—fingers tightly apposed, thumb flexed and adducted across the palm: the *main d'accoucheur* (*Fig.* 11.23). This indicates increased neuromuscular excitability, which may also cause laryngeal spasm and stridor. It may be demonstrated by two signs:

1. *Chvostek's sign*: elicited by tapping over the facial nerve as it emerges from the front of the parotid gland. This causes twitching of the upper lip and drawing up of the angle of the mouth. It is relatively non-specific and may be elicited in many normal people.

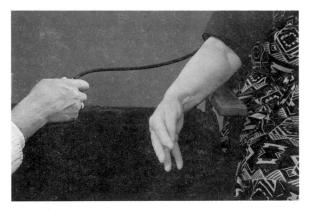

**Fig. 11.23** Trousseau's sign: main d'accoucher.

2. *Trousseau's sign*: involves eliciting latent carpopedal spasm by pumping a sphygmomanometer cuff above systolic pressure for up to three minutes. This is invariably uncomfortable but if the carpopedal spasm occurs the posture is unmistakable, and the spasm does not subside immediately on deflating the cuff, unlike the reaction seen with some hysterical subjects.

**Hyperparathyroidism** The hypercalcaemia may initially cause non-specific aching in limbs, anorexia or depression, thirst and polyuria. Gastrointestinal symptoms include dyspepsia, vomiting, abdominal pain and constipation. Renal and ureteric stones may be the mode of presentation and late cases develop renal failure and severe skeletal problems including painful bone swellings.

### Aetiological diagnosis

Hypoparathyroidism may result from previous neck surgery for goitre. The occurrence of operative damage to the recurrent laryngeal nerves makes the possibility of tetany potentially lethal. Idiopathic hypoparathyroidism is usually of autoimmune origin and may be associated with Addison's disease or thyroid disorder. The secretion of abnormal parathyroid hormone, which is biologically inactive, causes pseudohypoparathyroidism. These patients often have short fourth and fifth metacarpals so that on making a fist they have dimples in the place of knuckles.

Hyperparathyroidism is usually due to parathyroid adenoma. These are for all practical purposes too small to palpate. The one sign that can be useful is corneal calcification, best seen with a slit lamp but often also visible when shining a slanting pencil of light across the cornea where a thin white band may be seen in the 3 o'clock and 9 o'clock positions (as opposed to arcus senilis which is most marked at 12 and 6 o'clock). A convenient source of light is an auroscope bulb—using the instrument without an earpiece. The adjacent sclera often appears gritty and a little inflamed.

## PANCREATIC ISLET DISEASE

### Functional diagnosis

**Hypoglycaemia** This presents classically with symptoms of cerebral dysfunction and sympathetic activation. The former depend on the speed and severity of the hypoglycaemia and may cause coma of rapid onset with neurological changes such as extensor plantar responses and convulsions; hemiplegia may occur, usually rapidly reversible. Lesser degrees may cause mental confusion and amnesia and chronic hypoglycaemia may cause personality changes which can be hard to identify. The sympathetic features include palpitations, sweating and hunger.

**Hyperglycaemia** This causes thirst and polyuria because of the osmotic diuresis, weight loss often without anorexia and, especially in older women, pruritus vulvae. The underlying insulin lack can lead to diabetic ketoacidosis with vomiting, dehydration and hyperventilation due to air hunger, a ketotic odour on the breath, hypotension and drowsiness leading to coma. The complications of diabetes include retinopathy, cataracts, vascular insufficiency causing foot ulcers or gangrene (*Fig.* 11.24), peripheral neuropathy and nephropathy.

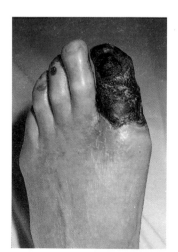

**Fig. 11.24**
Diabetic gangrene.

### Aetiological diagnosis

Hypoglycaemia is most frequently the consequence of overtreatment of diabetes mellitus with insulin or sulphonylurea drugs. Hyperinsulism as a result of islet cell tumour is rare and may present with hypoglycaemic symptoms in the fasting state or after exertion. The patient may learn to counteract symptoms with sugar-containing food and gain weight as a result.

Diabetes mellitus is generally of unknown origin but rarely may be due to excess insulin antagonists.

## ■ INVESTIGATION OF ENDOCRINE DISORDERS

### THYROID

#### Thyroid hormone levels

Total serum thyroxine (T4) and triiodothyroxine (T3) measured by radioimmunoassay may be raised in hyperthyroidism and low in hypothyroidism. Thyroid stimulating hormone (TSH) is especially valuable in hypothyroidism when a high value indicates thyroid gland insufficiency and a low value suggests a pituitary cause. Radioactive iodine/technetium scans are useful for imaging lumps but are not used as a first-line evaluation of thyroid status. Thyroid auto-antibodies are helpful in establishing thyroid auto-immunity: they are *not* a function test.

### PITUITARY

The insulin tolerance test (ITT) should only be performed in patients with no known cardiac disease or epilepsy and with normal basal morning cortisol levels. The induction of hypoglycaemia with insulin should stimulate ACTH and hence cortisol secretion.

Posterior pituitary function is screened by measuring plasma and urine (preferably early morning) osmolalities.

#### Diabetes insipidus

Water deprivation test: collect urine in hourly aliquots, measure urine and plasma osmolality; this is reduced in diabetes insipidus but increases in response to exogenous vasopressin analogue (DDAVP).

#### Hyperprolactinaemia

The best test is a series of three basal prolactin measurements. Women usually have higher levels than men.

#### Acromegaly

During an oral glucose tolerance test the growth hormone level is abnormally maintained above 4 mU/l and may even rise paradoxically. Bromocriptine test: 80 per cent of acromegalics show a marked fall in growth hormone after a 2·5 mg oral dose of bromocriptine.

### Radiology

Pituitary tumours may cause abnormalities of the pituitary fossa apparent on plain lateral or postero-anterior skull radiographs. CT scanning of the pituitary is useful for detecting small pituitary microadenomas (<1 cm diameter) as well as for delineating larger tumours.

### ADRENALS

In adrenal insufficiency the 0900 h cortisol level is reduced. The plasma ACTH is high in adrenal disease and low in hypopituitarism. The plasma urea and potassium are high and the plasma sodium may be low when compensatory mechanics fail.

### Synacthen test

Measure cortisol levels for 1 hour after a synacthen (ACTH) injection to assess adrenal reserve.

### Cushing's syndrome

Screen by measuring 0900 h cortisol after the patient has taken 2·0 mg dexamethasone at 2300 h the previous night. If the cortisol level is greater than 180 nmol/l, Cushing's syndrome is suspected. Fuller investigation includes ACTH measurement; this is undetectable in adrenal adenomas and carcinoma and in these disorders the circadian profile of plasma cortisol is also lost. High dose dexamethasone suppression of plasma cortisol is found in pituitary-dependent Cushing's syndrome and metyrapone tests may help in distinguishing these cases from those associated with carcinoma and ectopic ACTH production. Twenty-four hour urine estimations of free cortisol, 17-oxogenic and 17-oxosteroid measurements complement the plasma estimation of cortisol and ACTH.

### Conn's syndrome

The plasma potassium is abnormally low and the plasma aldosterone and renin levels are raised.

### Congenital adrenal hyperplasia

In this condition, raised levels of plasma 17-hydroxyprogesterone, urinary preganetriol and (in women) plasma testosterone are found.

### Assessment of adrenal size and morphology

This is best achieved by computerized tomography (CT) scanning. Radio-isotopic scanning may be useful, especially in adrenal tumours causing Cushing's syndrome and Conn's syndrome.

### Phaeochromocytoma

Raised levels of vanillylmandelic acid (VMA) and metadrenaline are found in 24-hour urine samples. Plasma noradrenaline is usually elevated but sampling and measurement requires specialized facilities. CT and radio-isotopic imaging may locate the tumour.

### GONADS

*Men*: measure plasma testosterone, FSH/LH.

*Women*: premenopausal: record basal body temperature and measure plasma oestradiol, progesterone and FSH/LH levels.

In suspected *virilization*: plasma testosterone.

In suspected *Klinefelter's* and *Turner's syndrome*: check karyotype.

### PARATHYROIDS

Measure total plasma calcium, albumen, inorganic phosphate and alkaline phosphatase, preferably fasting and in blood drawn without a tourniquet. In appropriate cases measure serum parathyroid hormone and vitamin D metabolites, also twenty-four hour urine calcium.

### PANCREAS

Diabetes mellitus is usually diagnosed on the basis of a high random or fasting plasma glucose. If in doubt, perform an oral glucose tolerance test.

*Diagnosis of insulinoma*: low fasting blood sugar with high insulin. A suppression test may be necessary using exogenous insulin and measuring C-peptide to check the patient's own pancreatic response. Sampling for insulin via a catheter passed percutaneously transhepatically along the splenic vein may be needed to localize the source of insulin in the pancreas.

CT scanning may be helpful in localizing tumours, which are often very small.

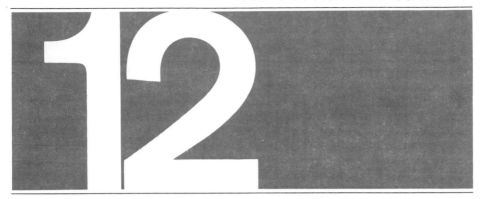

## Symptoms and signs in tropical diseases

HERBERT M. GILLES

The speed and convenience of modern travel together with the enormous boom in the tourist industry have resulted in more people becoming exposed to tropical diseases. Travellers, including immigrant labour moving from one part of the world to another, are altering the patterns and global distribution of disease so that today a tropical disease may present anywhere in a traveller or immigrant. Infected 'commuter' mosquitoes on incoming aircraft have transmitted malaria to persons working in or living around airports in Europe—'peri-airport malaria' (*Fig.* 12.1).

### ■ MEDICAL HISTORY

The basic principles of case-taking have already been fully described. Of vital additional importance in the diagnosis of tropical disease is the geographical history. Nowadays this point is as pertinent in temperate areas as in the tropics themselves. *In temperate areas* the questions 'Where have you come

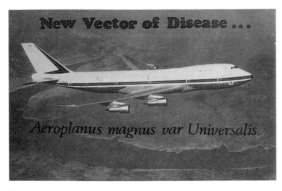

**Fig. 12.1**

from?' and 'When were you there?' are especially relevant when dealing with businessmen, civil servants, members of the teaching profession visiting or working overseas, schoolchildren who have been spending their holidays with parents or relatives in the tropics, seamen, air crews and individuals belonging to immigrant labour groups. The patient's vaccination and inoculation records should be enquired into, and the validity of the certificates checked. If the patient has taken antimalarial drugs, the doctor should find out which, when, for how long and how regularly. Any illness contracted recently abroad, especially if accompanied by fever or rashes, should be recorded.

*In the tropics* the pattern of disease can vary greatly from one country to another and even from one area of a country to another. A knowledge of conditions endemic in the area from which the patient comes is often the most important guide to pertinent questions. In some instances the religion is of some significance as in the case of fasting and pilgrimages. Specific dietary habits (e.g. raw fish) and social customs (e.g. pig feasting in New Guinea) are important. Dispensaries and clinics in many parts of the tropics operate at high pressure with long queues. Patients may be of different races or tribes and may speak different languages necessitating the use of interpreters. Long experience in the territory, a sound knowledge of the diseases to which the patient is likely to be exposed, a good brief medical history and a necessarily rapid, limited physical examination form the basis of diagnosis. It must also be remembered that simultaneous multiple infections are common; the doctor should therefore not be satisfied with having defined a single complaint.

## ■ FEVER

Fever is one of the most important manifestations of acute tropical disease. It is often associated with a *rapid pulse* and sometimes with *rigor*.

The classic intermittent fevers of tertian and quartan malaria are features of relapse rather than of the initial attacks. It is important to emphasize that the fever associated with a primary attack of malignant tertian malaria (*Plasmodium falciparum*) can be either continued or remittent. In *kala-azar* the intermittent or remittent fever may show a double diurnal rise, and there is a dissociation between the height of the fever and the subjective symptoms which are often mild. *Relapsing fever* is characteristic of infection with the *Borrelia* genus—louse borne or tick borne. Remittent or continued fever is present for several days, subsides suddenly and is followed by a variable interval of febrile calm and convalescence; the temperature then rises suddenly and the pattern of the first attack is repeated. In *dengue* a saddle-back temperature curve is often seen, characterized by two phases of high fever separated by a remission. A generalized morbilliform rash appears usually during the second febrile phase.

Associated with fever, a *rapid pulse* is usual, but an inverse relationship may be of clinical significance. Thus, in yellow fever the pulse rate is at first high but drops rapidly, so that a discrepancy between pulse and temperature develops— Faget's sign. On the other hand, the pulse rate may be very rapid and out of proportion to the temperature as in Chagas' disease and African trypanosomiasis. *Rigors* are common at the onset of many of the acute tropical diseases, particularly those associated with a dramatic and rapid rise of temperature, such as typhus and plague. In the relapses associated with malaria rigors recur intermittently in relation to the classic febrile patterns.

## ■ SKIN MANIFESTATIONS

Rashes of various kinds are common in tropical infections, either as part of the disease process or produced by treatment. Erythema and macular rashes are difficult to see in black skins. In the tropics, especially, many skin eruptions become complicated by scratching and secondary infection.

In kala-azar (the 'black sickness') increases in melanin occur, while in pellagra the skin is heavily pigmented on parts exposed to sunlight, e.g. the face, neck and back of hands and wrists. Diminished pigmentation is secondary to the lesions of yaws, leprosy and post kala-azar dermal leishmaniasis.

In onchocerciasis and leprosy the skin is coarsened and roughened, while local patches of transient oedema occur in loiasis (calabar swellings), trichiniasis, gnathostomiasis and American as well as African trypanosomiasis. Sweating is completely absent in heat stroke and loss of elasticity of the skin is associated with severe dehydration in cholera.

The rash of dengue is macular and bright red; that of African trypanosomiasis circinate. The macular lesions of leprosy are hypopigmented, slightly raised and later anaesthetic. Nodules are characteristically seen in onchocerciasis (*Fig.* 12.2). Ecchymoses occur in South-East Asian haemorrhagic fever (*Fig.* 12.3) while the characteristic 'eschar' due to the mite bite is pathognomonic of scrub typhus. Ulcers are commonly seen in the lower leg or, in the case of South American cutaneous leishmaniasis, in the pinna of the ear—chiclero ulcer. Creeping cutaneous eruptions are usually due to the presence of nematode larvae unnatural to man, e.g. hookworms of dogs and cats. Aberrant larvae of *Strongyloides stercoralis* (*Fig.* 12.4) are also responsible for similar lesions. In Britain this manifestation is seen in Far-Eastern ex-prisoners of war many years (over 30) after they have returned home. In tropical Africa furuncles may be caused by the larvae of the Tumbu fly (*Cordylobia anthropophaga*). The classic skin lesions of cutaneous leishmaniasis in the Middle and Near East are illustrated in *Fig.* 12.5 and the gross lymphoedema associated with filariasis in *Fig.* 12.6.

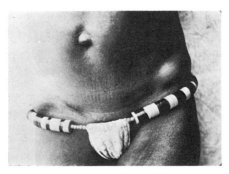

**Fig. 12.2**
Subcutaneous nodules in onchocerciasis.

Figs. 12.2, 12.3 and 12.7 are taken from *A Colour Atlas of Tropical Medicine and Parasitology*, 2nd ed., Ed. by W. Peters and H. M. Gilles, Wolfe Medical Publications, London, 1981.

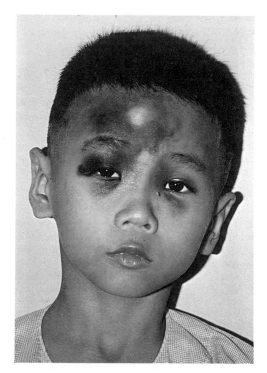

**Fig. 12.3** Facial ecchymoses in a boy with South-East Asian haemorrhagic fever.

Many diseases of the skin familiar in Europe and North America (e.g. pityriasis, erythema multiforme) are also common in the tropics.

## ■ GASTROINTESTINAL MANIFESTATIONS

### Symptoms

**Diarrhoea**   Diarrhoea is one of the most commonly encountered symptoms in tropical medical practice. Of a large number of causes, only a few examples can be mentioned here.

Amoebic dysentery is characterized by intermittent attacks of diarrhoea, and the patient may notice blood and slime in the stools. In acute bacillary dysentery the onset is often sudden with fever, colic and tenesmus, the stools become progressively smaller in amount until only blood and mucus together with pus cells and epithelial debris are passed. In tropical sprue the onset is often insidious with intermittent bouts of loose stools followed by the classic features of the malabsorption syndrome which are also encountered in giardiasis and strongyloidiasis (*see* p. 485). Malaria, especially in children, can be associated with diarrhoea although the causal relationship is difficult to prove. Profuse watery diarrhoea often associated with severe vomiting suggests cholera. Nausea and

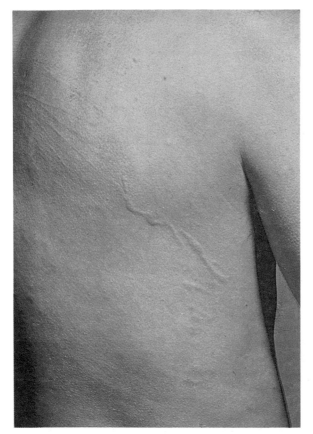

**Fig. 12.4** A 'creeping' elevation of the skin by the larvae of *Strongyloides stercoralis*.

vomiting associated with painful muscle cramps are prominent features of salt deficiency heat exhaustion.

**Abdominal pain**   Abdominal pain simulating an acute abdomen in an anaemic child should bring to mind the possibility of homozygous sickle cell disease (*see* Chapter 8) and laparotomy should not be undertaken until this possibility has been excluded. Pain, often referred to the shoulder, occurs in amoebic liver abscess, while pain in the left hypochondrium sometimes occurs in acute falciparum malaria and as a result of splenic infarction in sickle cell disease.

**Haematemesis and melaena**   Both are common in chronic intestinal schistosomiasis and occur in the terminal stages of yellow fever, Lassa fever, Ebola virus infection, and other viral haemorrhagic fevers.

**Jaundice**   Jaundice resulting from a combination of haemolysis and liver dysfunction is an important symptom of severe falciparum malaria.

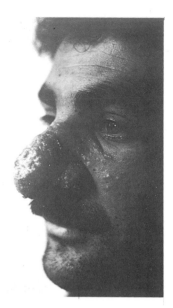

**Fig. 12.5**
Cutaneous leishmaniasis
involving the nose.

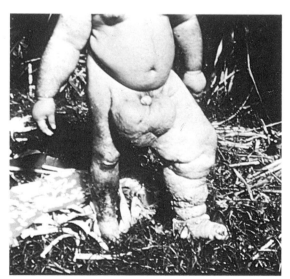

**Fig. 12.6** Lymphoedema of the leg and scrotum due to
filariasis ('elephantiasis').

## Signs

**The mouth** During hot and windy spells in dry climates the lips
are dry and may crack but this is not related to disease. On the other hand,
extreme dryness of the tongue and mouth are features of primary water depletion
and Ebola virus infection. Soreness of the lips with redness and crusting, and

commonly also fissuring at the angles of the mouth, are common in protein-energy-malnutrition and particularly in deficiency of the B group vitamins. In riboflavin deficiency there is inflammation of the lips and a magenta-coloured tongue (*see Fig.* 3.7, p. 40), while in pellagra (nicotinic-acid deficiency) and sprue the tongue is smooth and red due to loss of papillae. Painless enlargement of the parotid glands is often seen in protein-energy-malnutrition. Koplik's spots in an acutely ill febrile infant often gives the clue to the diagnosis of measles—a very serious disease in many parts of the tropics and one in which the rash is not easily seen.

**The intestines** The colon is thickened, palpable and tender in intestinal schistosomiasis and amoebic dysentery. In the latter, a hard tumour resulting from granuloma formation—amoeboma—can occasionally be palpated and may be mistaken for a colonic carcinoma. Severe trichuriasis in children is an important cause of rectal prolapse. Proctoscopy and sigmoidoscopy are useful ancillary diagnostic techniques in 'tropical' intestinal disease, e.g. in amoebiasis the first signs are often small yellowish mucosal papules containing thick pus while later, narrow-necked ulcers with undermined edges and a relatively 'normal' looking intervening mucosa are found. Specimens of mucus, scrapings or biopsy specimens will reveal amoebic trophozoites or, if the patient is suffering from intestinal schistosomiasis, schistosomal eggs and tubercles.

■  **HEPATOMEGALY**

Hepatic enlargement is common in the tropics. Some common causes of hepatomegaly of 'tropical' origin are given in *Table* 12.1.

| Table 12.1  **Some 'tropical' causes of hepatic enlargement** (*see also Table* 4.5, p. 98) | |
| --- | --- |
| *Tender enlargement* | *Painless enlargement* |
| Amoebic liver abscess | Bartonellosis |
| Beriberi | Clonorchiasis |
| Brucellosis | Fascioliasis |
| Chagas' disease | Hydatid disease |
| Hepatic veno-occlusive disease | Intestinal schistosomiasis |
| Leptospirosis | Leprosy |
| Malaria | Opisthorchiasis |
| Relapsing fevers | Plague |
| Sickle cell anaemia | Protein-energy-malnutrition |
| Thalassaemia | Trypanosomiasis |
| Toxocariasis | Visceral leishmaniasis |
| Virus hepatitis | Yellow fever |

In amoebic liver abscess the liver is tender on palpation, and screening will reveal diminished diaphragmatic excursion and usually a raised right hemidiaphragm, since most single abscesses are in the upper part of the right lobe. In chronic intestinal schistosomiasis all the classic features of portal obstruction are seen (*Fig.* 12.7).

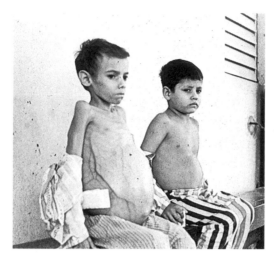

**Fig. 12.7** Chronic intestinal schistosomiasis. Note the abdominal distension due to ascites and splenomegaly and, in the nearest child, engorged abdominal veins, eversion of the umbilicus and cachexia.

# ■ SPLENOMEGALY

In many tropical areas splenomegaly is an extremely common finding. The physician has to decide whether the enlargement is related to the current illness of the patient or is merely a clinical manifestation of immunity to disease. In malarious areas of the world the endemicity of malaria in a community is measured by the 'spleen and parasite rate'. Thus, in holoendemic areas of malaria, splenomegaly may occur in 80 per cent of children and in 20 per cent of adults as a 'normal' finding. This clearly raises special problems in diagnosis. Hackett has described a method of recording the degree of splenomegaly, which has been widely used in the tropics, particularly in relation to malaria surveys, but which is also useful as a routine clinical method. The classification is as follows:

| Class of spleen | Findings on palpation |
|---|---|
| 0 | Spleen not palpable even on deep inspiration |
| 1 | Spleen palpable below the costal margin, usually on deep inspiration |
| 2 | Spleen palpable, but not beyond a horizontal line halfway between the costal margin and the umbilicus, measured in a line dropped vertically from the left nipple |
| 3 | Spleen palpable more than halfway to the umbilicus, but not below a line running horizontally through it |
| 4 | Spleen palpable below the umbilical level, but not below a horizontal line halfway between the umbilicus and the symphysis pubis |
| 5 | Spleen palpable, and extending lower than in Class 4 |

Some common causes of splenomegaly in the tropics are given in *Table* 12.2.

| Table 12.2 | **Some 'tropical' causes of splenomegaly** | |
|---|---|
| *Tender enlargement* | *Painless enlargement* |
| Brucellosis | Bartonellosis |
| Enteric fevers | Hydatid disease |
| Malaria | Intestinal schistosomiasis |
| Relapsing fever | Leprosy |
| Trypanosomiasis | Leptospirosis |
| Typhus fever | Sickle cell anaemia |
| | Thalassaemia |
| | Tropical splenomegaly syndrome |
| | Visceral leishmaniasis |

## ■ CARDIOVASCULAR SYSTEM (*see also* Chapter 7)

Cardiovascular manifestations occur in some of the tropical diseases. Furthermore, certain conditions of, as yet, undetermined origin, such as endomyocardial fibrosis and the cardiomyopathies, are common in many parts of the tropics.

Chagas' disease is a common cause of myocarditis in children in South America, and the condition is also associated with various dysrhythmias. Myocarditis also occurs in African trypanosomiasis, especially due to *Trypanosoma rhodesiense*, and has been described in toxoplasmosis, trichinosis, leptospirosis and balantidiasis.

Pericarditis occurs in amoebiasis, scrub typhus, African trypanosomiasis and yellow fever.

Cardiomegaly and cardiac failure have been described in association with Chagas' disease, schistosomiasis, hookworm disease, hydatid disease, endomyocardial fibrosis, protein-energy-malnutrition and beriberi.

## ■ RESPIRATORY SYSTEM (*see also* Chapter 6)

Coughing fits at night, eosinophilia and asthmatic paroxysms are allergic manifestations of the transpulmonary migration of a variety of nematode larvae such as ascaris, hookworm, strongyloides and toxocara. Symptoms are particularly marked for those larvae of which man is not a natural host, e.g. filarial worms of animal origin, which give rise to the syndrome known as 'eosinophilic lung'.

The Katayama syndrome of cough, fever, urticaria and eosinophilia occurs in the invasive stage of schistosomiasis. In the later stages, particularly of *Schistosoma mansoni* infections, the presence of eggs causes the formation of granulomas and eventually obliterative pulmonary arteritis, with consequent cor pulmonale and pronounced dyspnoea. In paragonimiasis the cough becomes chronic with bloodstained sputum ('endemic haemoptysis'). In hepatic amoebiasis there are often signs of inflammation at the base of the right lung, and there may be a pleural effusion or an embolic amoebic abscess of the lung. Signs of pneumonia with pleural friction rub and inspiratory crepitations may be elicited.

Pulmonary oedema may complicate severe falciparum malaria or result from excessive administration of fluid, by the intravenous route, to dehydrated patients with severe malaria; this often precedes the appearance of oedema elsewhere.

Single or multiple hydatid cysts can occur in the lung and African trypanosomiasis, especially rhodesiense infections, may cause pleural effusion.

■ **RENAL SYSTEM** (*see also* Chapter 5)

*Pain* associated with obstruction due to stones in the kidneys, ureters and bladder is common in the tropics. In North-East Thailand, for example, children are particularly prone to bladder stones. *Haematuria* occurs in association with *Schistosoma haematobium* infection, especially during the acute phase of the disease. In chronic infections there is dysuria with recurrent attacks of cystitis. Cystoscopic examination of the bladder reveals a variety of lesions depending on the intensity and duration of infection; these include hyperaemia, oedema, granulations, ulceration, fine sandy patches and polypi. When fibrotic stenosis of the ureters occurs, the resulting back pressure leads to hydronephrosis. *Chyluria* is a complication of filariasis (*Wuchereria bancrofti, Brugia malayi*). *Oliguria* and *anuria* due to acute renal failure from renal ischaemia may cause death in falciparum malaria. *Haemoglobinuria* may also complicate severe falciparum malaria; this is probably an immunological reaction resulting in a catastrophic haemolytic crisis. Gross *proteinuria*, oedema and ascites (nephrotic syndrome) are seen in association with quartan malaria (*Plasmodium malariae*).

■ **NEUROLOGICAL SYSTEM** (*see also* Chapter 10)

Delirium and coma are common in falciparum malaria, African trypanosomiasis and Japanese B encephalitis. Convulsions and various motor defects are seen in children with falciparum malaria, in cerebral schistosomiasis (*Schistosoma japonicum*), toxoplasmosis and kuru. Apparent clouding of the intellect and mental confusion are often observed in cerebral malaria.

Subjective sensory complaints may accompany vitamin deficiencies, e.g. the 'burning feet' syndrome of pellagra. Thiamine deficiency ('dry' beriberi) manifests itself with wrist-drop, foot-drop and marked wasting of the lower extremities.

In leprosy nerves are enlarged, hard and tender; the ulnar, posterior tibial and external popliteal nerves are the most commonly affected. Of the superficial sensory nerves, the most frequently involved is the great auricular (*see Fig.* 10.71, p. 409). Neural damage is followed by paralysis and anaesthesia, sometimes with trophic changes in the skin and neuropathic injuries to bones and joints.

Psychosomatic disorder is common in the tropics: weakness, sexual incapacity, feelings of hotness and coldness, 'worms under the skin' and paraesthesiae of various kinds are frequent symtoms.

■ **OCULAR SYSTEM**

The eyes are affected in a large number of tropical diseases and some, e.g. onchocerciasis and trachoma, are among the most serious causes of morbidity.

In leprosy there is loss of eyebrows and eyelashes and bacilliferous granulomas may be found in any structure. Quite distinct are the hypersensitivity reactions occurring in the uveal tract during the acute exacerbations of lepromatous leprosy, and the paralytic lagophthalmos (inability to close the eye) that leads to perforating corneal ulceration and its sequelae.

In onchocerciasis a whole variety of eye lesions are seen ranging from the 'snow flake opacities' to sclerosing keratitis and blindness. The appearance of small pale follicles in the palpebral conjunctiva of the upper lids, which must be everted before they are seen, are an early sign of trachoma. In vitamin A deficiency there is loss of lustre of the conjunctiva and dryness (xerophthalmia), Bitot's spots (white foamy spots lateral to the cornea), keratomalacia (softening), perforation of the cornea and finally blindness. Vascularization of the sclera with photophobia occurs in riboflavin deficiency. In loiasis the movement of the adult worm across the conjunctiva results in one of the most irritating and characteristic features of the condition. Subconjunctival haemorrhages are common in leptospirosis. Involvement of the posterior segment of the eye occurs in toxocara infection and the condition must be differentiated from a retinoblastoma. Retinal haemorrhages are common in falciparum malaria.

Unilateral palpebral and facial oedema is characteristic of Chagas' disease; it also occurs in African trypanosomiasis.

## ■ HAEMATOLOGICAL MANIFESTATIONS

Many of the parasites that are responsible for tropical disease are found in the blood and frequently a clinical diagnosis can be confirmed in this way.

### Parasitaemia

The appropriate parasite is found in the blood in the following tropical infections—(1) Malaria (*Plasmodium falciparum, P. vivax, P. malariae, P. ovale*). (2) Filariasis (*Wuchereria bancrofti, Brugia malayi, Loa loa, Dipetalonema perstans, Mansonella ozzardi*). (3) Trypanosomiasis (*Trypanosoma gambiense, T. rhodesiense, T. cruzi*). (4) Relapsing fevers (*Borrelia recurrentis, B. duttoni*). (5) Kala-azar (*Leishmania donovani, L. infantum, L. chagasi*); Bartonellosis (*Bartonella bacilliformis*).

### Eosinophilia

Eosinophils are increased in number in many parasitic infections, especially helminthic. This state is known as eosinophilia, and some of the conditions responsible are: (1) filariasis; (2) infections with non-human parasites (e.g. toxocara:animal hookworms); (3) loiasis; (4) acute schistosomiasis; (5) onchocerciasis; (6) acute migratory phase of intestinal nematodes (e.g. *Ankylostoma duodenale; Necator americanus; Ascaris lumbricoides*); (7) clonorchiasis; (8) strongyloidiasis; (9) trichinosis; (10) dracontiasis; (11) echinococciasis; (12) gnathostomiasis; (13) angiostrongyliasis.

### Leucopenia

Leucopenia is often associated with (1) kala-azar, (2) dengue, (3) yellow fever, (4) undulant fever, (5) typhoid and (6) malaria. Because of the frequency of concomitant secondary infections this finding is not as consistent as might be expected.

## ■ SIDEROOM DIAGNOSTIC TECHNIQUES*

Whereas sophisticated serological and other techniques have to be carried out in appropriate laboratories, the initial diagnosis of many tropical infections can and should be done in the hospital ward or clinic 'sideroom'.

### Blood

Small quantities suitable for examination on glass microscope slides may be obtained by pricking the finger, the lobe of the ear or, in children, the heel or big toe. The blood can then be examined as a fresh wet preparation, a thin smear or a thick film (*Fig.* 12.8).

**Wet preparation** The wet preparation is particularly useful when there are present certain motile protozoa, e.g. trypanosomes, or microfilarial helminth larvae, e.g. *W. bancrofti, L. loa, D. perstans, B. malayi.*

The drop of blood is placed on the centre of a clean coverslip which is then lowered drop downwards on to the surface of a thoroughly clean glass slide. The film should be examined as soon as possible. The areas in which movement is observed are examined under the 4 mm objective and trypanosomes, if present, are easily identifiable. Microfilariae are much larger and can be easily distinguished under the 16 mm objective.

**Thin films** (*Fig.* 12.8b) Prick the skin and put a small drop of blood near the end of the undersurface of a microscope slide and spread the film with the end of a second clean slide. The film should be allowed to dry thoroughly before staining with Leishman's or Giemsa's stain (for details see textbooks of parasitology or tropical medicine).

**Thick films** (*Fig.* 12.8c) Prick the skin and wait until a globule of blood has formed. Place the middle of the undersurface of a clean slide against the blood and remove it, then spread the blood quickly and evenly. After drying, the film can be stained with Giemsa's stain or Field's stain.

The blood should be examined on *several occasions* during a suspected attack of malaria, especially *P. falciparum*, because the number of parasites present at any one time varies greatly during the day. Since more blood goes into the making of a thick film, more parasites will be found per field under the 2 mm immersion objective than in thin films.

Thin films are useful for the differentiation of the various malaria parasites. In general, if small rings are present in large numbers and no other forms of the asexual parasites are seen, the infecting parasite is *P. falciparum*. The presence of large trophozoites in small numbers and a polymorphic appearance—e.g. rings, trophozoites, gametocytes—indicates infection with *P. vivax or P. malariae* (*Fig.* 12.9).

---

* For the morphological identification of the various parasites referred to in this section, the reader should consult *A Colour Atlas of Tropical Medicine and Parasitology* (1981), 2nd ed., Ed. W. Peters and H. M. Gilles, Wolfe Medical Publications, London.

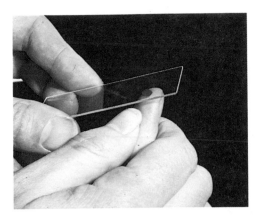

**Fig. 12.8**
*a*, Collection of blood from finger-prick.

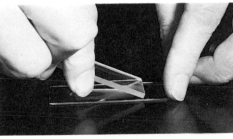

*b*, Preparation of thin film (*see text*).

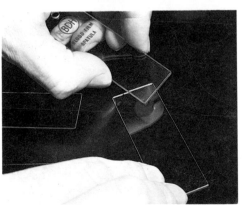

*c*, Preparation of thick film (*see text*).

Trypanosomes can be seen both in thick and thin stained films as can amastigotes of *Leishmania*, although the latter are more easily found in aspirates of the bone-marrow, spleen or liver. The characteristic microfilariae are found in the peripheral blood provided it is taken at the appropriate time, i.e. between 2200 and 0200 h for the nocturnal microfilariae, and around midday for the diurnal ones.

### Faeces

A portion of faeces is picked up on a bacterological loop or match-

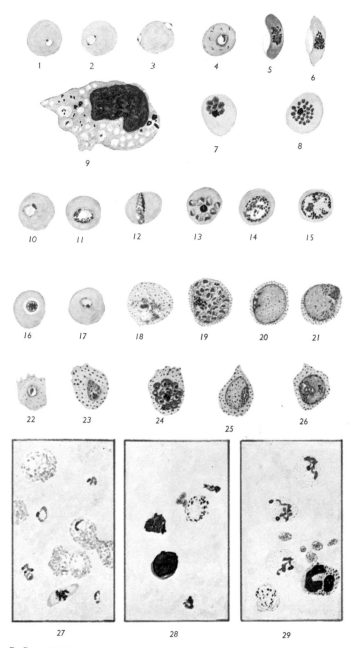

D. Dagnall del.

**Fig. 12.9** Malaria parasites. Nos. 1 to 26—thin films, Leishman's stain; Nos. 27 to 29—thick films, Field's stain. Smears made from peripheral blood unless otherwise noted. (×660.)

*Plasmodium falciparum* (malignant tertian malaria). (Nos. 1 to 9.) 1, Ring. 2, Ring with two chromatin dots. 3, Double infection of red cell. Marginal or accolé forms. 4, Ring in deeply stained cell showing coarse stippling (Stephen's and Christopher's dots). 5, Male sexual form. Gametocyte or crescent. Note purplish cytoplasm and scattered pigment. 6, Female sexual form. Gametocyte or crescent. Note slate-blue cytoplasm and compact pigment. 7, Half-grown asexual form from spleen smear of fatal case. 8, Fully grown asexual form (schizont) from spleen smear. 9, Macrophage containing ingested malarial pigment.

*Plasmodium malariae* (quartan). (Nos. 10 to 15.) 10, Ring. 11, 12, Trophozoites. Note compactness of cytoplasm and heavy pigment. No. 12 shows an equatorial form. 13, Schizont. Typical rosette form consisting of a central mass of pigment surrounded by 8 merozoites. 14, Male gametocyte. Shows diffusion of nucleus and scattered pigment. 15, Female gametocyte. Shows compactess of nucleus and pigment. 16, Blood-platelet superimposed on red cell. Often mistaken for a malarial parasite.

*Plasmodium vivax* (simple or benign tertian). (Nos. 17 to 21.) 17, Ring. 18, Trophozoite. Note amoeboid cytoplasm and paleness of red cell, which is enlarged and stippled with fine red dots (Schüffner's dots). 19, Schizont. Red cell enlarged, pale and stippled with Schüffner's dots. 20, Male gametocyte. 21, Female gametocyte. The gametocytes differ from those of quartan in being enclosed in enlarged, stippled cells, and in having finer pigment.

*Plasmodium ovale* (tertian). (Nos. 22 to 26.) 22, Ring. 23, Trophozoite. Differs from the trophozoite of *P. vivax* in being more solid, and is often found in an oval red cell with fimbriated edges. The stippling is heavier than in *P. vivax*. 24, Schizont. The number of merozoites (12) is less than in *P. vivax*, which has 16 to 24. 25, Male gametocyte. 26, Female gametocyte.

27, *P. falciparum*: thick film. Shows several rings lying at various angles, a gametocyte, and some blue-staining bodies, reticulocytes.

28, *P. malariae*: thick film. Shows two trophozoites and a schizont. Included in the field are blood platelets, a punctate basophil, and a lymphocyte.

29, *P. vivax*: thick film. Shows three trophozoites. Note apparent breaking up of cytoplasm, a typical feature. The outline of the infected red cells can be traced by the Schüffner's dots. Included are a neutrophil polymorphonuclear leucocyte, platelets and a reticulocyte.

stick and emulsified in a large drop of saline on a slide and covered with a coverslip. The specimen is examined systematically using the low-power objective (16 mm) with the light well cut down.

If adult worms or segments are present in the faeces they should be picked out and sent for detailed examination unless readily recognizable, e.g. ascaris worms.

During an attack of acute *amoebic dysentery* active vegetative amoebae are easily recognized provided that the preparation is fresh and is examined immediately; ingested red cells confirm the diagnosis. When the disease is quiescent the faeces are formed and contain only cysts.

Helminth ova if present in moderate numbers will also be detected in saline preparations.

### Urine

For the diagnosis of *S. haematobium* infection, a 24-hour specimen should be used but if random samples only are available, those collected around the middle of the day (1000–1400 h) are likely to contain the most eggs. The urine specimens are allowed to stand for half an hour in a conical flask or are centrifuged at 1500 rpm for 5 min. Samples of the wet sediment are transferred to microscope slides and examined under the 16 mm objective with the light cut down. The characteristic eggs of *S. haematobium* can be identified easily. Eggs of *S. mansoni* and more rarely *S. japonicum* may also be found in the urine, although they are much more commonly excreted in the faeces.

### Skin

The best method for the parasitological diagnosis of onchocerciasis is the skin snip. In Africa the best site is just above the iliac crest; in Central America over the scapula or iliac crest and in the Yemen over the lower calf. The snip is transferred immediately to a drop of normal saline on a microscope slide. If no microfilariae are seen at first, the snip is teased and re-examined after 30 min.

---

### ■ ILLUSTRATIVE DISEASES

By way of summary will be described two tropical diseases likely to be encountered in the tropics or in the Western world—malignant tertian malaria and amoebic dysentery.

### Malignant Tertian Malaria (*P. falciparum*)

Falciparum malaria is a tropical medical emergency since it may be fatal if treatment is inadequate or delayed. The majority of infections diagnosed in Europe develop within 30 days of arrival from endemic areas and in most instances patients have either not taken prophylactic drugs or have stopped taking them on arrival.

Falciparum malaria is protean in its manifestations. It may be symptomless in the tropics among immune subjects or may present as an influenza-like fever, jaundice, anaemia or encephalitis. Fever in primary attacks is often remittent or continued, *not* intermittent and tertian. Headache, malaise, nausea, vomiting and generalized joint pains may be the only additional presenting symptoms of an *uncomplicated* attack. On physical examination there may be hepatospleno-megaly and a variable degree of anaemia.

The more dramatic 'pernicious' manifestations are (i) cerebral malaria characterized by confusion, delirium, convulsions or coma; (ii) renal insufficiency or failure presenting as oliguria and later anuria; (iii) malarial anaemia usually haemolytic in character; (iv) gastrointestinal malaria manifested by severe vomiting, diarrhoea and jaundice; (v) hyperpyrexia; (vi) algid malaria producing a shock syndrome with or without septicaemia (vii) hypoglycaemia and (viii) malarial haemoglobinuria. These patients will usually also be febrile, dehydrated and pale and examination of the blood reveals a dense parasitaemia.

The crucial single factor in the diagnosis of malaria is that it should be thought

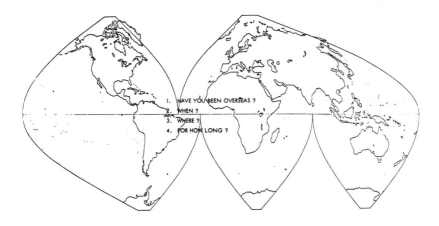

**Fig. 12.10** The geographical history is very important.

of as a cause of illness in any patient who lives in or has visited an endemic area. The geographical history is extremely important (*Fig.* 12.10).

### Amoebic Dysentery

The patient usually gives a history of dysentery or intermittent diarrhoea. Constitutional disturbance is slight with pyrexia either absent or mild. Three to ten dysenteric stools are passed daily. The caecum and descending colon are sometimes palpable.

Parasitological examination should be performed on a *freshly* obtained specimen of faeces. The presence of motile amoebae containing red blood cells is pathognomonic of invasive amoebiasis. On sigmoidoscopy the typical amoebic ulcers are seen usually in the lower rectum.

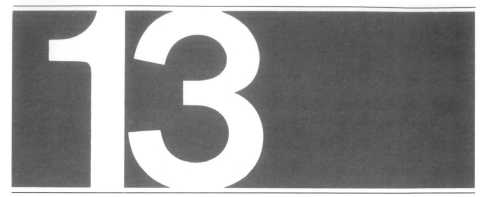

## The examination of children

## F. Harris

The examination of the infant and child is dealt with in three sections, namely, the newborn infant and neonate, the infant and toddler and the schoolchild and adolescent. Throughout infancy, childhood and adolescence there is a continuum of growth and development. During these years the physical growth of the young subject is an important marker of personal health and environment. For this reason there will be repeated references to accurate measurement of height and weight. The study of growth and development through childhood has rightly been described as the basic science of paediatrics.

Clinical examination of the young always includes examination, by interrogation and inspection, of the parents; for parents and family are, to a lesser or greater extent, part of the clinical picture.

Skill in examining the young comes only from repeated contact with young patients. Most experienced clinicians are able to complete a thorough examination of the young child using less physical contact with the patient than the corresponding examination requires in an adult. In paediatrics considerable importance is placed on continuous inspection and observation, not only of the patient, but also of the parent's reaction to the clinical procedures.

## ■ THE EXAMINATION OF THE NEWBORN INFANT AND NEONATE

The newborn infant is examined at birth and again more fully prior to discharge when a few days old. The clinical priorities depend on when the examination is performed. The primary purpose of the examination at birth is to ensure that vital functions have been established, that there are no life-threatening congenital malformations and that birth trauma has not been sustained. The examiner should take into account the history of maternal health during pregnancy and the conduct of labour and delivery. As the immediate postnatal progress will be related to the infant's maturity an assessment of gestational maturity is necessary.

If the examination is carried out immediately at birth, the infant's general condition is recorded at 1 min and then again at 5 min after delivery. This assessment follows the standard pattern devised by Virginia Apgar and is based on a scoring system of five signs which indicate the status of vital functions (*Table* 13.1). Although equal weighting is given to all five clinical indices, it is important to consider not only the total score but also how the individual indices scored. Low or high scores on 'heart rate' and 'respiration' are of more clinical significance than similarly low scores for colour and reflex irritability. The ideal score is 10 and a score of less than 7 indicates a significant (albeit often temporary) degree of depression of vital functions. However, if the Apgar score is still low at 5 min, then the infant may have sustained damaging intrapartum asphyxia, cerebral birth injury or be depressed from maternal analgesia given during labour. In preterm infants particularly (gestation less than 37 weeks and weight less than 2500 g) the prognosis for survival worsens with a lowering of the Apgar score. If no resuscitation is required and the initial Apgar score has been obtained, then further clinical examination is deferred until the infant has been adequately swaddled or brought to a source of heat. The importance of avoiding heat loss by the infant during the clinical examination cannot be overstressed.

| Table 13.1 | **The Apgar score** | | |
|---|---|---|---|
| | 0 | 1 | 2 |
| Colour | Blue or pale | Body pink<br>Hands and feet blue | Completely pink |
| Heart rate | Absent | <100 | >100 |
| Respiration | Absent | Slow, irregular | Strong cry |
| Reflex irritability | No response | Grimace | Cry |
| Muscle tone | Limp | Some flexion of limbs | Active |

## Inspection, palpation, auscultation

The further assessment starts with thorough inspection of the infant and is followed by palpation and auscultation. With experience the examiner should be able to observe and palpate simultaneously. The routine clinical examination therefore proceeds with a visual appraisal of the whole infant noting especially the *posture* which in fullterm babies is normally one of partial flexion. The preterm infant adopts the 'frog' position when lying supine (*Fig.* 13.1). The thighs are widely abducted with the knees flexed and the relatively large head turned to one side. This position is the result of the hypotonia and weakness that is characteristic of the preterm. An initial assessment should be made of the infant's *state of wakefulness*, which significantly influences certain aspects of physical examination and in particular the neurological assessment. During this period of visual appraisal the quality and strength of the infant's *cry* should be noted, e.g. weak, high pitched. Any *spontaneous movements* should be noted to determine whether they are bilateral, rhythmic, coarse or fine. The only clinical evidence of

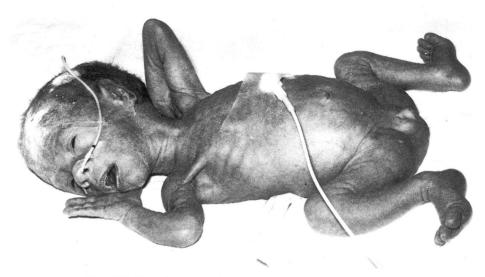

**Fig. 13.1** Typical posture of a preterm infant in the frog position.

a generalized seizure in a newborn infant may be the intermittent clenching of one fist.

## Skin

If the examination is carried out prior to bathing, the skin will be covered with vernix caseosa. Note should be taken of meconium staining which may signify that the baby experienced intra-uterine distress. The foul odour of an intra-uterine pyogenic infection will not be missed easily. After bathing the baby the presence of a persistent odour may signify an inborn error of metabolism. Infants with inherited short chain fatty acid disorders and some amino acid disorders often have a characteristic body or urine odour.

The majority of newborns will have pale pink capillary haemangiomas of no clinical significance on the nape of the neck ('storkbite') and eyelids. Infants with one or two coloured parents commonly have slate grey areas of pigmentation (Mongolian blue spots) over the buttocks, back and occasionally on the upper limbs and face (*Fig.* 13.2). These pigmented areas need to be distinguished from bruising which has occurred during delivery. White pinhead lesions (milia) over the nose are very common and are normal. Larger white or yellow vesicles surrounded by erythema (erythema toxicum) occur frequently. These vesicles contain eosinophils and have no clinical significance, but they need to be distinguished from the pus-containing bullae of staphylococcal skin sepsis. Petechiae may be present on the forehead and face of the baby following delivery. However, more widespread petechiae should be taken as an indication of purpura from an underlying thrombocytopenia due to transplacental intrauterine infection such as toxoplasmosis, rubella, cytomegalovirus and herpes (acronym TORCH). Purpura may occur with acute bacterial infections acquired from the birth canal

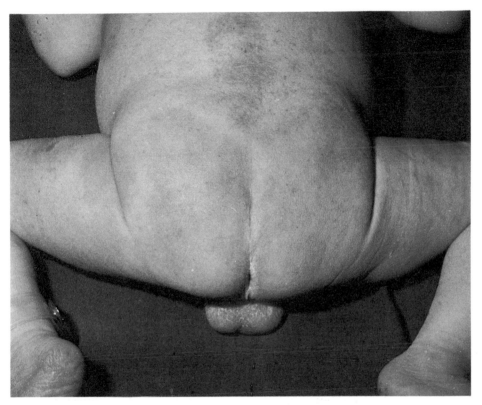

**Fig. 13.2** Mongolian blue spots.

and also with severe haemolytic disease of the newborn, particularly due to Rh incompatibility.

Skin pallor either denotes severe asphyxia with peripheral circulatory failure or a degree of anaemia which requires urgent transfusion. The latter may be due to isoimmune haemolytic disease, feto-maternal bleed or intrapartum placental abruption with intra-uterine fetal haemorrhage.

**Jaundice** The presence of jaundice should be sought routinely and preferably in natural light. The yellow skin pigmentation characteristically first becomes visible on the nose and forehead. Jaundice appearing within the first 24 h after birth strongly indicates a 'pathological' underlying cause such as haemolytic disease of the newborn, sepsis or galactosaemia. Physiological jaundice or so-called 'jaundice of immaturity' does not appear so soon after birth. Physiological jaundice prolonged beyond 7 days in the fullterm and 10 days in the preterm infant is a feature of congenital hypothyroidism. The passage of pale stools and dark urine by a jaundiced infant is found in the 'neonatal hepatitis' syndrome, which includes transplacental intra-uterine infection (rubella, cytomegalovirus and toxoplasmosis), alpha$_1$-antitrypsin deficiency and biliary atresia. In this syndrome there is considerable firm enlargement of the liver and spleen.

**Cyanosis** Newborn babies may have marked peripheral cyanosis; the feet and hands may be dark purple. This by itself is rarely of any significance, whilst cyanosis of the tongue and lips is always significant and may indicate cardiopulmonary or intra-cranial pathology. The presence of an audible grunt and tachypnoea is an important sign of respiratory distress. The pliability of the newborn thoracic cage makes obvious any difficulty with breathing and retraction of the sternum and intercostal spaces will be seen. Thus the cardinal clinical features of *respiratory distress* in a newborn infant are tachypnoea (respiratory rate >60 per min sustained for 1 h), grunting respiration, sternal recession and central cyanosis. In the presence of these clinical signs the more common life-threatening conditions requiring urgent treatment should be sought by immediate further clinical examination. Life-threatening clinical conditions presenting as respiratory distress and which are amenable to treatment include:

Pneumothorax
Lobar emphysema
Diaphragmatic hernia
Transposition of the great vessels
Choanal atresia
Meningitis
Hypoglycaemia

### Ears and facies

During the routine examination of the newly born infant, particular attention should be given to the ears and facies. The diagnosis of Down's syndrome (mongolism) can be suspected from the first look at the infant's whole face before inspecting more individual features (*Fig.* 13.3). The *ears* should be examined for normal formation of the external auricle and the presence of an external meatus. The position of the whole ear should be observed relative to a line drawn though the canthi of the eye. Malformed and low set ears are often associated with occult malformations such as hypoplastic kidneys, and may also be a marker of autosomal trisomy.

### Head and scalp

Following the general inspection, the infant's head and scalp should be inspected and palpated for any swellings. Immediately after birth generalized scalp oedema particularly involving the presenting part at delivery is quite common (Caput succedaneum) and may be accompanied by moulding where the parietal bones override the occipital and frontal bones. Both the caput succedaneum and moulding disappear spontaneously during the first week. A more tense scalp swelling which appears some hours or days after birth and is localized over individual cranial bones (usually one) is a cephalhaematoma. This is due to subperiosteal bleeding which uncommonly causes anaemia and may contribute towards hyperbilirubinaemia. The haematoma will resolve spontaneously and usually disappears during the first 2 months of life. After resolution a firm margin can often be felt and radiographs at this time will show calcification at the edges (*Fig.* 13.4).

The patency and pressure of the anterior and posterior fontanelles should be assessed. Normal pulsation of the anterior fontanelle may be felt synchronous with the apex beat. The posterior fontanelle is frequently very small or closed at

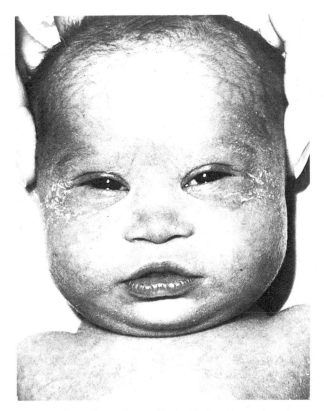

**Fig. 13.3** Down's syndrome. Typical facies. Note epicanthus and upward slant of the eyes.

birth. The head circumference should be measured at the level of the largest diameter and plotted on an appropriate chart (*Fig.* 13.5). The interpretation of this measurement must take into account the gestational maturity and birth weight. The midline of the scalp and nape of neck should be inspected for any small swellings or dimples. Scalp and posterior midline anomalies are sometimes connected to the central nervous system. Similarly, anterior midline cervical swellings or sinuses may be related to the thyroid gland. Lateral neck swellings may be due to a cystic hygroma, bronchial cyst or a sternomastoid tumour.

### Mouth

The mouth should be inspected for the presence of a cleft palate and the roof of the mouth should be palpated for a submucous cleft. White nodules on the palate are frequently seen and represent an accumulation of epithelial cells (Epstein's pearls) which are a normal finding. However, these white spots should be differentiated from moniliasis ('thrush') in any infant who is a few days old.

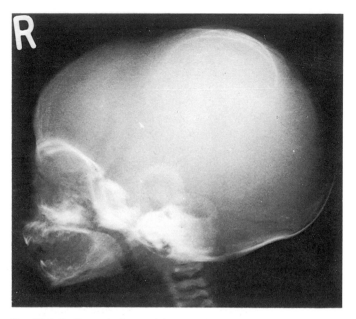

**Fig. 13.4** Radiograph of a resolving cephalhaematoma with a rim of calcification present.

## Chest

Inspection of the chest movement in the newly born commonly will reveal an irregular respiratory rhythm with a rate of about 40 per min. A rate of more than 60 per min sustained for 1 h is taken as tachypnoea. An increased respiratory rate due to a congenital heart lesion may be indistinguishable on inspection from tachypnoea due to cerebral haemorrhage or hyperventilation from metabolic acidosis. Grunting respiration is always significant of respiratory distress. Mild sternal recession, particularly in preterm infants, is often seen. With the infant's head in the midline, the chest should be inspected for symmetry. Gentle percussion can be used in the larger neonate to detect pneumothorax or displacement of cardiac dullness. Chest percussion in the preterm infant is of little use and is not recommended for these very small babies.

On auscultation the normal breath sounds are harsh and when present crepitations are fine. Localization of such abnormal breath sounds can be difficult as the thin chest wall permits wide conduction of added sounds. The heart rate, like the respiratory rate, varies considerably with a wide range from 80 to 180 per min. Systolic murmurs are frequently heard but they do not necessarily indicate congenital heart disease, and conversely congenital heart disease may exist in the absence of murmurs. The presence of the femoral pulse should be confirmed and note made of the pulse volume. A patent ductus arteriosus is a common occurrence in preterm infants but the murmur is not typically continuous. More often only a systolic murmur is heard but a full or bounding pulse is a valuable clue to the diagnosis.

## Abdomen

Examination of the abdomen should include careful inspection of the umbilical cord or stump. The cut surface of the umbilical cord is examined to confirm the presence of three vessels, namely two umbilical arteries and one vein. A single umbilical artery may be associated with occult malformations of the viscera. The abdomen often looks slightly distended. The liver edge can sometimes be felt 2 cm below the costal margin, but under normal circumstances the consistency is soft. The kidneys and occasionally the spleen may be palpable in a normal infant. Most normal infants (93 per cent) will have passed urine by 24 h. The finding of a distended bladder when urine has not been voided may indicate lower urinary tract obstruction. The perineum is inspected for the position and patency of the anus. Over 90 per cent of newborns will pass meconium by 24 h after birth. If by 36 h there has been no passage of meconium and the anus is patent, some form of intestinal obstruction should be suspected. Fresh blood may be seen mixed with the early meconium stools. The commonest source is ingested maternal blood. This can be confirmed by demonstrating the presence of HbA which is not resistant to decolorization by sodium hydroxide (Abt test).

## Genitalia

The genitalia are examined, especially in males for descent of the testes into the scrotum. In the preterm infant, the testes do not descend into the scrotum before the 36th week and inguinal herniae are common. At term the testes are either in the scrotum or can be manipulated into the scrotal sac in 98 per cent of male infants. Note should be taken of any abnormal pigmentation around the scrotum and penis. No attempt should be made to retract the prepuce. In the presence of any abnormality of the prepuce, the glans is inspected for the position of the urethral orifice. In females the labia are palpated for any mass and the size of the clitoris noted. The labia minora are prominent in the newborn. A trace of blood from the vagina usually signifies the effect of maternal oestrogen withdrawal. At this stage it is convenient to examine the inguinal regions for the presence of hernia and to confirm the presence of normal femoral artery pulsation.

## Thighs and lower legs

Both thighs and lower legs are palpated to detect any abnormality in the subcutaneous tissue and bone; the feet are examined for the presence of talipes or supernumerary digits. It is essential to examine the hips of every newborn in order to detect subluxation. As the procedure usually is resented by the infant, it should be left to the end.

## Back

The infant is now placed prone and the back carefully inspected for a midline sinus or hairy patch. If the sinus is above the level of S2 it probably communicates with the theca and requires surgical excision. Other major defects such as encephalocele or myelomeningocele will be obvious.

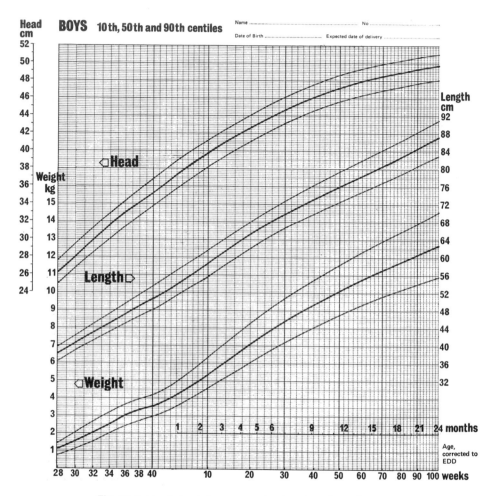

**Fig. 13.5** Head circumference, supine length and weight charts. Charts prepared by Dr D. Gairdner and Dr J. Pearson. (*Published and distributed by Castlemead Publications, Gascoyne Way, Hertford, Herts, 1971, Ref. GPB (Boys) and GPG (Girls).*)

## Nervous system

The examination of the nervous system in the newborn requires an entirely different approach from the conventional neurological examination. Nervous system function in the newborn is mainly brainstem and spinal cord (subcortical), and abnormalities found on examination rarely have any localizing significance. An obvious exception is the finding of unilateral lower motor neuron signs in the limbs such as arises with brachial plexus damage. Thus the examination of the newborn's central nervous system is based on an assessment of the general level of responsiveness, tone and the symmetry of the primitive reflexes.

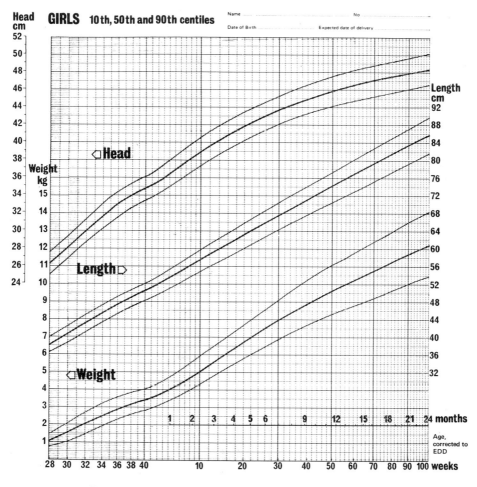

**Head cm** **GIRLS** 10th, 50th and 90th centiles

Name

No

Date of Birth

Expected date of delivery

Length cm

Head

Weight kg

Length

Weight

months

Age, corrected to EDD

weeks

Fig. 13.5

The general attitude of the infant should be observed. Marked lethargy with depressed primitive reflexes may denote a central nervous system disorder due to birth trauma, hypoxia, hypoglycaemia or infection. Paradoxically, the same conditions can cause irritability with fine tremor of high amplitude and exaggerated reflexes ('jittery baby'). Typical *grand mal* convulsions in the newborn are rare, and focal fits should always be interpreted as evidence of a generalized seizure. In the preterm infant particularly, a fit may present as an apnoeic episode with or without cyanosis and poor peripheral circulation. Convulsions in the newborn are due usually to cerebral birth injury, malformations of the brain or metabolic aberrations such as hypoglycaemia or hypocalcaemia.

**Tone** Tone can be assessed by noting the position that the infant adopts in ventral suspension. The baby is suspended by the examiner's hand under his abdomen and the position of the head is noted relative to the plane of the spine. Normal term infants maintain the head in the plane of the spine and only intermittently raise it above. Persistence of an extended neck suggests increased tone of the spine extensors.

The tone of the limbs is tested by observing the resistance to passive movements. Only persistent abnormalities or asymmetries of tone are usually significant of neuromuscular dysfunction.

**Reflexes** Deep tendon reflexes can be elicited in the neonate by briskly tapping the appropriate tendon using the flexed middle finger or a small patella hammer.

Whilst formal fundoscopy is not practised as a routine in the newborn, the 'red reflex' should be elicited. If the infant is held upright the eyes will often open spontaneously. The red retinal tissue can be visualized easily with an ophthalmoscope and congenital cataract may be excluded. Retinal haemorrhages are found in about 20 per cent of normal newborns.

In the newborn, the presence of primitive reflexes lends a unique aspect to the neurological examination at this stage. These reflexes have been aptly described as 'a diagnostic window which will soon close' (R. C. MacKeith). The infant's level of arousal can affect the test responses and the ideal state for examination is a wide awake baby with large movements. When testing for the primitive reflexes the head of the infant should be in the midline.

The *Moro Reflex* is present at birth and disappears by 4–5 months. It is abnormal if present after 6 months. This response is elicited by holding the baby in the supine position supported by the examiner's right arm and hand, and cradling the occiput in the examiner's left hand. The head is allowed to fall a few centimetres only. The Moro response is abduction of the infant's upper arms, extension of the elbows and fingers, followed by adduction and flexion.

If the Moro reflex is absent or decreased it may signify central nervous system depression. If asymmetrical and the head is in the midline the infant may have sustained birth injury to an upper limb, e.g. nerve palsy or fracture. An exaggerated Moro response may indicate cerebral irritation from birth injury, meningitis or a metabolic disturbance such as hypoglycaemia or hypocalcaemia.

The *Rooting Reflex* is present at birth and disappears after 2–4 months. It can be elicited by gently caressing the cheek near the angle of the mouth. The infant responds by turning the head towards the stimulated side, opening the mouth and protruding the tongue. The absence of such a response may signify central nervous system depression.

The *Sucking Reflex* is present at birth and is elicited by inserting a clean finger into the baby's mouth. A poor or absent sucking response may indicate cerebral birth injury or depression of central nervous system function. The rooting and sucking reflex can be tested as a single manoeuvre.

The *Palmar Grasp Reflex* is present at birth and disappears by 3–4 months. It can be elicited by placing the finger across the palmar surface of the baby's hand. The infant's fingers will rapidly flex around the examiner's digit. The plantar grasp similarly can be elicited by pressure at the head of the metatarsals of the infant's foot. The toes will flex. The examiner should remember that a persistent plantar grasp may override a positive Babinski sign if the eliciting stroke crosses the metatarsal heads. The plantar grasp disappears at 9–12 months.

Absent grasp reflexes may signify cerebral depression whilst persistent grasp reflexes may be important evidence of brain damage.

The *Asymmetrical Tense Neck Reflex* is present at birth and usually disappears after 4 months. With the infant supine this reflex is elicited by rotating the head to one side. The ipsilateral arm is extended and the contralateral knee flexed. Persistence of the reflex after the age of 6 months is found in infants with spastic cerebral palsy.

### Clinical assessment of gestational maturity

The clinical course of the low birth weight infant (weight less than 2500 g) during the neonatal period differs not only from the fullterm but there are also important differences between low birth weight infants who are preterm (less than 37 weeks' gestation) and those who are small for dates (SFD). The SFD infant has a birth weight less than the 10th centile or is more than 2 standard deviations below the mean weight for gestational age (*Fig.* 13.6). Preterm infants are predisposed to hyaline membrane disease, intraventricular haemorrhage, hyperbilirubinaemia, apnoeic attacks and necro-tizing enterocolitis, whereas SFD babies are liable to meconium aspiration, severe hypoglycaemia and polycythaemia. Intra-uterine infections such as toxoplasmosis, rubella and cytomegalovirus infections and congenital malfor-mations are important causes of intra-uterine growth failure. It is therefore important to assess accurately the gestational maturity of infants weighing less than 2500 g, as a newborn weighing 2000 g could be preterm, SFD or both.

An accurate, widely used and clinically orientated assessment of maturity is that devised by Dubowitz in 1960. It is based on a score from 10 neurological observations (*Fig.* 13.7) and 11 physical features (*Table* 13.2). The gestational age accurate to within ± 2 weeks is determined from a graph relating the total score obtained to gestational age (*Fig.* 13.8).

### Weight, head circumference, length

Under ordinary circumstances every newborn infant should be accurately *weighed*. The largest head circumference and the supine length should be measured and recorded on a Gairdner–Pearson-type chart (*see Fig.* 13.5). As there may be considerable scalp oedema the head circumference should be re-measured on a later occasion but prior to discharge. The supine length can be measured readily using a neonatometer. These measurements can be left until the end of the initial examination but should not be deferred in a normal infant as the parents are often reassured and interested to hear the weight and length of their infant.

### Hip joint

At the end of the examination the stability of the hip joints is tested (*Fig.* 13.9). With the infant lying supine and facing the examiner, the hips are flexed to a right-angle with the knees fully flexed. The examiner holds the knees with the middle finger of each hand over the greater trochanter and the thumb over the inner side of the thigh opposite the lesser trochanter. Whilst the thighs are abducted the middle finger is used to apply pressure over the greater trochanter in a forward direction. Where the hip is dislocated, the head of the femur can be

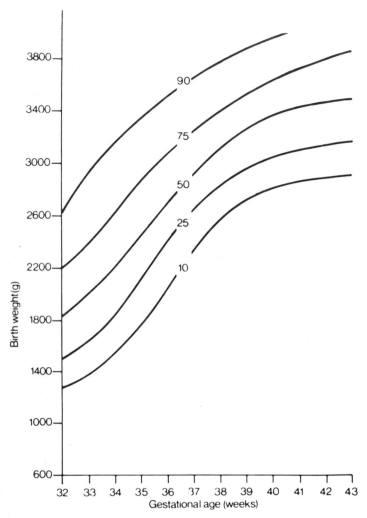

**Fig. 13.6** Birth weight plotted against gestational age.
*Figs.* 13.6–13.8 by kind permission of Dr Victor Dubowitz.
Reproduced from the *Journal of Pediatrics*, 1970, **77**, pp. 1–10,
by permission of C. V. Mosby, St Louis.

felt slipping forwards in the acetabulum and a coarse click will be elicited. The examiner now proceeds to push backwards and upwards with the thumb on the inner side of the thigh. If the head moves out over the posterior lip of the acetabulum and returns with release of pressure whilst the hips are abducted, then the hip is dislocatable, that is unstable (Barlow's manoeuvre).

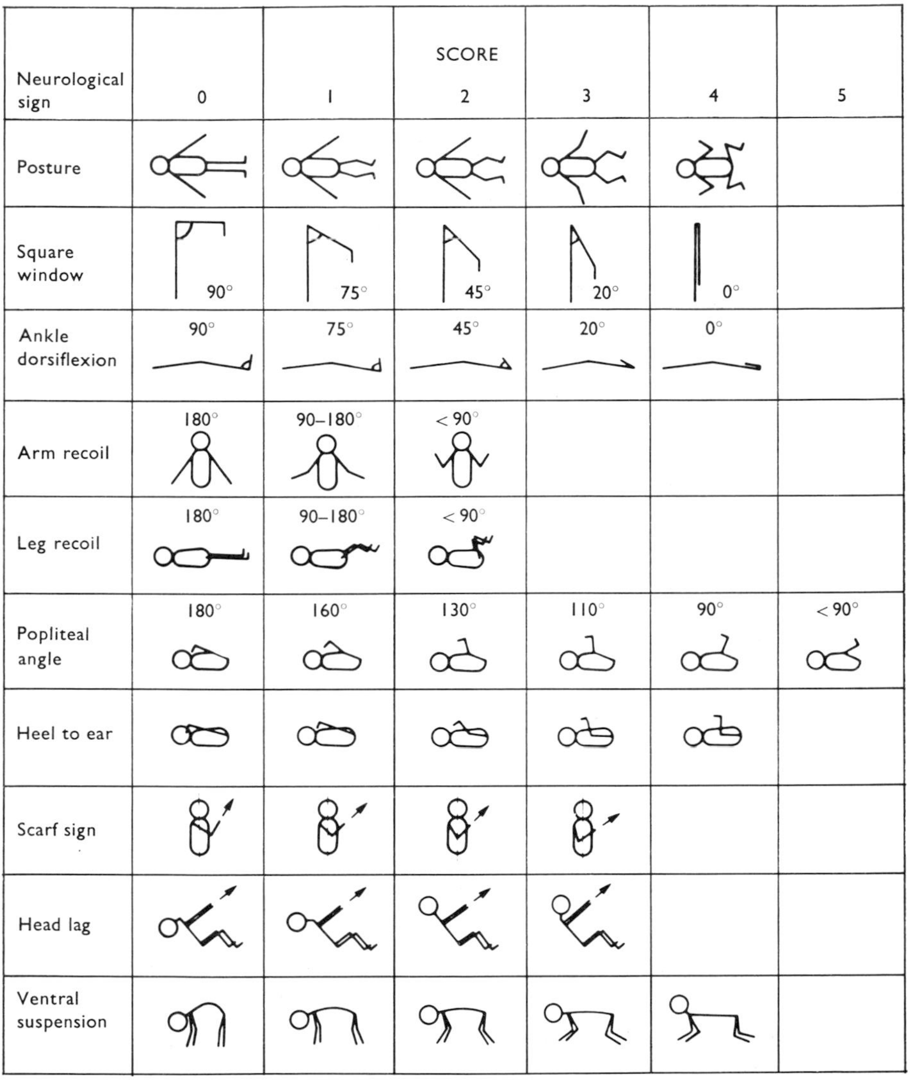

| Neurological sign | SCORE | | | | | |
|---|---|---|---|---|---|---|
| | 0 | 1 | 2 | 3 | 4 | 5 |
| Posture | | | | | | |
| Square window | 90° | 75° | 45° | 20° | 0° | |
| Ankle dorsiflexion | 90° | 75° | 45° | 20° | 0° | |
| Arm recoil | 180° | 90–180° | < 90° | | | |
| Leg recoil | 180° | 90–180° | < 90° | | | |
| Popliteal angle | 180° | 160° | 130° | 110° | 90° | < 90° |
| Heel to ear | | | | | | |
| Scarf sign | | | | | | |
| Head lag | | | | | | |
| Ventral suspension | | | | | | |

*Posture*. Observe with infant quiet and in supine position.

*Square window*. Flex hand on the forearm. *Ankle dorsiflexion*. Dorsiflex foot on to the anterior aspect of leg.

*Arm recoil*. Flex forearm for five seconds, then fully extend and release.

*Leg recoil*. Flex hip and knees for five seconds, then fully extend and release.

*Popliteal angle*. Hold thigh in the knee–chest position, then extend leg.

*Heel-to-ear*. Draw the foot near to head. Observe degree of extension of knee and distance between foot and head.

*Scarf sign*. Draw hand towards opposite shoulder. Grade position of elbow according to illustration. *

*Head lag*. Pull up slowly from supine position, grasping hands.

*Ventral suspension*. Suspend in prone position, holding under the chest.

**Fig. 13.7** Neurological criteria for determining gestational age.

Table 13.2    Physical criteria for determining gestational age

| External sign | | Score | | | |
|---|---|---|---|---|---|
| | 0 | 1 | 2 | 3 | 4 |
| Oedema | Obvious oedema hands and feet; pitting over tibia | No obvious oedema hands and feet; pitting over tibia | No oedema | | |
| Skin texture | Very thin gelatinous | Thin and smooth | Smooth; medium thickness. Rash or superficial peeling | Slight thickening. Superficial cracking and peeling esp. hands and feet | Thick and parchment-like: superficial or deep cracking |
| Skin colour (infant not crying) | Dark red | Uniformly pink | Pale pink: variable over body | Pale. Only pink over ears, lips, palms or soles | |
| Skin opacity (trunk) | Numerous veins and venules clearly seen, especially over abdomen | Veins and tributaries seen | A few large vessels clearly seen over abdomen | A few large vessels seen indistinctly over abdomen | No blood vessels seen |
| Lanugo (over back) | No lanugo | Abundant; long and thick over whole back | Hair thinning especially over lower back | Small amount of lanugo and bald areas | At least half of back devoid of lanugo |
| Plantar creases | No skin creases | Faint red marks over anterior half of sole | Definite red marks over more than anterior half; indentations over less than anterior third | Indentations over more than anterior third | Definite deep indentations over more than anterior third |

| External sign | Score |  |  |  |
|---|---|---|---|---|
|  | 0 | 1 | 2 | 3 | 4 |
| Nipple formation | Nipple barely visible; no areola | Nipple well defined; areola smooth and flat; diameter <0·75 cm | Areola stippled, edge not raised; diameter <0·75 cm | Areola stippled, edge raised; diameter >0·75 cm | |
| Breast size | No breast tissue palpable | Breast tissue on one or both sides <0·5 cm diameter | Breast tissue both sides; one or both 0·5–1·0 cm | Breast tissue both sides; one or both >1 cm | |
| Ear form | Pinna flat and shapeless, little or no incurving of edge | Incurving of part of edge of pinna | Partial incurving whole of upper pinna | Well defined incurving whole of upper pinna | |
| Ear firmness | Pinna soft, easily folded, no recoil | Pinna soft, easily folded, slow recoil | Cartilage to edge of pinna, but soft in places, ready recoil | Pinna firm, cartilage to edge, instant recoil | |
| Genitalia (male) | Neither testis in scrotum | At least one testis high in scrotum | At least one testis right down | | |
| Genitalia (female) (with hips half abducted) | Labia majora widely separated, labia minora protruding | Labia majora almost cover labia minora | Labia majora completely cover labia minora | | |

By kind permission of Dr Victor Dubowitz. Reproduced from the *Journal of Pediatrics*, 1970, **77**, pp. 1–10, by permission of C. V. Mosby, St Louis.

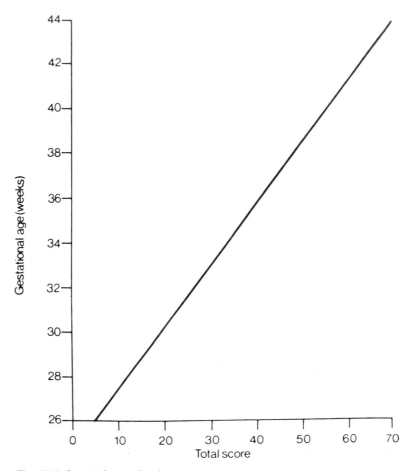

**Fig. 13.8** Graph of gestational assessment score (*see Table* 13.2 and *Fig.* 13.7).

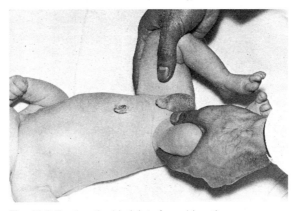

**Fig. 13.9** Testing the hip joints for subluxation.

## ■ THE INFANT AND TODDLER

The term 'infant' generally applies to babies between 28 days and 1 year of age. At this age the examination is usually conducted in the presence and with the assistance of the mother. A history should be obtained of symptoms as perceived by the parent and care must be taken to avoid accepting the parent's diagnoses instead of symptoms. Enquiry must be made of the pregnancy, delivery and infant's behaviour during the neonatal period, with specific reference to cyanotic attacks, fits and jaundice. The quality of the pregnancy should be assessed by enquiring closely whether the mother smoked, drank alcohol or took drugs from whatever source; her occupation should also be noted. This information is always relevant and, in the context of the symptoms, may be significant. A history of feeding should be obtained, and if the infant is artifically fed, the details of the milk formula and administration of any mixed feeding are elicited. The family history should be determined with particular reference to genetic disease and the health of parents and siblings. The immunization status of the infant must be established and this opportunity taken to promote the value of the procedure.

### Assessment of development

During the first year the normal infant will have achieved certain *milestones in development*. There can be wide variations between infants, but nevertheless the sequence is similar (*Fig.* 13.10). Marked delay in one aspect of

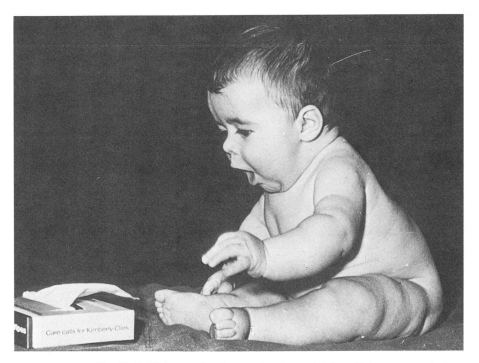

**Fig. 13.10** Eight-month milestone in a 6-month infant. Sitting unsupported.

development or more moderate delay in all milestones requires careful and repeated assessment, as there may be a specific handicap or global retardation present.

An outline of the sequence of normal development is shown in *Table* 13.3.

The assessment of development is always part of the routine examination in the first year of life. The following should be borne in mind:

1.  Allowance must be made for prematurity.

2.  Acute illness or lack of stimulation through prolonged stay in hospital or emotional deprivation may have a very marked, albeit temporary, delaying effect on milestones.

3.  Personal–social milestones (alert responsiveness) and fine motor milestones (use of hands) are more significant markers than gross motor activities such as sitting or walking.

4.  There is a fairly wide range of normality around each milestone. Moderate delay of all milestones can be more significant of mental retardation than marked

| Table 13.3 | Cardinal milestones in development in the first year |
| --- | --- |
| 4–6 weeks | Smiles responsively at mother |
| 6 weeks | Ventral suspension – head held up momentarily in the same plane as rest of body. Some extension of hips and flexion of knees and elbows. Prone – pelvis largely flat, hips mostly extended |
| 8 weeks | Gurgles responsively with smile, and eyes follow objects or person |
| 3 months | Holds rattle placed in hand.<br>Turns head to sound in same plane as ear |
| 5 months | Reaches for object and gets it |
| 6 months | Supine – lifts head spontaneously. Rolls prone to supine.<br>Pulled to sitting position with no head lag.<br>Sits supported by hands forward on floor.<br>Transfers cube from hand to hand. Plays with toes.<br>Primitive reflexes have disappeared |
| 7 months | Briefly sits on floor unsupported.<br>Rolls supine to prone. Feeds self with biscuit |
| 8 months | Sits unsupported.<br>Turns head to sound in plane above ear |
| 9 months | Pulls self to stand or sit. Crawls on abdomen |
| 9–10 months | Index finger pointing to object. Finger–thumb apposition |
| 10 months | Waves bye-bye and plays pat-a-cake.<br>Helps to dress by holding out arm for coat or foot for shoe |
| 11 months | Offers object to mother. Walks with support.<br>Says single word with meaning |
| 1 year | Two or three words with meaning. Walks with one hand held.<br>Casting objects begins. Gives brick to mother |

By kind permission of Professor R. S. Illingworth. After his table in *Basic Developmental Screening*, 2nd edition, published by Blackwell Scientific Publications, Oxford, 1977.

delay in a single milestone which may be a pointer either to a specific handicap or to a normal variant.

5. Under ordinary circumstances the objective developmental assessment should agree with the history of the baby's development. However, parents may sometimes offer a developmental history that they feel the baby should have achieved rather than what has been achieved. This may occur particularly when the parents themselves suspect mental retardation in their infant.

Thus the assessment of development is based partly on the history and partly on objective findings during the physical examination of the infant and toddler.

### General examination

Considerable information can be obtained from the attitude and behaviour of the parent during the history taking and subsequent examination. Not all symptoms volunteered will reflect organic pathology in the infant. Therefore in some circumstances the clinician must consider the possibility that symptoms are being offered as a cry for help from parents unable to cope.

Prior to the physical examination the infant should be weighed and measured (*Fig.* 13.11). This should be interpreted using the appropriate chart and taking into account the birth weight and any other previous weights (*see Fig.* 13.5).

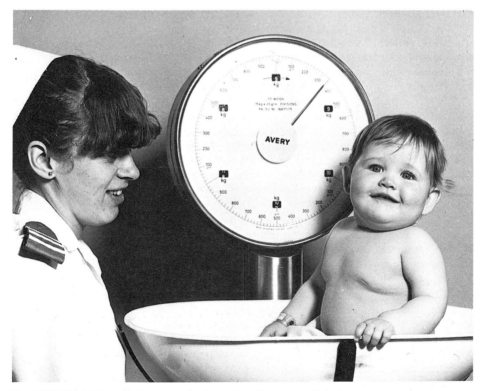

**Fig. 13.11** Weighing an infant. A well-tolerated and important clinical procedure.

The infant's general demeanour should be noted. Acute and chronically ill infants may either ignore the examiner and the subsequent proceedings or react with undue irritability, distress or restlessness.

Rapid movement should be avoided and the examiner should sit at the side of the couch and not loom over the patient. The examiner may maintain useful social contact with the young subject through softly spoken words in a reassuring tone, whilst in the toddler and pre-school child gentle chatter about siblings and pets often helps to contain the patient's fear and uncertainty. Well-intentioned but forceful loud overtures of friendship may rapidly reduce the young to tears. At all times during the examination the face must be watched for signs of pain, apprehension or distress. However, sustained eye contact may be threatening and upset the infant.

The infant and the younger child is usually less disturbed by continuous contact of the examiner's whole hand than by intermittent palpation with the fingers. For this reason a regional approach to clinical examination is better received than examinations by systems that require large movements by the examiner.

A regional examination usually begins with *palpation of the abdomen* and placing the whole hand on the skin and gently palpating the superficial structures. The liver and spleen, even when enlarged, are frequently of such soft consistency that forceful palpation may not detect the organ edge. Throughout early childhood the lower edge of the liver may be felt below the costal margin, but the consistency under normal circumstances is always soft. This part of the examination includes palpation of the inguinal region for hernias, glands and the presence of femoral pulses. The genitalia are inspected and in males the presence of both testes in the scrotum confirmed.

*The lower limbs* are inspected for abnormal bruising. The condition of the feet and toenails gives a reasonable indication of the standard of hygiene.

The presence of occult malformations of the internal organs may be suspected from inspection of the *face, ears and hands of infants*. The presence of unusual facies, maldeveloped and malpositioned ears accompanied by abnormalities of the hands and fingers are an indication for chromosome analysis. The type of abnormalities found in association with the unusual facies include fingerlike thumbs, proximally placed thumbs, overlapping fingers, abnormally short or long fingers accompanied by unusual palmar and digital crease patterns.

There are over 200 recognizable syndromes characterized by abnormal facies with or without other more generalized clinical signs and so it is no longer possible to present a list that could be comprehensive enough to be useful. Recourse must be made to compendia on dysmorphogenetic syndromes or to a suitably programmed computer. An isolated finding of a 'funny' looking face may be a familial physical feature of no more than aesthetic significance.

Amongst the more commonly encountered disorders in childhood which have characteristic facies and other specific stigmata are Down's syndrome (1 in 660 newborns), Turner's syndrome (about 1 in 2500 female births) (*see Fig.* 11.22) and congenital hypothyroidism (about 1 in 4000 births) (*Fig.* 13.12). Whilst Down's syndrome (Mongolism) always should be diagnosed at birth, both congenital hypothyroidism and Turner's syndrome may present difficulties in the early clinical diagnosis.

Milder instances of 'congenital' hypothyroidism may take some months before

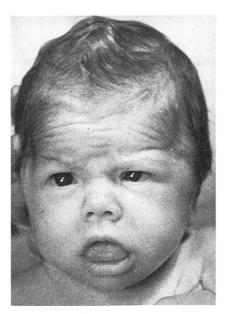

**Fig. 13.12**
Severe hypothyroidism in a
2-month-old infant whose
mother had received
antithyroid drugs during
pregnancy. Note the coarse
features, wrinkled brow and
thick tongue.

| Table 13.4 | **Clinical features of hypothyroidism in infants** |
|---|---|
| *Symptoms* | *Signs* |
| 'Sleeps all day' | Pallor |
| 'Feels cold and dry' | Sparse hair. Cool, dry skin |
| 'Motionless body' | Puffy eyes |
| 'Constipated' | Protruding (enlarged) tongue |
| 'Hoarse cry' | Thick neck |
| 'Noisy breathing' | Large abdomen |
| | Umbilical hernia |
| | Infantile proportions |
| | Prolonged tendon reflex relaxation time |
| | Bulky muscles |
| | Delayed and defective dentition |

the classic clinical features appear (*Table* 13.4). By this time growth failure will
be present because the growing skeleton is very sensitive to lack of thyroxine.
The toddler, whilst short, will have retained the infantile proportions of a longer
upper segment. It should be rare to have the diagnosis delayed so late that all the
features of cretinism are present. There is a known association between Down's
syndrome and hypothyroidism. The widespread routine use of the biochemical
screening of newborns for congenital hypothyroidism (and phenylketonuria) will
reduce but not entirely eliminate the need for a high index of suspicion for this
disorder which is so easily treated if diagnosed early.

Turner's syndrome in the very young can be suspected in infants and toddlers who are short and who have presented with puffiness of hands and toes, deepset nails, low posterior hairline and multiple naevi. There should be no difficulty in the diagnosis if the young patient has a webbed neck. Coarctation of the aorta is the commonest associated cardiac defect, and therefore the femoral pulses should be examined with particular care. This syndrome has both a variable genotype and phenotype and therefore enters the clinical differential diagnosis in any girl with short stature and/or sexual infantilism. The assessment of growth and puberty is dealt with later (pp. 532–3).

### Skull

It is not unusual to find some degree of skull asymmetry in the normal infant. However, premature fusion of sutures will lead to striking abnormalities in cranial shape. Premature fusion of the sagittal suture leads to a long narrow skull (scaphocephaly) with a prominent ridge in the anteroposterior axis. Early closure of the coronal suture produces elevation of the vertex and a backward sloping frontal bone (oxycephaly). Bossing of the frontal and parietal bones due to vitamin D deficiency rickets is now uncommon but may be seen in children with chronic haemolytic anaemias (sickle cell disease or thalassaemia).

The tension of the anterior fontanelle is a guide to intracranial pressure. This fontanelle normally closes round about 18 months with a range of about 9 months to 27 months. A tense or bulging fontanelle is found in meningitis, hydrocephalus, cerebral tumours and other causes of raised intracranial pressure. The fontanelle will feel tense in a crying infant. Significant dehydration causes a sunken fontanelle. Pulsation in the fontanelle is a normal finding.

Transillumination of the skull in a darkened room using a rubber torch closely applied to the skin can yield useful information. Increased luminescence will be found in hydrocephalus and hydranencephaly. A fibre optic source of light may reveal areas of decreased light transmission and indicate subdural blood.

In older children raised intracranial pressure causing diastasis of the sutures can be detected by the 'cracked pot' note on percussion of the skull.

An early sign of rickets is softening of the skull bones which is most easily detected by thumb pressure over the parietal bones. The bone will indent and spring back like a table tennis ball (craniotabes). Craniotabes may be found occasionally in normal infants under 3 months of age.

The maximum head circumference should always be measured and related to the infant's weight. A large head may be a normal variation (familial) or be found in a big baby and grows at a normal rate. Megalencephaly and hydranencephaly also cause the head to be large. In hydrocephalus the head is not only large but serial measurements at short intervals will show an increased rate of growth so that the head circumference ascends through centile channels.

A noticeably small head may be due to a normal variation, i.e. familial feature or small baby, but the growth rate will be normal. Both in mental deficiency and craniostenosis the head is small but the growth rate will be poor.

### Spine

Throughout infancy and childhood the spine should be inspected for obvious abnormalities such as deep dimples and tufts of hair, as they may connect to the theca. Toddlers and other children should be examined for scoliosis by having the patient flex the spine with the arms hanging down and palms touching. Postural deformities will correct in this position and any curvature and rib hump are signs of a structural scoliosis.

### Nutrition and hydration

The state of nutrition and hydration can be assessed by inspection and palpation. Tissue loss must be differentiated from fluid loss (dehydration). Recent weight loss should be suspected from redundant skin folds on the medial surface of the thighs, axillae and wasted buttocks. The face is often spared and young subjects do not commonly have the typical cachectic look of adults who have lost a lot of weight.

The signs of fluid loss are both quantitative and qualitative. in the presence of sunken eyes and fontanelle, loss of skin turgor and intact peripheral circulation the fluid loss is between 5 and 10 per cent of body mass. If there is accompanying peripheral circulatory failure, fluid loss exceeds 10 per cent of body mass. Skin turgor is assessed best by picking up the skin (over the chest, abdomen or thighs) between thumb and forefinger and gently compressing it. In dehydration the skin only slowly regains its original position. In hypertonic (hypernatraemic) dehydration the skin has a peculiar rubbery or doughy feel and the patient has varying somnolence and irritability. The sensorium in isotonic dehydration usually is lethargic.

The signs of frank dehydration may occur in the absence of diarrhoea and vomiting and result from increased insensible water loss (tachypnoea and sweating) or third compartment sequestration (fluid exudation into small bowel) of fluid prior to the passage of loose stools. Thus relatively mild abdominal distension may be an indication of a potential site for accumulation of large amounts of extracellular fluid.

When dehydrated infants present without a history of diarrhoea and vomiting and no other source of loss, a rectal examination should be done. Withdrawal of the finger may be accompanied by an explosive passage of watery stools if the cause of the dehydration has been fluid loss into distended loops of bowel.

### Heart

Examination of the heart begins with inspection and palpation. Congenital cardiac malformation leading to hypertrophy of the ventricles in early life will cause precordial bulge. The apex beat is rarely visible in normal children. If the chest wall is thin and the patient apprehensive, ventricular activity may be seen. In many children the apex beat is not palpable. Note should be made of any thrills, and as young children, particularly infants, breathe at a faster rate, care should be taken to distinguish palpable vibration arising from secretions within the respiratory tree from cardiac thrills. As the chest wall is thin, cardiac thrills may be widely conducted and thus difficult to localize. Ventricular septal defects cause a systolic thrill at the lower left sternal border. Left basal systolic thrills may arise from a patent ductus arteriosus and pulmonary stenosis. Aortic stenosis may be associated with a systolic thrill palpable at the base and in the suprasternal notch. The heart impulse and thrills may be palpable through the diaphragm in the epigastric notch of young children who have cardiomegaly.

Gentle percussion of the precordium in infants and toddlers can establish the site and extent of cardiac dullness.

The heart sounds in infancy have a sharper quality than in later life and the resting heart rate is faster. The pulmonary second sound is normally accentuated and frequently split, being more marked during inspiration. 'Innocent' or functional murmurs are common in infancy and childhood. They are always systolic, ejection in type and soft. They vary with posture and may disappear in the erect position. During inspiration functional murmurs decrease in intensity. The patient is free of symptoms and there is no cardiomegaly.

A further entirely innocent auscultatory finding is a venous hum which is heard at the base of the heart and mimics a continuous or machinery murmur. The venous hum always disappears with gentle compression of the jugular veins.

Detailed analysis of abnormal cardiac sounds and murmurs is given in the chapter on Cardiovascular Disease (*see* p. 201). Attention should be paid to the special importance in infancy and childhood of auscultating below the left clavicle for a patent ductus arteriosus. In some instances the murmur may be heard only in systole and localized to below the left clavicle.

*Blood pressure measurement* in toddlers is often neglected because of assumed technical difficulties. Given patience and the right cuff size it is quite feasible to obtain blood pressure measurements in most young subjects who require a general examination. It is a procedure that should be left towards the end of the clinical examination. The cuff should cover at least two-thirds of the upper arm. An inappropriately small cuff size will give a spurious reading in the hypertensive range.

## Central nervous system

Toddlers and pre-school children may be unwilling to co-operate in a systematic examination of the *central nervous system*. Fortunately it is possible by inspection of the child's activities in the examination room to determine the presence of gross deficits in the long tracts concerned with power of muscle groups, position sense and co-ordination of the arms and legs.

The toddler or child should be encouraged to roam around the examination room, handle toys (including building bricks) and climb on to the couch unassisted. Once the child is supine he should be allowed to sit up without assistance. If the young patient is able to clamber on to an examination couch, go from sitting to supine and from supine to sitting, all without assistance, it is highly unlikely that significant weakness exists in the limbs or trunk. The manipulation of blocks 2·5×2·5 cm is not only an index of cortico-visio-spatial perception but also a test of fine movements of the hand and fingers. The child with a spastic upper limb will exhibit the characteristic fanning of the fingers and external rotation of the wrist as he reaches towards an object.

Long-standing local neuromuscular deficits in the growing child will be accompanied by differences in growth when the two parts are compared. The parents may confirm the differences in glove or shoe size between the two sides.

The presence of a Babinski reflex may be masked by the persistence of the plantar grasp reflex. This can be avoided by testing for the Babinski reflex in two discrete movements using the thumb or a rounded blunt end of a patella hammer. Car keys and latch keys should not be used as the young child's skin on the sole of the foot is very soft and extremely sensitive. The purpose of the test is not to cause extreme discomfort to the patient. The first part of the test is to stroke the lateral border of the foot starting at the heel and working up to the fifth toe. The second movement is firm stroking towards the medial border of the foot across the sole at the base of the toes. A child with a spastic diplegia may have an extensor response with the first component but the presence of a grasp reflex elicited by the horizontal movement may then cause the toes to flex.

In the floppy infant syndrome the differentiation between hypotonia and weakness is very important. As infants cannot co-operate in conventional tests of power, it is necessary to determine the presence of any spontaneous movement by inspection and also by response to mildly unpleasant stimuli applied to the limbs. Hypotonic infants without weakness will exhibit intermittent spontaneous or withdrawal movements of varying amplitude. It may be possible in this group of infants to demonstrate that the limb can be held against gravity.

### Measurement of growth

Abberrations in *growth* through childhood and adolescence are sensitive clinical markers of disease. There are considerable normal variations in growth. The examiner must take into account the family history, duration of pregnancy, birth weight and past illnesses. Charts of height and weight are available and have facilitated the interpretation of both cross-sectional and longitudinal measurements.

The clinical value of the measurements depends entirely on the accuracy with which they are carried out and recorded. The accompanying illustration (*Fig.* 13.13) shows the child standing in bare feet with the back against the measuring scale and the head held in the Frankfurt plane with gentle upwards pressure on the mastoids. Supine length requires two persons to carry out the manoeuvre (*Fig.* 13.14). The infant's head is held with the occiput on the backplate and the crown of the head touching the baseplate. One leg is extended and the moveable footplate brought up to make contact with the sole of the patient's foot which should be at right angles to the lower leg. It is necessary to repeat this manoeuvre three or four times and take the average of the readings. Whilst the correct measurement of supine length may be time consuming and require two operators, the alternative use of a tape measure next to the infant is so inaccurate as to be useless.

Significant short stature is defined as a height for age below the 3rd centile (*Fig.* 13.15). As the 3rd centile is less than two standard deviations below the mean, some charts have an additional shaded grey area below the 3rd centile which covers three standard deviations below the mean. Young patients whose height falls below the shaded area should be investigated to determine the cause of their short stature. Those children whose height falls within the grey area should, in the absence of any clinical signs denoting disease, be remeasured over a 1-year period. This will enable the growth velocity to be determined.

### Ears

*Inspection of the eardrums* should precede examination of the mouth and throat, which is generally left to the end of the clinical examination. The use of an auriscope or spatula is likely to be resented by an otherwise co-

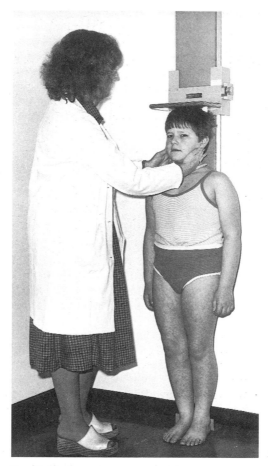

**Fig. 13.13** Measurement of standing height with the head held in the Frankfurt plane using a stadiometer.

operative young patient. It is most important that the infant and toddler be restrained adequately as there is a real risk of hurting a struggling young subject during the examination of the ears and mouth. Secure yet gentle restraint can be obtained by having the toddler seated on the mother's lap with one arm placed around the child's chest (pinning the arms) whilst the other hand firmly holds the forehead pressing the child's head against her chest. The child's lower legs are secured between her knees (*Fig.* 13.16). Older toddlers are more often likely to co-operate if their consent is sought to examine the ears by asking which ear should be examined first.

After first inspecting the external auditory meatus the aural speculum is inserted carefully. The auditory canal is both shorter and straighter in infants and only slight retraction of the auricle is necessary. The normal tympanic membrane is pale grey and translucent with a bright cone of light in the lower half. An

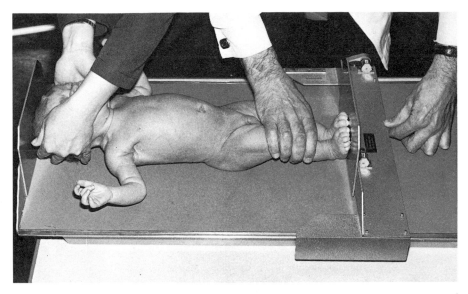

**Fig. 13.14** Measurement of supine length using an infant measuring board.

inflamed eardrum may be pink or bright red with loss of the light reflex and may bulge. Following a serous otitis media the tympanic membrane loses its lustre and light reflex and may be retracted.

A number of young children have some deficit of *hearing* albeit temporary and often mild. Therefore in infancy some assessment of hearing should be done. Free field testing can be carried out by standing behind the infant and using familiar sounds (rattle, rustling paper, small bell, spoon inside a cup and a soft voice from about a metre). By the age of 3–4 months the normal infant will respond by turning the head to various sounds. By 9 months the infant should localize the side and whether above or below the level of the ear.

### Nostrils

The nostrils should be inspected. In gross posterior nasal obstruc-
due to adenoidal hypertrophy, the nostrils tend to be small, pinched and ante-
verted. Infants with unilateral choanal atresia may have chronic nasal discharge, whilst in toddlers a foreign body is a common cause of a unilateral nasal discharge.

### Mouth and throat

The final procedure is the clinical examination of the *mouth and throat*. It always is worth attempting to visualize as much as possible without introducing any instruments. A co-operative toddler will often open the mouth wide enough for complete examination without the need for inserting a spatula. Some older children may prefer to depress the base of the tongue with their fingers rather than have a spatula inserted. Young infants commonly have a sucking pad in the centre of the upper lip. This is entirely normal. In young patients the

Name..................................

Date of Birth..................................

Reg.No..................................

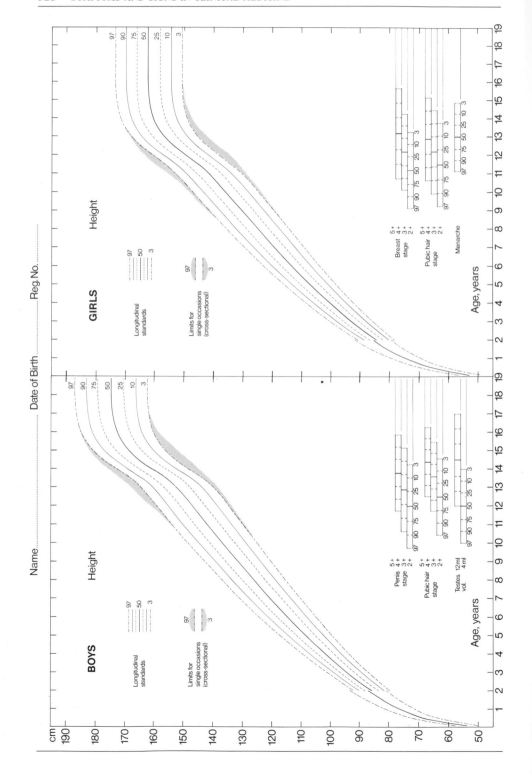

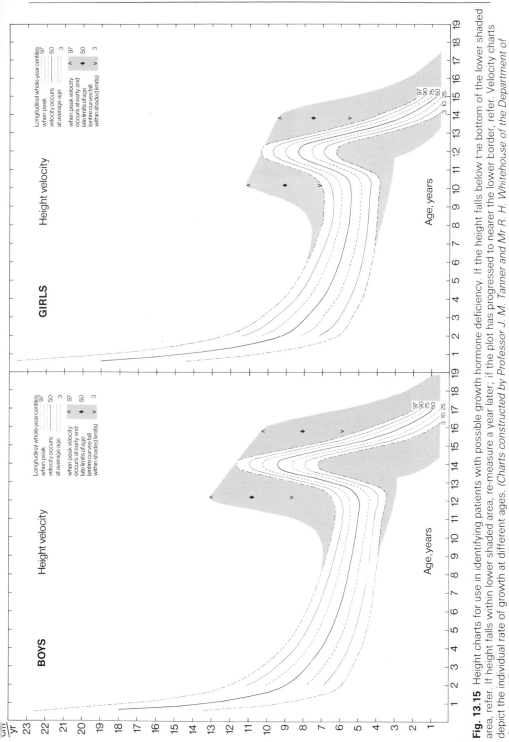

**Fig. 13.15** Height charts for use in identifying patients with possible growth hormone deficiency. If the height falls below the bottom of the lower shaded area, refer. If height falls within lower shaded area, re-measure a year later; if the plot has progressed to nearer the lower border, refer. Velocity charts depict the individual rate of growth at different ages. (Charts constructed by Professor J. M. Tanner and Mr R. H. Whitehouse of the Department of Growth and Development, Institute of Child Health, London. Published with copyright by Castlemead Publications, Gascoyne Way, Hertford, Herts.) Ref. LBH1A (Boys) and LGH3A (Girls).

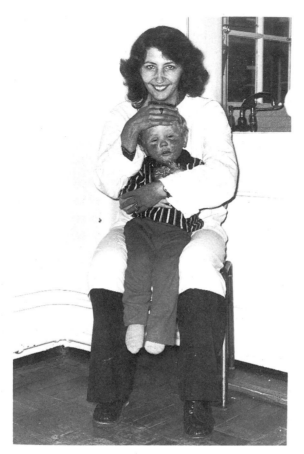

**Fig. 13.16** Method of holding a child for examination of the ears and mouth.

commonest cause of vesicles and ulceration of the lips, gums and tongue is primary herpes simplex gingivostomatitis. This infection is accompanied by significant constitutional upset, and the child will appear ill and febrile. Moniliasis (thrush) should not be confused with herpes simplex infection as vesicles and frank ulceration are not seen with oral thrush. Monilial infection is characterized by white plaques inside the mouth on the buccal mucosa and on the tongue (*see Fig.* 4.7, p. 71). Thrush does not cause fever or significant constitutional upset but may lead to difficulty in feeding.

Infantile scurvy is such a rare cause of bleeding gums that it should never be diagnosed unless other more common causes such an non-accidental injury (child abuse) and haematological disorders have been excluded.

The teeth should be examined for their number and quality. Dental caries is a significant clinical finding and appropriate advice should be given. Tetracycline given to the mother during pregnancy or to the child less than 7 years of age will discolour the teeth a yellow or green, and they may have defective enamel leading to premature shedding (*see Fig.* 4.2, p. 67). The oral mucosa should be examined as it is commonly involved in childhood infectious diseases. The enanthema of measles (Koplik's spots) are greyish white dots on the buccal mucosa and resemble grains of sea sand. This finding is pathognomonic and is best sought opposite the lower molars. In children with mumps there is often oedema and redness in the buccal mucosa around the opening of Stensen's duct. Petechiae on the soft palate frequently occur in infectious mononucleosis. Herpangina due to Coxsackie A virus causes petechiae on the posterior third of the palate and fauces.

The anginose form of infectious mononuclcosis has a pseudomembrane covering the tonsils and needs to be distinguished from confluent septic tonsillitis where the exudate is more easily scraped from the tonsil. If the patient has not been immunized, diphtheria enters the differential diagnosis especially in endemic areas.

The tonsils normally are relatively larger in children than in later life and it is doubtful if tonsillar size alone has any clinical significance apart from such rarities as neoplastic involvement and Tangier disease (analphalipoproteinaemia). In the latter disorder the lipid laden tonsils are a bright orange colour. However, in an acutely ill child a unilateral tonsillar swelling may indicate a peritonsillar abscess (quinsy).

If a young patient has stridor (croup) the oropharynx should be examined with great circumspection as the cause of the airway obstruction may be acute epiglottitis. In this disorder the epiglottis is inflamed, bright red, oedematous and upright. It may cause complete obstruction as a result of inserting a spatula into the mouth. Under these circumstances the oropharynx is best examined in a situation where an emergency airway can be provided if necessary. Retropharyngeal abscess is an uncommon cause of stridor, dysphagia and neck extension and may lead to considerable difficulty in examining the oropharynx. The diagnosis is best made by palpating with the finger a soft fluctuant mass on the posterior pharyngeal wall.

## ■ EXAMINATION OF THE OLDER CHILD

Although the clinical technique and format of examination used can be similar to the adult, older children and adolescents do require a reassuring approach. The presence of a parent during the clinical examination of the adolescent is a matter for individual judgement. In general, the young adolescent should be given an opportunity to be alone with the examiner.

Many of the symptoms presenting at this age have an emotional basis and the real cause for the symptoms may not become apparent unless the history is taken under conditions favourable to the young person.

At and around the age of 12–15 years parents and adolescents may become aware of an unusual pattern of physical growth and pubertal development. Whilst measurement of height and weight is recommended as part of the routine examination throughout childhood, it is particularly important that accurate measurements be made at this age. First, the equipment should be reliable and capable of accurate results and, secondly, the examiner must use the standard technique referred to earlier.

## Pubertal status

In this age group it is necessary to assess the pubertal status. This is done by examining for the presence of secondary sexual characteristics and grading the findings according to the scheme devised by Tanner (*Tables* 13.5–13.7). In both girls and boys the amount and quality of the pubic hair is recorded. In girls the staging of breast development and in boys the development of the penis and scrotum is examined. Additionally, in males the testicular volume is assessed using a Prader orchidometer (*Fig.* 13.17). If the testicular volume is greater than 4 ml, further obvious pubertal changes are incipient. In normal boys the increase in testicular volume may begin between 9·5 years and 13.5 years and even later in some. The growth spurt generally starts approximately a year after the enlargement of the testes and reaches peak height velocity about 2 years after

| Table 13.5 | Stages of pubic hair development in boys and girls |
|---|---|
| Stage 1 | No pubic hair. Pre-adolescent |
| Stage 2 | Sparse growth of long, slightly pigmented downy hair, straight or slightly curled, mostly at the base of the penis or along the labia |
| Stage 3 | Considerably darker, coarser and more curled. Hair spreads sparsely over the junction of the pubis |
| Stage 4 | Adult type hair but less profuse |
| Stage 5 | Adult in type and quantity |

| Table 13.6 | Stages of breast development in girls |
|---|---|
| Stage 1 | Pre-adolescent. Elevation of papilla only |
| Stage 2 | Breast bud stage and projection of breast and papilla as a small mound. Areola enlarged |
| Stage 3 | Breast and areola enlarged and elevated more than in Stage 2. No separation of contours |
| Stage 4 | Areola and papilla project above the contour of the breast as a secondary mound |
| Stage 5 | Mature stage. Papilla only projects |

| Table 13.7 | Stages of genital development in boys |
|---|---|
| Stage 1 | Pre-adolescent. Scrotum and penis same size as in early childhood |
| Stage 2 | Slight englargement of scrotum and testes (>4 ml) with some redness of scrotal skin. Penis shows little growth |
| Stage 3 | Lengthening of penis and further enlargement of testes and scrotum |
| Stage 4 | Further enlargement of penis in breadth, length and development of glans. Testes and scrotum enlarge further than Stage 3. Scrotal skin darker |
| Stage 5 | Adult genital stage |

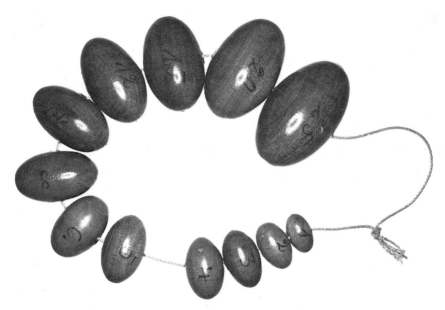

**Fig. 13.17** Prader orchidometer for the assessment of testicular volume.

testicular enlargement then the penis is obviously growing and pubic hair is at stage 3–4.

In girls pubertal changes begin with the development of the breast bud (stage 2). This occurs between 9·0 and 13 years in the majority of normal girls. The onset of menstruation follows after peak height velocity has been reached, and the average age for onset of menstruation is about 13 years, with a range of 11–15 years.

At puberty most boys will have palpable breast tissue and even if unilateral this is normal. A small number of adolescent males develop conspicuous gynaecomastia which may require investigation and treatment. Neoplasia of the male breast at this age is excessively rare.

Whilst it is known that pre-pubertal children may be sexually active, it is nevertheless very uncommon, and consequently symptoms and signs of sexually transmitted disease are encountered rarely. On the other hand, sexual activity to a lesser or greater extent is a feature of the pubertal and post-pubertal teenage years. There should be no inhibition, but always sensitivity, to the examination of the genitalia in teenage patients when the symptoms are interpreted as indicating sexually transmitted disease and signs of pregnancy sought when there is a history of sexual activity. Similarly, the complex of non-specific symptoms such as mood change and unusual behaviour should raise the possibility of drug abuse and the appropriate questions should be asked, again with sensitivity.

There are few clinical signs of drug abuse in the early stages. Solvent abuse (glue sniffing) may give rise to perioral excoriation. Heroin sniffing (snorting) can be associated with chronic changes in the nares whilst the obvious evidence of multiple needle marks must be taken as pathognomonic of intravenous drug usage.

Smoking is now accepted as a very significant cause of morbidity and increased mortality. Consequently, clinical evidence of cigarette smoking in older children and teenagers should be sought from nicotine stains on the fingers and teeth.

Certain groups of disorders are prevalent in teenage children and are very uncommon in pre-pubertal subjects. Thyroid disease due to auto-immune thyroiditis is the commonest cause of goitre in adolescence and enlargement of the thyroid gland should be sought routinely.

Idiopathic adolescent scoliosis, as the name implies, must be examined for in older children and teenagers.

Both thyroid disease and idiopathic scoliosis are much more common in girls.

# Index

## J